MINIMAL ACCESS
SURGICAL ANATOMY

MINIMAL ACCESS SURGICAL ANATOMY

CAROL E. H. SCOTT-CONNER, M.D., Ph.D., M.B.A.

Professor and Head
Department of Surgery
University of Iowa College of Medicine

Staff Physician
Department of Surgery
University of Iowa Hospitals & Clinics
Iowa City, Iowa

PROFESSOR SIR ALFRED CUSCHIERI, F.R.S.E., M.D., Ch.M., F.R.C.S.Ed., F.R.C.S.Eng., F.R.C.S.Glas., F.R.C.S.I.

Professor of Surgery
Head, Department of Surgery and Molecular Oncology
University of Dundee
Ninewells Hospital and Medical School
Scotland, United Kingdom

FIONA J. CARTER, Bsc. (Hons.)

Research Assistant
Department of Surgery and Molecular Oncology
University of Dundee
Ninewells Hospital and Medical School
Scotland, United Kingdom

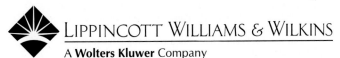

LIPPINCOTT WILLIAMS & WILKINS
A **Wolters Kluwer** Company

Philadelphia · Baltimore · New York · London
Buenos Aires · Hong Kong · Sydney · Tokyo

Acquisitions Editor: Lisa McAllister
Developmental Editor: Gina Gerace
Production Editor: Elaine Verriest
Manufacturing Manager: Tim Reynolds
Cover Designer: Lynn Amft
Compositor: Maryland Composition

© 2000 by **LIPPINCOTT WILLIAMS & WILKINS**
530 Walnut Street
Philadelphia, PA 19106-3780 USA
LWW.com

Printed and bound in China

Library of Congress Cataloging-in-Publication Data

Scott-Conner, Carol E. H.
  Minimal access surgical anatomy / Carol E.H. Scott-Connor, Sir Alfred Cuschieri,
Fiona Carter.
    p. ; cm.
  Includes bibliographical references and index.
  ISBN 0-397-51459-X
    1. Laparoscopic surgery—Atlases.   2. Human anatomy—Atlases.   3.
Abdomen—Endoscopic surgery—Atlases.   I. Cuschieri, A. (Alfred) II. Carter, Fiona. III.
Title.
  [DNLM: 1. Anatomy, Regional—Atlases.   2. Surgical Procedures,
Laparoscopic—methods—Atlases. WO 517 S425m 2000]
  RD33.53   .S35 2000
  617′.05—dc21   99-053181

Care has been taken to confirm the accuracy of the information presented and to describe generally accepted practices. However, the authors and publisher are not responsible for errors or omissions or for any consequences from application of the information in this book and make no warranty, expressed or implied, with respect to the currency, completeness, or accuracy of the contents of the publication. Application of this information in a particular situation remains the professional responsibility of the practitioner.

The authors and publisher have exerted every effort to ensure that drug selection and dosage set forth in this text are in accordance with current recommendations and practice at the time of publication. However, in view of ongoing research, changes in government regulations, and the constant flow of information relating to drug therapy and drug reactions, the reader is urged to check the package insert for each drug for any change in indications and dosage and for added warnings and precautions. This is particularly important when the recommended agent is a new or infrequently employed drug.

Some drugs and medical devices presented in this publication have Food and Drug Administration (FDA) clearance for limited use in restricted research settings. It is the responsibility of the health care provider to ascertain the FDA status of each drug or device planned for use in their clinical practice.

10 9 8 7 6 5 4 3 2 1

CONTENTS

CONTRIBUTING AUTHORS

Wendy Gram Brick, M.D.   Fellow, Section of Hematology/Oncology, Department of Medicine, Medical College of Georgia, 1120 15th Street, Augusta, Georgia 30912

Gene L. Colborn, Ph.D.   Department of Cellular Biology and Anatomy, Medical College of Georgia, School of Medicine, Augusta, Georgia 30912

Sean P. Hedican, M.D.   Department of Urology, University of Iowa Hospitals and Clinics, 200 Hawkins Drive, Iowa City, Iowa 52242

INTRODUCTION

Successful surgery starts in the anatomy laboratory. Without a sound knowledge of surgically relevant anatomy, the practicing surgeon will get into trouble over and over again. Thus, this book is a primer, the foundation of laparoscopic surgery. All students of surgery, residents, attendings, and consultants must start here. Like so many starting points in life, it helps to return for refreshment periodically.

Unless we revisit basic anatomy and the way it influences our operations, we risk several problems. The most obvious risk is that we may divide a vessel, a duct, or a nerve that we ought to preserve. This is not a common problem, as most operations are designed to avoid such transgressions. Unfortunately for surgeons, anatomy is not constant and operations are designed for the most common anatomical considerations. Unless one understands the variations in anatomy, even well performed common operations may lead to catastrophe. For example, one must understand all the variations in cystic duct and hepatic artery anatomy to successfully perform laparoscopic cholecystectomy. But where does one turn to attain this information? Anatomic concerns relevant to the surgeon are often believed to be too arcane for textbooks and atlases of anatomy. Manuals of surgical technique tend to seek a simple explanation of complex procedures, and overlook anatomic pitfalls. A second risk concerns the high posterior wall of the stomach that is invariably supplied by several vessels which we call the posterior gastric vessels. If the surgeon does not divide these vessels, gastric fundus mobilization is incomplete. If the surgeon does not know what they are, he or she may mistakenly identify these vessels as branches of the left gastric artery and leave them *in situ*. These vessels and their surgical relevance are discussed in this text. I challenge the reader to find a detailed description of these important structures in a standard anatomic text or manual of surgical technique.

Occasionally, it is necessary for a surgeon to alter the operative plan to overcome a problem presented by the pathology or by the medical condition of the patient. Under these circumstances, creativity and improvisation are mandatory attributes of the surgeon. Before he or she can exercise creativity, the surgeon must have a firm command of regional anatomy. The superb photographs and line drawings that accompany each chapter in this text provide all the information necessary to exercise creativity with care and confidence.

This text provides something fresh and different. As I have alluded earlier, it is not either an anatomy text or a manual of surgical procedures. It is both. By discussing the relevant anatomy in the context of minimal access surgical procedures, the authors have brought anatomy to life. Nothing could be more interesting (and more important to operative outcome) than learning new information about old operations. I have performed nearly a thousand laparoscopic operations on the gastroesophageal junction, yet it was enjoyable and eye-opening to read the authors' description of the anatomy relevant to such procedures—a description that noted structures I had not thought about in years because they are out of the endoscopic field of vision, structures which are never seen, because getting too close may cause damage to them. As such, this text is more than a weighty reference for the bookshelf. It is to be read by the novice and the maven, alike. It will provide new insight on old procedures.

John G. Hunter, M.D.
Department of Surgery
Emory University School of Medicine
Atlanta, Georgia

PREFACE

This atlas is intended as a comprehensive guide to the keyhole world of laparoscopic surgery. It is organized regionally. Within each region, the reader will find material dealing with surgical exposure, topographic anatomy, and specific surgical procedures. Each chapter is illustrated with carefully selected color photographs paired with labeled line drawings indicating specific anatomic features. Two hundred twenty color photographs were collected from the authors' collections of laparoscopic videotapes. For Chapter 10 entitled "Inguinal Region," we chose to utilize photographs of cadaver dissections rather than laparoscopic images in order to portray crucial anatomic structures with maximal clarity. For this chapter, each carefully prepared dissection was photographed from the laparoscopic point of view and an accompanying line drawing was produced.

This book was written by practicing minimal access surgeons for practicing surgeons. Think of it as a bridge between the anatomy text and the laparoscopic surgical technique books and articles. We have tried to be concise yet complete. The table of contents guides the reader to the chapter where anatomy relevant to specific surgical procedures may be found. A bibliography at the end of each chapter lists references the authors have found particularly helpful—articles that describe additional techniques and provide further detail on the anatomy.

The chapters are designed to provide a working knowledge of laparoscopic surgical anatomy. While *Nomina Anatomica* terms were used whenever possible, in several instances (e.g. "adrenal gland" rather than "suprarenal gland") the terms in common surgical usage were substituted. Readers desiring to supplement this with traditional anatomic views of the areas as seen during open surgery are referred to Scott-Conner and Dawson, *Operative Anatomy.*

Carol E. H. Scott-Conner
Professor Sir Alfred Cuschieri
Fiona J. Carter

ACKNOWLEDGMENTS

The concept of this book originated with Dr. David Dawson, and the authors gratefully acknowledge his contributions throughout the preparation of the manuscript. The assistance, patience, and wise counsel of our editor, Lisa McAllister, is gratefully acknowledged. The majority of the color images in the book were contributed by Dr. Cuschieri and Ms. Carter. The following individuals generously contributed additional color images used in this book: Gene Colborn, Ph.D.; Sean Hedican, M.D.; James Howe, M.D.; Richard Koehler, M.D.; James Maher, M.D., Barry Salky, M.D.; and Siroos Shirazi, M.D. The line drawings were created by Mary Shirazi. Finally, we wish to acknowledge the patience of our students, our colleagues, and our families.

MINIMAL ACCESS
SURGICAL ANATOMY

1

ANTERIOR ABDOMINAL WALL

GENERAL PRINCIPLES OF ACCESS TO THE ABDOMEN AND PREPERITONEAL SPACES

This chapter describes the anatomy of the anterior abdominal wall as it pertains to access to the peritoneal cavity and preperitoneal space and to laparoscopic ventral hernia repair. The inguinal region is described separately in Chapter 10. The laparoscopist is really concerned with just two aspects of the anterior abdominal wall: the anatomy as seen from the outside in as it pertains to laparoscopic access and the anatomy from the inside out as it pertains to laparoscopic ventral hernia repair. The organization of this chapter reflects that principle.

After a brief review of the relevant anatomy, the structure of the abdominal wall midline and considerations related to trocar placement for initial laparoscopic access are described in depth. The most common site for initial puncture is the umbilicus, because of its central location and because the abdominal wall is usually thinnest at this site.

The lateral abdominal wall is described next. Secondary cannulae are commonly placed through sites above and below the umbilicus, lateral to the midline. Proper trocar placement significantly improves access and exposure; conversely, improper placement can render even a simple laparoscopic procedure difficult. General principles applicable to all procedures are discussed in this chapter. Special considerations related to trocar placement are given throughout this book as the anatomy of specific laparoscopic procedures is described.

Finally, the anatomy of the preperitoneal and peritoneal spaces is described, followed by anatomic considerations for laparoscopic ventral hernia repair. Laparoscopic ventral hernia repair is emerging as a useful technique in the management of selected patients. Knowledge of the abdominal wall from the inside out facilitates accurate repair, and anatomic considerations related to this procedure are discussed at the end of the chapter.

ANATOMY AND SPECIFIC SURGICAL PROCEDURES

Muscles and Fascia

Structural strength of the anterior abdominal wall comes from the muscles and fascia that span the space between the costal margin superiorly, the spine and muscles of the back posteriorly, and the pelvis inferiorly. There are three large, flat muscles (external oblique, internal oblique, and transversus abdominis) and one long vertically oriented segmental muscle (rectus abdominis) on each side (Fig. 1-1A). The flat muscles are muscular laterally and are aponeurotic medially.

The most superficial flat muscle, the external oblique, is also the largest. It originates as eight muscular slips arising from the lower eight ribs and interdigitating with serratus anterior. Muscle fibers then course from above downward "as if putting one's hands in one's pockets" (Fig. 1-1A). Medially, fibers of this muscle give way to a broad, flat aponeurosis that forms the anterior rectus sheath and decussates in the midline at the linea alba (discussed later).

The next muscle layer is the internal oblique. Fibers arise from the pelvis and then sweep anteriorly and forward, almost perpendicular to the direction of the fibers of the external oblique. Medially, the internal oblique becomes aponeurotic as well, contributing to the anterior and posterior rectus sheaths and the linea alba (Fig. 1-1).

The deepest muscle is the transversus abdominis (Fig. 1-1). Its fascia, the transversalis fascia, provides the strong lining and inner stabilizing layer of the musculoaponeurotic walls of the abdominal cavity. The transversalis fascia is actually that portion of the endoabdominal fascia that covers the transversus muscle. Hernias of the abdominal wall begin as weaknesses in the endoabdominal fascia. The aponeurotic portion of the transversus abdominis contributes to the rectus sheaths.

The paired rectus abdominis muscles attach to the fifth, sixth, and seventh costal cartilages and the xiphoid process of the sternum above and to the superior ramus of the pubis, symphysis pubis, and linea alba below. These segmental, vertically oriented muscles are enclosed in sheaths that derive components from the aponeuroses of all the flat muscles previously mentioned. Above the umbilicus, the anterior and posterior sheaths are well developed (Fig. 1-1B) and derive from fibers of the external oblique aponeurosis (anteriorly), the internal oblique aponeurosis (anteriorly and posteriorly), and the transversus abdominis (posteriorly). Below the linea circumlinearis (of Douglas), the posterior rectus sheath is flimsy and is composed only of transversalis fascia. Because the exact location of the linea circumlinearis varies considerably, it is simplest to regard the posterior rectus sheath as unreliable below the umbilicus. Above the umbilicus, the anterior rectus sheath is formed from fibers of the aponeuroses of the external and internal oblique muscles. Decussation of fibers from the anterior and posterior rectus sheaths forms the linea alba. Below the umbilicus, the recti become closer together, and the sheaths and linea alba are less well defined. The lateral border of the rectus sheath forms a visible groove (the linea semilunaris) in slender, muscular individuals.

Arteries, Veins, and Nerves

Four major arteries on each side form an anastomotic arcade that supplies the abdominal wall. The superior and inferior epigastric artery and their branches provide the major blood supply to the rectus abdominis muscle and the medial structures of the abdominal wall. These vessels run within the rectus sheath just posterior to the rectus muscle. The superior epigastric artery and vein descend on each side of the midline to anastomose the inferior epigastric artery and vein. The inferior epigastric artery and vein arise lateral to the rectus and enter the rectus sheath at the linea semicircularis.

Of the vessels supplying the abdominal wall, the one most significant for the laparoscopist is the inferior epigastric artery with its accompanying veins (Fig. 1-2A). Fortunately, these vessels are fairly constant in location and can be avoided by placing trocars outside the lateral border of the rectus. The superior epigastric vessels are smaller and are much more variable in location and number. Although these vessels are generally found inside the rectus sheath, trocar sites frequently must traverse the rectus muscle in the subcostal region for optimum exposure and manipulation of instruments. Bleeding may be encountered and must be dealt with using standard laparoscopic techniques.

Laterally, the musculophrenic artery descends to anastomose with the deep circumflex iliac artery arising from below. These vessels supply the lateral abdominal wall structures. They are of little laparoscopic significance.

Motor and sensory innervation is segmental (Fig. 1-2B). Numerous cutaneous and muscular nerves derive from the six lower thoracic and upper lumbar spinal nerves and run in the plane between the internal oblique and transversus abdominis muscles. Overlap between the territory of adjacent nerves makes it possible largely to disregard these nerves when abdominal incisions (or laparoscopic trocar sites) are selected.

Umbilicus and Midline Abdominal Wall

The umbilicus is the scar remaining after the umbilical cord withers and detaches. At the umbilicus, skin, fascia, and peritoneal cavity are in close apposition with a minimum amount of intervening fat. A small fascial defect may be encountered unexpectedly, and it is easily closed at the conclusion of the laparoscopic procedure.

Several peritoneal ligaments remain as reminders of the original purpose of the umbilicus as conduit to and from the placenta. These are the ligamentum teres hepatis with its associated falciform ligament and the median and medial umbilical ligaments.

The ligamentum teres hepatis passes from the superior margin of the umbilicus to the liver and contains the obliterated umbilical vein. Dilated venous collaterals, including a patent umbilical vein, are noted in patients with portal hypertension and should be anticipated and avoided. The falciform ligament is a peritoneal reflection that covers the ligamentum teres and attaches it to the diaphragm. In obese patients, preperitoneal fat dips down into the falciform ligament. The falciform ligament is then thick, and it is easy to bury a trocar in its depth. The laparoscopist should avoid the ligamentum teres by making the initial puncture within the actual umbilical ring rather than superior to it.

The median and medial umbilical ligaments are less significant and pose less of a risk. These ligaments of the lower anterior abdominal wall are described in detail later.

The linea alba is formed by the decussation of fibers from the anterior and posterior rectus sheaths. At the midline, it is the only musculofascial layer encountered. Just lateral to the midline are the paired rectus abdominis muscles. The linea semilunaris delineates the lateral edge of the recti.

A small, inconstant triangular muscle, the pyramidalis, attaches to the symphysis pubis and inserts on the linea alba. With this exception, the midline is purely fascial, as previously mentioned.

Choice of Laparoscopic Trocar Sites

The midline is free of muscle fibers, nerves, and vessels except at its inferior edge where the pyramidalis muscle is sometimes found. This small, inconstant muscle lies superficial to the linea alba. The umbilicus is the scar that marks the site of the umbilical cord. Generally skin, fascia, and peritoneum are closely applied at this point. This feature makes it an excellent choice for initial laparoscopic entry (Fig. 1-3).

Beyond the linea semilunaris, the structure of the abdominal wall is more complex. Three musculofascial layers can be identified, but they are of minimal clinical significance. Trocar sites in these locations rarely cause significant bleeding, but they may be difficult to close securely. The colon attaches to the lateral abdominal wall along both gutters. One should make secondary punctures only under direct laparoscopic visual control, to avoid visceral injury.

Alternate puncture sites are useful under special circumstances. An old midline scar or prior umbilical hernia repair may render umbilical puncture unwise. Left and right subcostal sites are sometimes used under this circumstance, and some laparoscopists prefer and use these sites routinely, particularly in massively obese patients. Advanced procedures such as splenectomy or adrenalectomy (performed in the lateral position) generally require the use of alternate puncture sites.

The left subcostal site is chosen approximately 2 cm below the costal margin (Figs. 1-3A to C). The costal margin provides excellent resistance as the needle is introduced. A similar choice of right subcostal puncture site is less commonly required (Figs. 1-3 to 1-7). Multiple layers of the abdominal wall must be traversed to enter at this site, and it may be difficult to detect when peritoneal entry has been accomplished.

When puncture sites lateral to the midline are used, it is prudent to choose locations lateral to the linea semilunaris to avoid the inferior and superior epigastric vessels, as previously mentioned. Bleeding from epigastric vessels is more of a problem below the umbilicus, because the inferior epigastric vessels are larger than their counterparts above the umbilicus. If the linea semilunaris are not visible in an obese patient, the location can be approximated by a curved line joining the pubic tubercles (two fingerbreadths' lateral to the midline at the pubis) inferiorly to the costal margin at the midclavicular line superiorly.

Preperitoneal Space and Peritoneum

The preperitoneal space lies between the endoabdominal fascia and the peritoneum. The only contents are remnants of the umbilical arteries and vein, the urachus, and the inferior epigastric vessels. This space contains a variable amount of fat, and in individuals of average build, it may be simply a potential space.

Glistening parietal peritoneum lines the abdominal wall. In the upper abdomen, the prominent ligamentum teres hepatis divides the space into two compartments (see Fig. 1-5). The ligamentum teres converges on the umbilicus, as previously noted. The muscle and central tendon of the diaphragm are visible cephalad boundaries of the peritoneal cavity. Laterally, attachments of the right and left colon are seen and must be avoided when trocars are placed (see Figs. 1-6 and 1-7).

In the lower abdomen, five peritoneal folds converge on the underside of the umbilicus. These form excellent landmarks. The median umbilical fold ascends in the midline from the dome of the bladder to the underside of the umbilicus. It is the remnant of the obliterated urachus. It is rarely seen laparoscopically because the peritoneum frequently flattens out with insufflation and with collapse of the bladder around an indwelling catheter. When present, it is easily recognized by its midline location. Occasionally, this duct remains patent and may be injured during laparoscopy.

The next pair of folds comprises the two medial umbilical folds, which correspond to the obliterated umbilical arteries (Figs. 1-8 to 1-11). The bladder lies between these folds. Lateral to these, the less prominent lateral umbilical folds mark the location of the inferior epigastric artery and vein. Gonadal, iliac, and inferior epigastric vessels are commonly seen through the peritoneum (Figs. 1-10 to 1-14). The lateral umbilical folds are rarely appreciated laparoscopically. Any of these folds or ligaments may be inconspicuous or, alternatively, fat-laden and prominent. Careful inspection of the entire pelvic peritoneum comparing landmarks and symmetry combined with palpation and indentation of the abdominal wall at external landmarks will establish the anatomy in each individual case.

Between these folds are three fossae. The paired medial supravesical fossae, bounded laterally by the median umbilical folds, contain the bladder at the base. Frequently, the median fold is imperceptible, and the supravesical fossa appears as a single space (see Figs. 1-9 to 1-11). Just lateral are the paired medial inguinal fossae (site of direct inguinal hernias), bounded medially by the medial umbilical folds and laterally by the lateral umbilical folds (see Figs. 1-8, 1-13, and 1-14). The most lateral paired fossae are the lateral inguinal fossae, which lie lateral to the inferior epigastric vessels (and hence lateral to the lateral umbilical folds). These are the sites of indirect inguinal hernias (see Chapter 10).

Preperitoneal Access

Access to the preperitoneal space is gained by penetrating almost all the layers of the abdominal wall but stopping short of peritoneal entry. Many laparoscopists prefer to use a blunt-tipped Hassan cannula for this, because the initial preperitoneal dissection can be accomplished with a finger after incising the fascia with a scalpel. The thinness of the peritoneum is demonstrated in many of the figures in this chapter, in which the underlying muscles of the abdominal wall are clearly seen through the peritoneum. It is emphasized in Fig. 1-15, which shows the peritoneum tented over a trocar as it enters the peritoneal space. Accurate dissection in the preperitoneal space requires leaving this thin membrane intact.

Ventral Hernia Repair

Ventral hernias are easily fixed with a laparoscopic approach. The characteristic appearance of a ventral hernia defect is shown in Fig. 1-16. The parietal peritoneum extends into the defect forming the sac. Adhesions to adjacent viscera must be divided to define the defect. Closure is usually achieved with a patch, and several techniques have been described (see Bibliography).

Spigelian hernias occur at the intersection of the linea semilunaris and linea semicircularis. These hernias are difficult to diagnose because the hernia sac may not protrude as a visible bulge (as a result of overlying muscles). Laparoscopy is thus doubly useful to establish the diagnosis and to exclude other causes of pain. Repair of the hernia then proceeds in a routine fashion.

BIBLIOGRAPHY

Anatomic References

1. Blichert-Toft M, Koch F, Neilson OV. Anatomic variants of the urachus related to clinical appearance and surgical treatment of urachal lesions. *Surg Gynecol Obstet* 1973;137:51–54.
2. MacVay CB, Anson BJ. Composition of the rectus sheath. *Anat Rec* 1940;77:213–217.
3. Milloy FJ, Anson BJ, McAfee DK. The rectus abdominis muscle and the epigastric arteries. *Surg Gynecol Obstet* 1960;110:293–298.
4. Orda R, Nathan H. Surgical anatomy of the umbilical structures. *Int Surg* 1973;58:454–464.
5. Weibel MA, Majno G. Peritoneal adhesions and their relation to abdominal surgery: a post mortem study. *Am J Surg* 1973;126:345–353.

Surgical References

1. Amendolara M. Videolaparoscopic treatment of spigelian hernias. *Surg Laparosc Endosc* 1998; 8:136–139.
2. Bertelsen S. The surgical treatment of spigelian hernia. *Surg Gynecol Obstet* 1966;122:567–572.
3. Felix EL, Michas C. Laparoscopic repair of spigelian hernias. *Surg Laparosc Endosc* 1994;4:308–310.
4. Halpern NB. The difficult laparoscopy. *Surg Clin North Am* 1996;76:603–613.
5. Hashizume M, Migo S, Tsugawa Y, et al. Laparoscopic repair of paraumbilical ventral hernia with increasing size in an obese patient. *Surg Endosc* 1996;10:933–935.
6. Holzman MD, Puret CM, Reintgen K. Laparoscopic ventral and incisional hernioplasty. *Surg Endosc* 1997;11:32–35.
7. Linos D, Mitropoulos F, Patoulis J, et al. Laparoscopic removal of urachal sinus. *J Laparoendosc Adv Surg Tech A* 1997;7:135–138.
8. McLucas B, March C. Urachal sinus perforation during laparoscopy. *J Reprod Med* 1990;35:573–574.
9. Oshinsky GS, Smith AD. Laparoscopic needles and trocars: an overview of designs and complications. *J Laparoendosc Surg* 1992;2:117–125.
10. Spangen L. Spigelian hernia. *Surg Clin North Am* 1984;64:351–366.
11. Yong EL, Prabhakaran K, Lee YS, et al. Peritonitis following diagnostic laparoscopy due to injury to a vesicourachal diverticulum. *Br J Obstet Gynaecol* 1989;96:365–368.

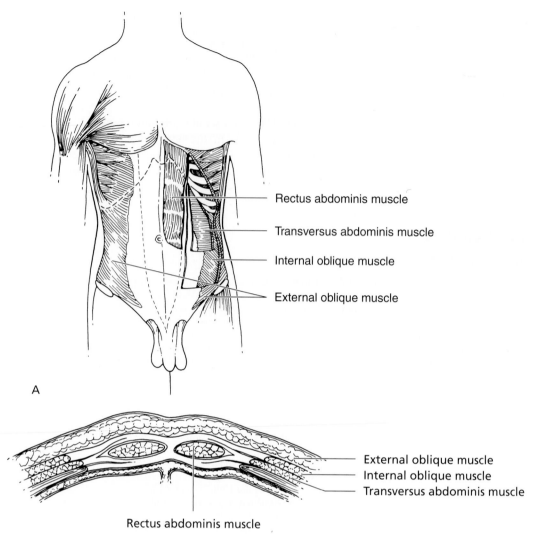

Rectus abdominis muscle

Transversus abdominis muscle

Internal oblique muscle

External oblique muscle

A

External oblique muscle
Internal oblique muscle
Transversus abdominis muscle

B   Rectus abdominis muscle

Fig. 1-1. Muscle layers of the anterior abdominal wall. **A.** This frontal view of the torso shows the muscle layers and the direction of their fibers. The left side of the figure shows the outermost layer, the external oblique muscle, and its aponeurosis. Fibers from this muscle run diagonally down and forward. The strong aponeurosis of the external oblique muscle forms part of the anterior sheath of the rectus muscle (medially) and inferiorly forms the roof of the inguinal canal. The inferior rolled edge of the aponeurosis forms the inguinal ligament. The right side of the figure shows the rectus sheath cut away to reveal the rectus abdominis muscle (medially) and the internal oblique and transversus abdominis muscles (laterally). **B.** A cross-section through the anterior abdominal wall above the umbilicus demonstrates how aponeuroses of the external oblique, internal oblique, and transversus abdominis muscle contribute to the rectus sheaths. The midline fascia is formed by decussating fibers from both sheaths. (From Scott-Conner CEH, Dawson DL. *Operative Anatomy.* Philadelphia: JB Lippincott, 1993:273, with permission.)

Fig. 1-2. Arteries and nerves of the anterior abdominal wall. **A.** The major blood vessels of the anterior abdominal wall can cause troublesome bleeding if injured when trocars are placed. Knowledge of the position of these vessels may help the surgeon to avoid injuring the patient. Two vascular arcades provide blood supply to the anterior abdominal wall. Medially and most important, the superior epigastric artery and inferior epigastric artery (with accompanying veins) may be avoided by keeping trocar sites outside the rectus sheath. The rectus abdominis muscle is shown to indicate its location relative to the vessels, which generally run posterior to the muscle within the rectus sheath. Because the inferior epigastric artery is generally larger and more constant in location than the superior epigastric artery, this is an especially important concern below the umbilicus. Laterally, the musculophrenic artery (from above) and the deep circumflex iliac artery (from below) are rarely encountered or endangered. **B.** The major nerves are segmentally distributed. Overlap between adjacent nerves allows sacrifice of these when incisions are made. These numerous nerves are disregarded when trocar sites are chosen. The right side of the figure shows the approximate segmental distribution of the cutaneous nerves of the anterior abdominal wall. These run superficial to the external oblique muscle. The left side of the figure shows major segmental nerves that run in the plane superficial to the transversus abdominis muscle to supply abdominal wall muscles. (From Scott-Conner CEH, Dawson DL. *Operative Anatomy.* Philadelphia: JB Lippincott, 1993:273, with permission.)

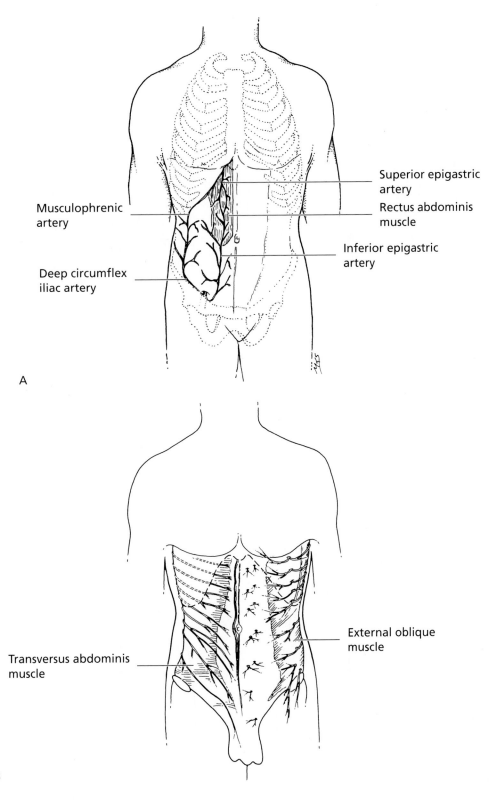

Superior epigastric artery

Rectus abdominis muscle

Inferior epigastric artery

Musculophrenic artery

Deep circumflex iliac artery

A

External oblique muscle

Transversus abdominis muscle

B

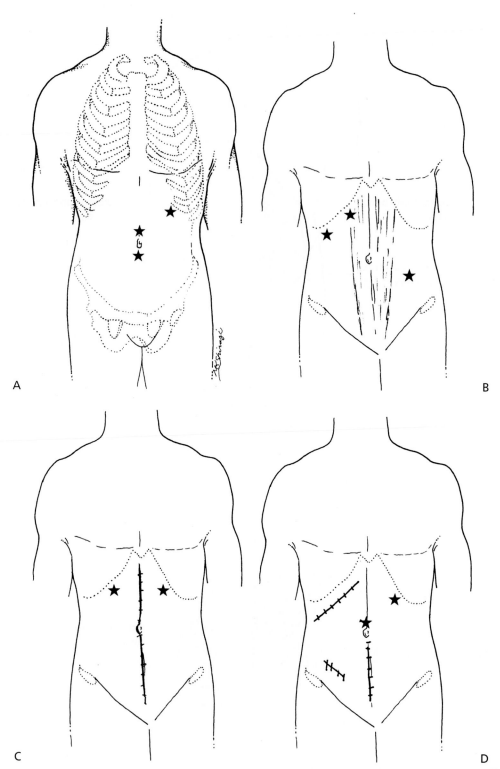

Fig. 1-3. Standard and alternate trocar sites for initial and secondary puncture, sites to avoid. (The *star* indicates the trocar site.) **A.** Periumbilical or midline sites are generally chosen for initial puncture. Alternatively, a subcostal site allows the ribs to give support and may provide easier access in the obese patient or when a lateral position is used. **B.** Secondary puncture sites are chosen to facilitate access to the operative site. Choice of secondary puncture sites is discussed in the chapters that follow, as individual anatomic regions are discussed. The rectus abdominis muscles are shown to emphasize that below the umbilicus, secondary trocar sites should be placed outside the lateral border of the rectus abdominis muscle to avoid injury to the inferior epigastric vessels. General principles of choice of trocar sites are discussed in Chapter 2. **C.** Trocar sites in the previously operated abdomen. Generally, a site remote from any scar is chosen for initial entry. When a long midline incision is present, the alternate subcostal sites provide a possible choice for closed entry into the abdomen. **D.** Other alternate trocar sites that avoid subcostal, right lower quadrant, or lower midline scars.

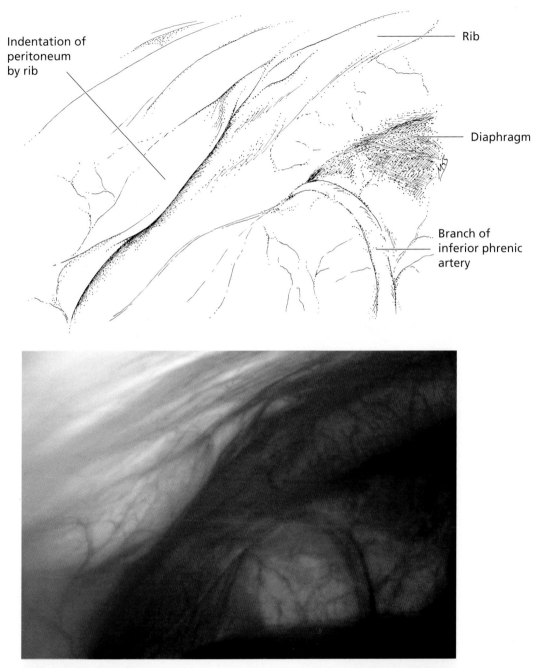

Fig. 1-4. Laparoscopic view of the right subphrenic space showing the lateral abdominal wall and diaphragm. In the foreground, the transversalis fascia may be seen through the translucent peritoneum and minimal preperitoneal fat. Laterally, fat associated with the right colon becomes visible and underscores the importance of visualizing the colon attachments before placing lateral trocars. Ribs can be seen indenting the peritoneum. Superiorly, the diaphragm and associated phrenic neurovascular bundles are seen. The liver has dropped down away from the diaphragm and is glimpsed near the bottom of the picture.

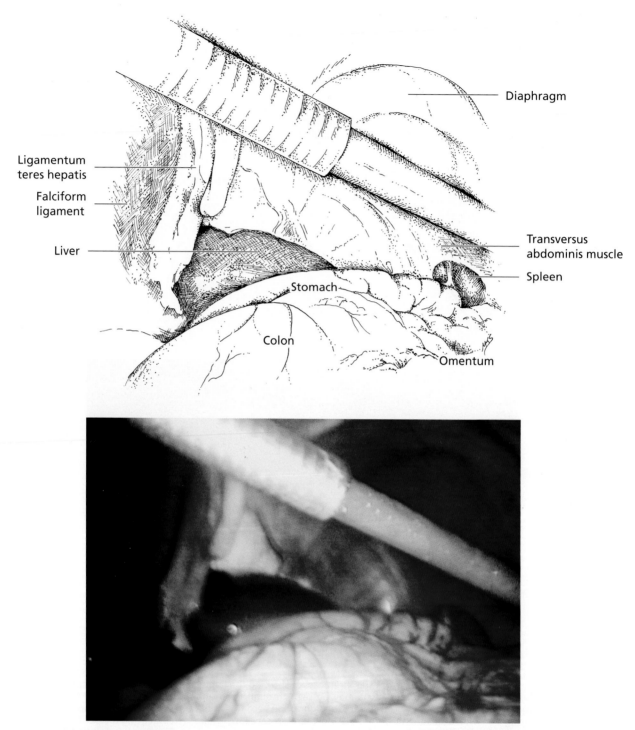

Fig. 1-5. Falciform ligament and left subphrenic space. This view of the left subphrenic space demonstrates how the falciform ligament connects the liver to the underside of the abdominal wall, with the ligamentum teres hepatis coursing to the umbilicus. It is being retracted by a trocar and grasper. The left subphrenic space with diaphragm and phrenic neurovascular bundle are seen. Stomach, spleen, colon, and omentum are glimpsed in the foreground.

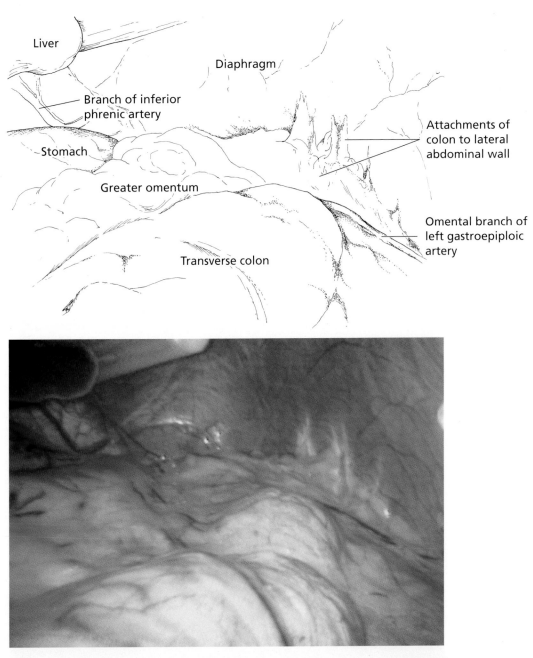

Fig. 1-6. Left lateral abdominal wall. The attachments of the left colon to the anterior abdominal wall are seen in this view of the left lateral abdominal wall. Preperitoneal fat is minimal, and the transversalis fascia and transversus abdominis muscle fibers are seen through the translucent peritoneum, as are randomly oriented small vessels. The diaphragm forms the cephalad border of the working space, and a branch of the inferior phrenic artery, with its accompanying veins and nerve, is noted. The liver, stomach, greater omentum, and transverse colon are seen in the foreground. The omental branch of the left gastroepiploic artery is noted descending along the left-hand border of the greater omentum.

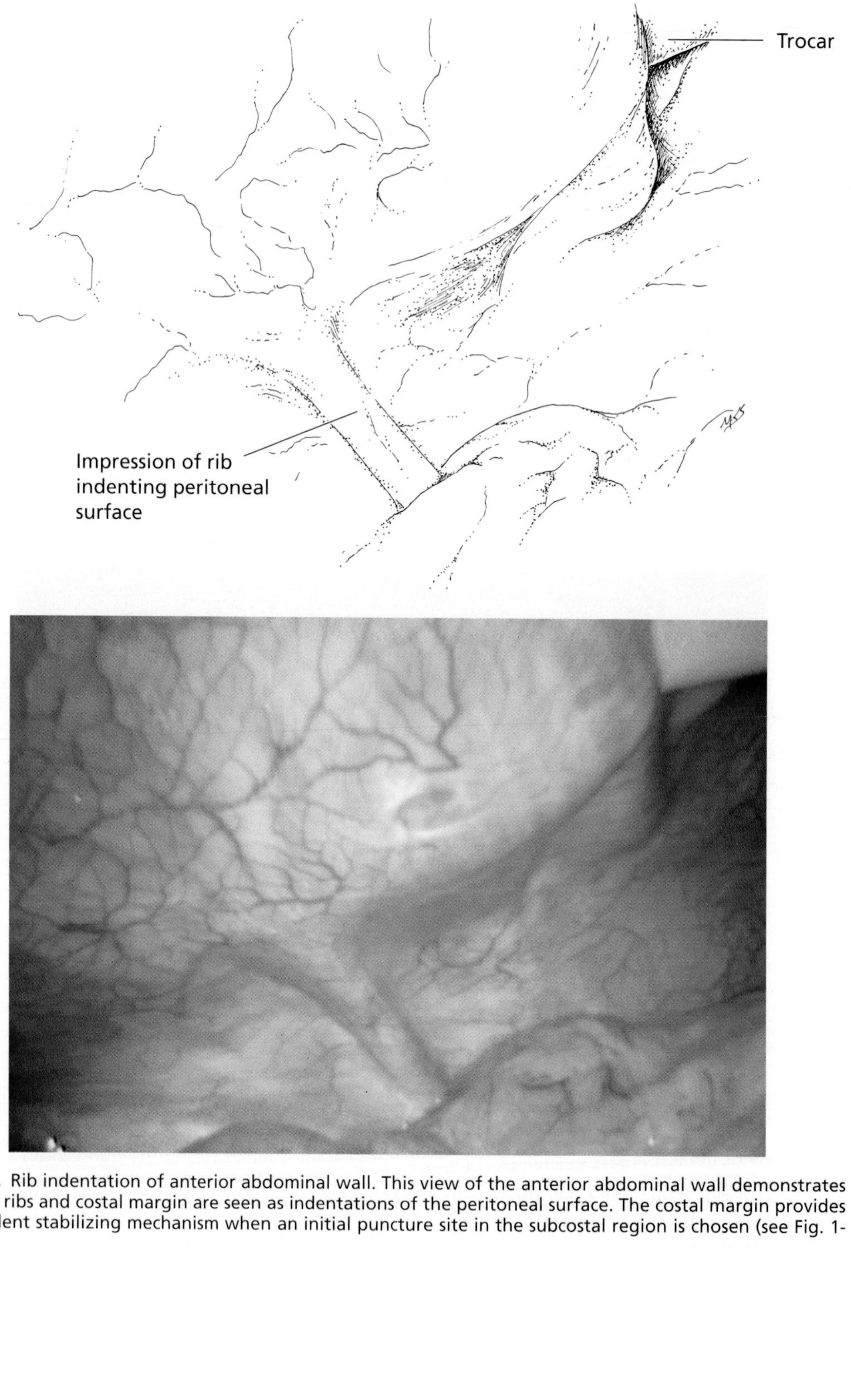

Trocar

Impression of rib
indenting peritoneal
surface

Fig. 1-7. Rib indentation of anterior abdominal wall. This view of the anterior abdominal wall demonstrates how the ribs and costal margin are seen as indentations of the peritoneal surface. The costal margin provides an excellent stabilizing mechanism when an initial puncture site in the subcostal region is chosen (see Fig. 1-3A).

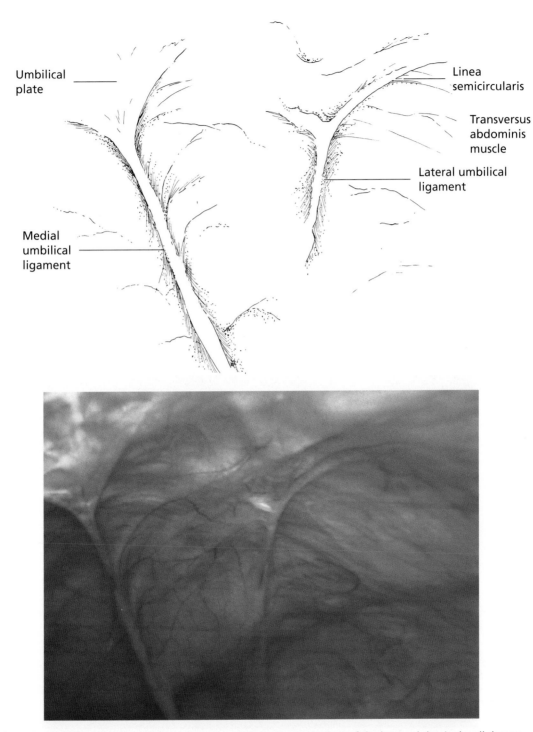

Umbilical plate

Linea semicircularis

Transversus abdominis muscle

Lateral umbilical ligament

Medial umbilical ligament

Fig. 1-8. Medial and lateral umbilical ligaments. This laparoscopic view of the lower abdominal wall demonstrates the medial and lateral umbilical ligaments on the right side. The medial umbilical ligament is seen to terminate in a broad attachment on the umbilical plate in the foreground. The lateral umbilical ligament terminates indistinctly at the linea semicircularis, which is quite cephalad in this individual. Above the linea semicircularis, the posterior sheath of the rectus abdominis muscle obscures visualization of the epigastric vessels, which appear to be dividing at their termination. The transversalis fascia and transversus abdominis muscle are visible laterally. The supravesical fossa is seen to the left, and the median inguinal fossa lies between the medial and lateral umbilical folds. The lateral inguinal fossa lies to the right of the lateral umbilical fold.

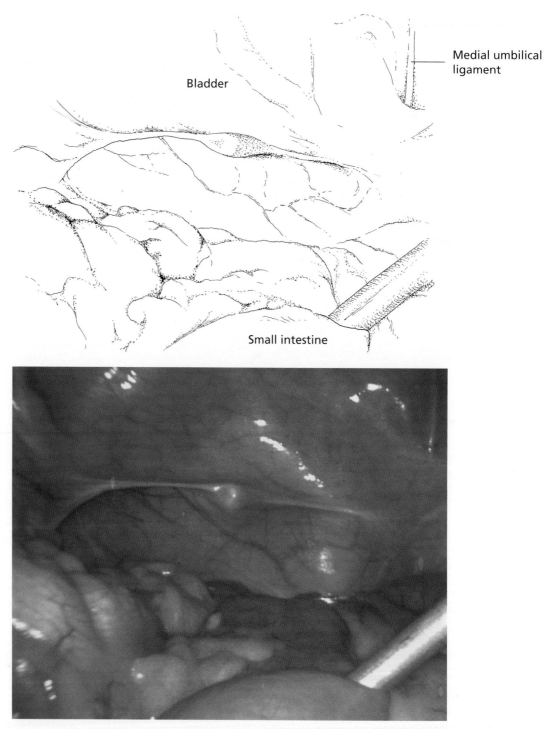

Fig. 1-9. Medial umbilical ligament, supravesical fossa, and bladder. In this view of the pelvis, the bladder is seen collapsed around the balloon of an indwelling catheter (which creates the appearance of a small mound with transverse radiating folds). The right medial umbilical ligament is seen. Small intestine occupies the foreground. The supravesical fossa is seen as a single space. Commonly, as in this example, the median umbilical fold (obliterated urachus) is not appreciated in the distended abdomen.

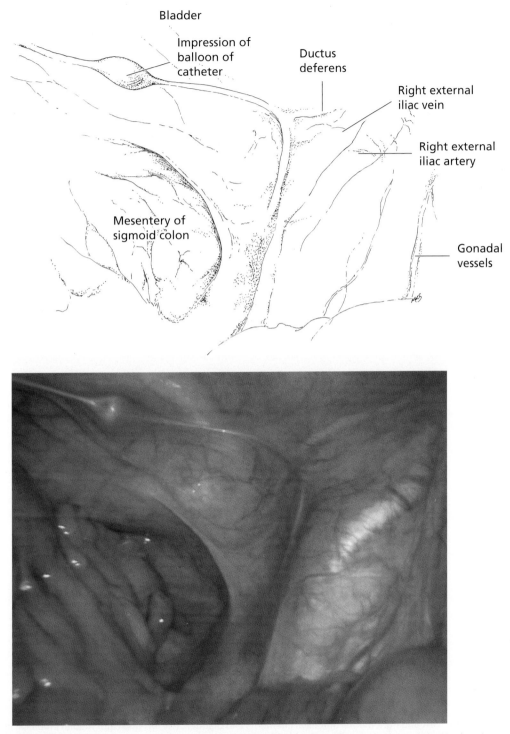

Fig. 1-10. Medial umbilical ligaments, ductus deferens, external iliac artery. This view of the abdominal cavity on the right side shows peritoneal folds and structures visible through the peritoneum. The bladder is collapsed around an indwelling catheter. The balloon of the catheter is visible through the bladder wall. The laparoscope is being directed down to visualize the external iliac artery and vein on the right. The ductus deferens and gonadal vessels are clearly seen. In the foreground, the mesentery of the sigmoid colon is noted.

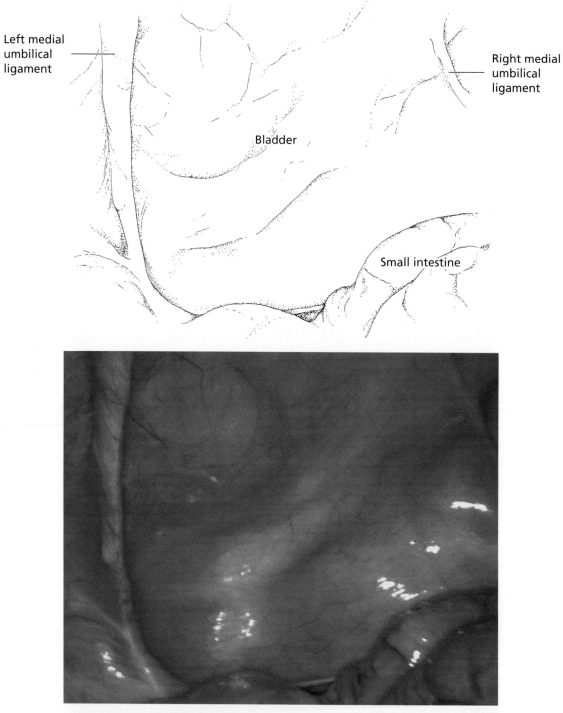

Fig. 1-11. Left and right medial umbilical ligaments and bladder. The left and right medial umbilical ligaments delineate the peritoneum overlying the bladder (the supravesical fossa). The median umbilical ligament, the remnant of the obliterated urachus, would arise from the dome of the bladder, but it is too close to the laparoscope to be seen. The small intestine occupies the foreground.

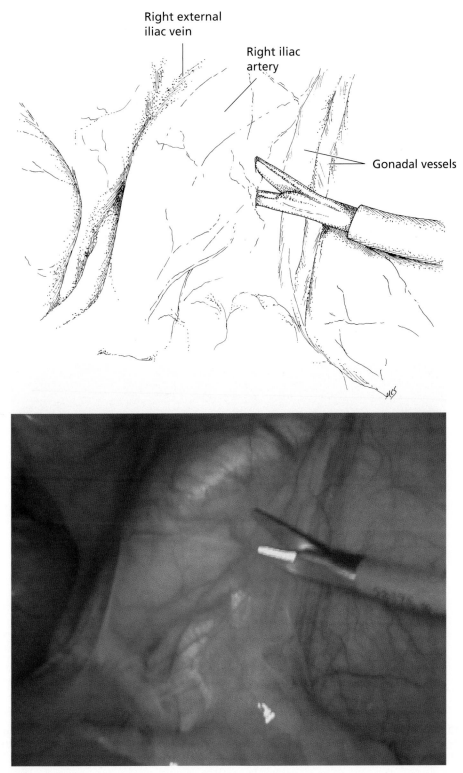

Fig. 1-12. The right external iliac artery and vein and gonadal vessels. An incision is being made to expose underlying lymph nodes.

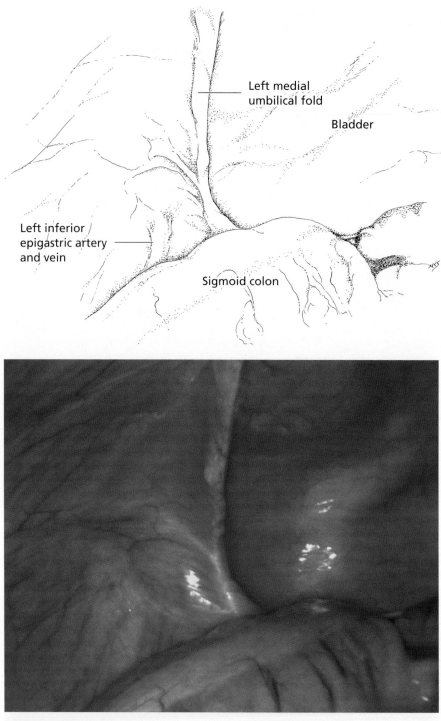

Fig. 1-13. The left medial umbilical ligament and inferior epigastric artery and vein. The left medial umbilical ligament and bladder are shown, with the sigmoid colon in the foreground. The left inferior epigastric artery and vein are seen.

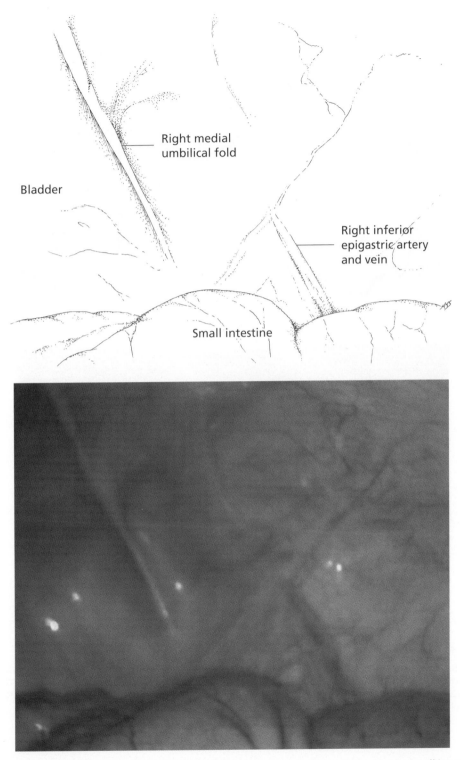

Fig. 1-14. The right medial umbilical ligament and right inferior epigastric artery and vein. Small intestine occupies the foreground.

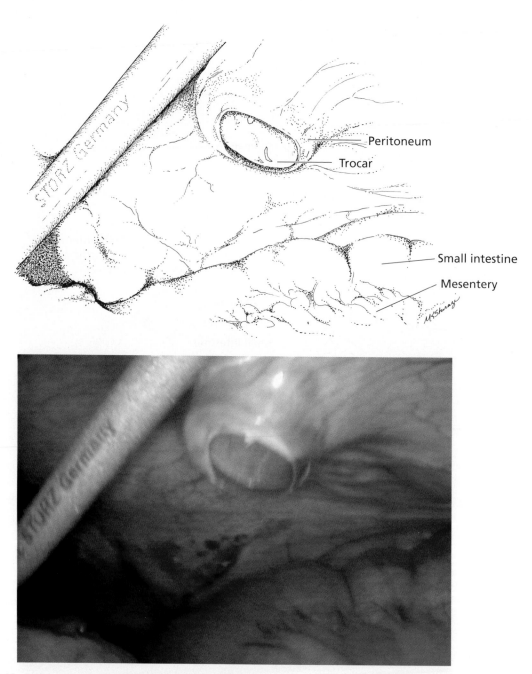

Fig. 1-15. Peritoneum. A trocar is shown advancing into the peritoneal cavity. The peritoneum is tented upward. Dissection in the preperitoneal space must avoid inadvertent entry through the flimsy peritoneum. As this figure illustrates, the peritoneum is often closely applied to the transversalis fascia without significant intervening fat or areolar tissue.

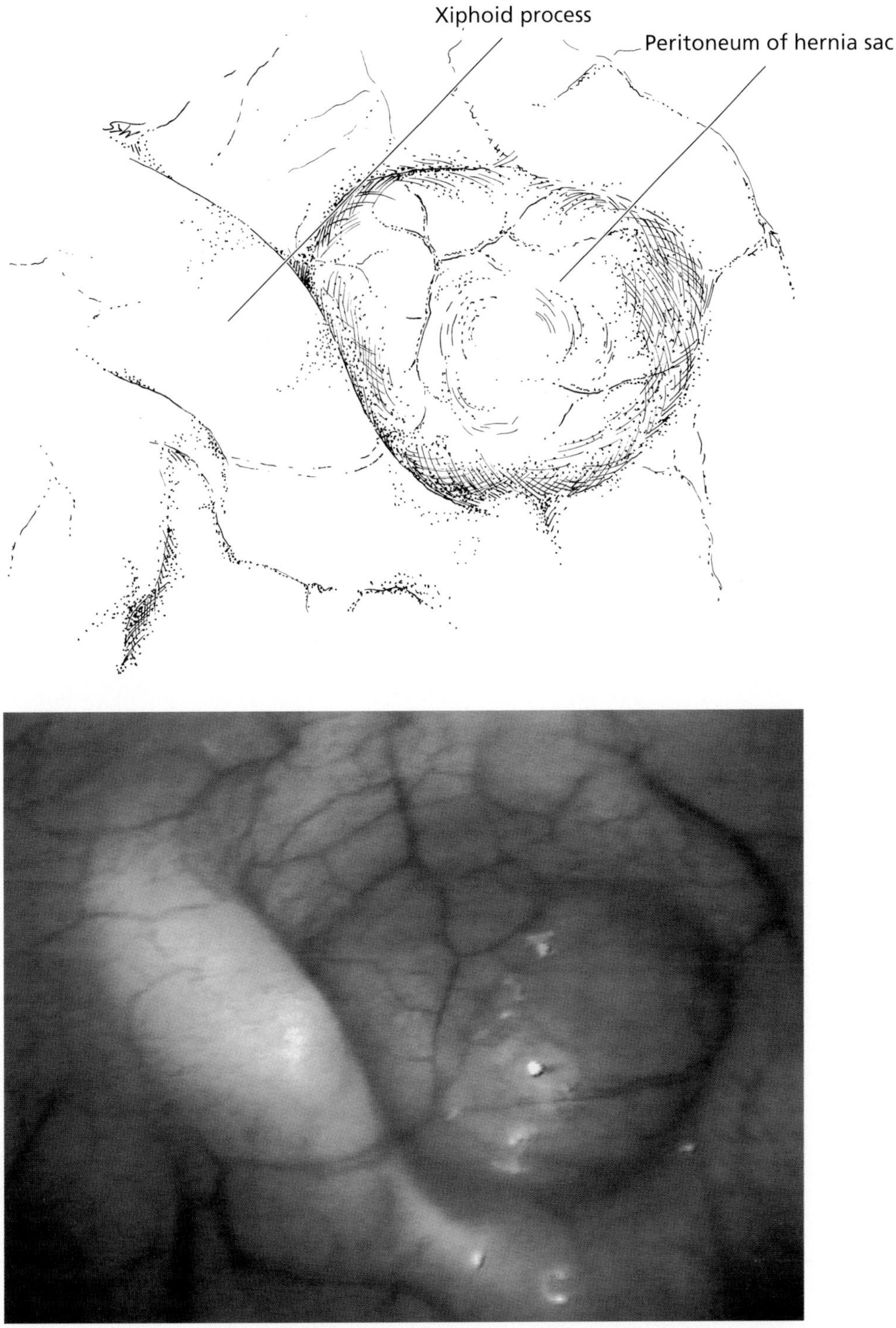

Xiphoid process

Peritoneum of hernia sac

Fig. 1-16. Xiphoid process and hernia defect. A prominent xiphoid process is seen indenting the upper anterior abdominal wall. A hernia defect adjacent to the xiphoid (from prior open heart surgery) is seen. This is the typical laparoscopic appearance of a ventral hernia and demonstrates how the peritoneum of the hernia sac is simply a continuation of the parietal peritoneum.

2

PERITONEAL CAVITY

INITIAL LAPAROSCOPIC VIEW AND PRINCIPLES OF EXPOSURE

The first step in diagnostic or therapeutic laparoscopy is thorough exploration, just as during laparotomy. The room, monitors, and patient should be positioned for the planned procedure and probable site of pathologic features. Preservation of the eye-hand-video monitor alignment prevents paradoxic movement and enhances dexterity. A systematic approach to exploration aids in ensuring that nothing is missed. This chapter briefly outlines such a systematic approach and provides an overview of the topographic anatomy of the abdominal cavity as seen by the laparoscopist. The anatomy of specific regions is discussed in detail in the chapters that follow.

The peritoneal reflections are described first, because these divide the peritoneal cavity into a series of communicating compartments. Understanding these topographic relationships facilitates thorough exploration. A brief topographic survey of the viscera follows. More detailed laparoscopic anatomy is given in later chapters. Retroperitoneal structures are described in Chapters 6 and 11.

ANATOMY AND SPECIFIC SURGICAL PROCEDURES

The rotation of the gut provides the key to understanding basic peritoneal topography. During embryonic development, the gut elongates and leaves the abdominal cavity. The loop of gut that is formed then rotates around the axis of the superior mesenteric artery and returns to the abdominal cavity. This net 270-degree counterclockwise rotation determines the ultimate position of the various viscera, which become fixed to a varying degree in their final positions. The blood supply (with the exception of that of the esophagus and rectum) comes from posterior, and various mesenteries form where the gut does not become adherent to the abdominal parietes. The duodenum passes behind the superior mesenteric artery and tunnels through the transverse mesocolon to emerge slightly to the left of midline at the ligament of Treitz. The mesentery of the small intestine progresses from left to right, from cephalad to caudad. The cecum comes to rest in the right lower quadrant, with the remainder of the colon draped like a picture frame around the inframesocolic viscera. Usually, the duodenum and ascending and descending colon become adherent to the posterior abdominal wall through a series of peritoneal attachments. Because the cecum is the last portion of the gut to rotate and attach, it is most subject to variation, and varying degrees of mobility are common.

Peritoneal Reflections

Parietal and visceral peritoneum lines the abdominal cavity. As this lining conforms to the shape of the structures it covers, folds and reflections (where the peritoneum is sharply bent back or reflected on itself) are created. The peritoneal folds of the anterior abdominal wall are described in Chapter 1. As the parietal peritoneum curves around to enfold the viscera, a more complex series of peritoneal reflections is formed (Fig. 2-1). These essentially compartmentalize the abdominal cavity. A basic understanding of these reflections is crucial because a thorough exploration may require inspecting all compartments.

In the upper abdomen, the attachments of the liver divide the space into a left and a right subphrenic space (Fig. 2-2). The right subphrenic space communicates laterally and anteriorly with the subhepatic space and through the epiploic foramen with the lesser sac.

The transverse colon and its mesentery effectually divide the abdomen into two compartments. The supramesocolic compartment contains all the viscera that lie above the transverse colon, its mesentery, and the greater omentum; the inframesocolic compartment contains the remaining viscera, which lie below these structures. The remaining peritoneal reflections are those of the mesentery of the small intestine and sigmoid colon.

Supramesocolic Viscera

The peritoneal cavity above the transverse colon is divided into left and right subphrenic spaces and a subhepatic space that connects through the epiploic foramen with the lesser sac or omental bursa. On the left, the esophagus exits the mediastinum through the esophageal hiatus of the diaphragm. It is essentially invisible at initial exploration, covered with the phrenoesophageal ligament and with glistening peritoneum. Elevation of the liver displays this region (Fig. 2-3). The anterior surface of the stomach is usually obvious and may be distinguished from colon by its color, absence of taeniae, and the greater omentum, which hangs like an apron from the greater curvature. Generally only the tip or medial border of the spleen is visible. Decompressing the stomach with an indwelling nasogastric or orogastric tube and applying gentle medial traction to the fundus of the stomach facilitate exposure. The spleen is tethered in the left upper quadrant by a series of peritoneal folds or ligaments, and full exposure requires atraumatic division of these folds (see Chapter 6). Segments II and III of the liver (sometimes termed the lateral segment of the left lobe) cover the lesser curvature of the stomach and lesser omentum and must be elevated to display these structures.

The epiploic foramen is the anatomic connection between the subhepatic space and the lesser sac. The hepatoduodenal ligament, containing the hepatic artery, the portal vein, and the common duct, forms the margin of this foramen. Surgical or laparoscopic access to the lesser sac is obtained by dividing the greater omentum and reflecting the stomach upward or by opening the transparent avascular portion of the lesser omentum. This procedure is described in more detail in Chapters 4 and 6.

The falciform ligament is an obvious dividing point between the left and right upper quadrants. In the right upper quadrant, the liver, gallbladder, and a portion of transverse colon and omentum are generally visible (Figs. 2-4 to 2-7). When the subhepatic space is opened by elevation of the gallbladder or liver, the pylorus and first portion of the duodenum may be seen (Figs. 2-5 and 2-6).

Inframesocolic Viscera

The greater omentum must be elevated and swept into the upper abdomen to explore the inframesocolic viscera adequately. The transverse colon is adherent to the underside of the greater omentum. The hepatic flexure is relatively easy to visualize (Fig. 2-7); the splenic flexure may be deep and cephalad, and it is most easily visualized with the patient in a steep lateral position (Fig. 2-8). The descending colon on the left (Fig. 2-9) and ascending colon on the right occupy the peritoneal gutters.

In the root of the transverse mesocolon, the ligament of Treitz (Fig. 2-10), is noted and the fourth portion of the duodenum may be visible as it makes the transition into jejunum. Paraduodenal fossae are relatively common and may be sites of internal herniation. Five such sites have been identified. Of these, the superior and inferior duodenal fossae are the most common. Because the anatomy is variable and the anatomic boundaries of these defects may include major vessels, care is warranted when approaching these anomalies.

From the ligament of Treitz, the small intestine (Fig. 2-11) progresses caudad and to the right to terminate in the ileum (Fig. 2-12). The appendix is variable in position, but it is reliably located by following the cecum and/or terminal ileum. The mesentery of the appendix tethers it posteriorly, and it is necessary to elevate the cecum or appendix to see the appendiceal base (Fig. 2-13).

The left lower quadrant contains primarily sigmoid colon (Fig. 2-14). Laparoscopic inspection of the pelvis is generally limited to that portion above the peritoneal reflection. The uterus and adnexal structures in female patients occupy the space between the bladder and the rectum (Fig. 2-15).

Exploratory Laparoscopy

Successful diagnostic laparoscopy requires careful attention to detail. A best guess is made about the quadrant in which pathology is likely to be found, and the video monitors and surgeon are positioned to allow direct view into this quadrant. Thus, if the supramesocolic compartment is thought to be the site of pathologic features, monitors are positioned at the head of the table. Conversely, pathology thought to be intramesocolic or in the pelvis mandates positioning the monitors near the foot of the table. If the site of pathology is truly unknown, then positioning the monitors on each side of the patient and moving them cephalad and caudad as needed give the greatest flexibility.

General survey of the abdomen usually begins with inspection through a periumbilical port. If the region of interest is in the midabdomen (such as an omental cyst), this may place the laparoscope too close to the lesion, and a more oblique approach through a lateral port will prove easier. Selective use of an angled laparoscope facilitates visualization of all structures.

At initial laparoscopic inspection, the greater omentum and transverse colon usually obscure visualization of the inframesocolic viscera. Hence it is easiest and most convenient to inspect the upper abdomen first. A systematic approach ensures that no area is overlooked (Fig. 2-16). Experienced surgeons commonly examine the area of anticipated pathology last, particularly if perforation or abscess is suspected; this may require beginning in another quadrant.

Initial inspection of the left upper quadrant is greatly facilitated by placing the patient in a steep reverse Trendelenburg position and decompressing the stomach with a nasogastric or orogastric tube. The diaphragm and segments II and III of the liver are readily seen. Gentle manipulation of the stomach and liver allows full inspection of the anterior surface of the stomach. The posterior surface of the stomach can only be seen by entering the lesser sac, either through the lesser omentum or, preferably, by division of the gastrocolic omentum. The pancreas is hidden behind the stomach. Gentle medial traction on the stomach elevates the spleen. The spleen is attached posteriorly, superiorly, and inferiorly by peritoneal reflections; hence such traction must be done with caution.

In the right upper quadrant, pneumoperitoneum and gravity cause the liver to fall away from the diaphragm, revealing the subphrenic spaces, the diaphragmatic surface of the liver, and the diaphragm. The subhepatic space can only be seen by elevating the liver (see Chapter 5). Frequently, the tip of the gallbladder is visible under the edge of the liver.

The greater omentum must be swept cephalad to expose the inframesocolic compartment. A neutral position facilitates inspection of the small intestine. Running the small bowel requires two-hand coordination using two atraumatic clamps (such as Babcock clamps) placed through lateral ports. It is simplest to select a place in the middle of the small intestine and run the bowel proximally or distally (it is not always easy to tell which way one is going). Running the bowel proximally eventually reveals the ligament of Treitz. Distally, the terminal ileum is recognized by a fatty stripe on the antimesenteric border. The entire small intestine can then be inspected by reversing the progression.

The table can then be placed in the Trendelenburg position and the patient's cecum, right colon, and appendix can be visualized. The appendix is located posterior to the juncture of the ileum and cecum. Adequate exposure of a retrocecal appendix may necessitate mobilization of the right colon. Full visualization of the colon requires rotating the table from side to side so the side of interest is elevated. Exposure of the splenic and hepatic flexures requires mobilization of the colon, and it is rarely done unless specific pathology in this region is suspected.

The pelvic viscera are exposed by placing the patient in a steep Trendelenburg position and gently sweeping the small intestine and omentum cephalad, assisted by gravity. The pelvic peritoneum is a common site of tumor studding and should be carefully inspected. The adnexae (in the female) may be displayed by gently elevating the uteroovarian ligaments and fallopian tubes (see Fig. 2-15).

Omentum

The greater omentum descends from the greater curvature of the stomach and folds over to attach to the taenia omentalis of the transverse colon. Structurally, it is a double sheet of peritoneum folded on itself. The fusion of the resulting four layers of peritoneum and intervening connective tissue forms a functionally single layer that may contain significant fat depots.

The blood supply of the omentum comes from the left and right gastroepiploic arteries, which send descending omental branches. Although the omentum is adherent to the transverse colon, only minor blood supply comes from the middle colic artery or its branches. Two anastomotic arcardes provide collateral circulation between the left and right gastroepiploic arteries. The first arcade is the most obvious, because it is generally within 2 cm of the greater curvature of the stomach and parallel to it. The second arcade (sometimes termed the arc of Barkow) is found in the posterior leaf of the greater omentum a variable distance from the transverse colon.

Omental Resection or Harvest

Laparoscopic diagnosis and resection of omental torsion or cysts are straightforward and do not require special attention to anatomic details. Branches of the left or right gastroepiploic arteries are secured and divided as needed. The transverse colon is adherent to the underside of the omentum and must be avoided. Occasionally, the greater omentum is adherent to the transverse mesocolon as well as to the taenia omentalis. The laparoscopic surgeon must exercise care to avoid injury to the middle colic artery in this circumstance.

Harvest of a viable omental pedicle for use in reconstructive surgery depends on knowledge of vascular anatomy. Either the left or right gastroepiploic artery and its accompanying vein are preserved. A considerable length of well-vascularized omentum can be harvested by preserving the left or right gastroepiploic artery and one of these arcades. Generally when a long pedicle of omentum is required, the subgastric arcade is divided, and the arc of Barkow is preserved; the omentum can then be extended on a long pedicle of right (or left) gastroepiploic artery. There is considerable individual variation, and laparoscopic Doppler ultrasound is a useful adjunct.

BIBLIOGRAPHY
Anatomic References

1. Alday ES, Goldsmith HS. Surgical technique for omental lenthening based on arterial anatomy. *Surg Gynecol Obstet* 1972;135:103–107.
2. Gray SW, Skandalakis JE. The small intestines. In: Gray SW, Skandalakis JE, eds. *Embryology for surgeons.* Philadelphia: WB Saunders, 1972:129–147.
3. Marschall MA, Cohen M. The use of the greater omentum in reconstructive surgery. *Surg Annu* 1994;26:251–254.
4. McVay CB. The abdominal cavity and contents. In: McVay CB, ed. *Anson and McVay surgical anatomy,* 6th ed. Philadelphia: WB Saunders, 1984:585–730.
5. Michels NA. Blood supply of the great omentum and the transverse mesocolon. In: Michels NA, ed.

Blood supply and anatomy of the upper abdominal organs with a descriptive atlas. Philadelphia: JB Lippincott, 1955:274–279.

6. Willwert BM, Zollinger RM Jr, Izant RJ Jr. Congenital mesocolic (paraduodenal) hernia. *Am J Surg* 1974;128:358–361.

Surgical References

1. Asencio-Arana F. Laparoscopic access to the lesser sac in gastric cancer staging. *Surg Laparosc Endosc* 1994;4:438–440.
2. Berci G, Sackier JM, Paz-Partlow M. Emergency laparoscopy. *Am J Surg* 1991;161:332–335.
3. Brandt CP, Priebe PP, Eckhauser ML. Diagnostic laparoscopy in the intensive care patient: avoiding the nontherapeutic laparotomy. *Surg Endosc* 1993;7:168–172.
4. Childers JM, Balserak JC, Kent T, Surwit EA. Laparoscopic staging of Hodgkin's lymphoma. *J Laparoendosc Surg* 1993;3:495–499.
5. Conlon KC, Dougherty EC, Klimstra DS. Laparoscopic resection of a giant omental cyst. *Surg Endosc* 1995;9:1130–1132.
6. Corral CJ, Prystowsky JB, Weidrich TA, Harris GD. Laparoscopic-assisted bipedicle omental flap mobilization for reconstruction of a chest wall defect. *J Laparoendosc Surg* 1994;5:343–346.
7. Cuatico W, Vannix D. Laparoscopically guided peritoneal insertion in ventriculoperitoneal shunts. *J Laparoendosc Surg* 1995;5:309–311.
8. Cuschieri A, Hall AW, Clark J. Value of laparoscopy in the diagnosis and management of pancreatic carcinoma. *Gut* 1978;19:672–677.
9. Easter DW, Cuschieri A, Nathanson LK, Lavelle-Jones M. The utility of diagnostic laparoscopy for abdominal disorders: audit of 120 patients. *Arch Surg* 1992;127:379–383.
10. Ishitani MB, DeAngelis GA, Sistrom CL, Rodgers BM, Pruett TL. Laparoscopic ultrasound-guided drainage of lymphoceles following renal transplantation. *J Laparoendosc Surg* 1994;4:61–64.
11. Julian TB, Ribeiro U. Laparoscopic removal of a displaced ventriculoperitoneal shunt. *J Laparoendosc Surg* 1995;5:55–58.
12. Kim HB, Gregor MB, Boley SJ, Kleinhaus S. Digitally assisted laparoscopic drainage of multiple intraabdominal abscesses. *J Laparoendosc Surg* 1993;3:477–479.
13. Lowy AM, Mansfield PF, Leach SD, Ajani J. Laparoscopic staging for gastric cancer. *Surgery* 1996;119:611–614.
14. Nagy AG, James D. Diagnostic laparoscopy. *Am J Surg* 1989;157:490–493.
15. Saltz R. Endoscopic harvest of the omental and jejunal free flaps. *Clin Plast Surg* 1995;22:747–754.

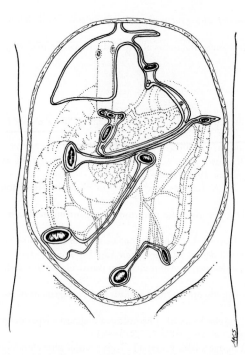

Fig. 2-1. Peritoneal reflections of the posterior abdominal wall. Most of the viscera have been removed for clarity. Note how the lesser sac communicates the subhepatic space through the epiploic foramen. The transverse colon and its mesentery divide the abdomen into a supramesocolic and inframesocolic compartment. The mesentery of the small intestine attaches along a line that runs from left to right from cephalad to caudad. In the pelvis, the sigmoid colon has a mesentery.

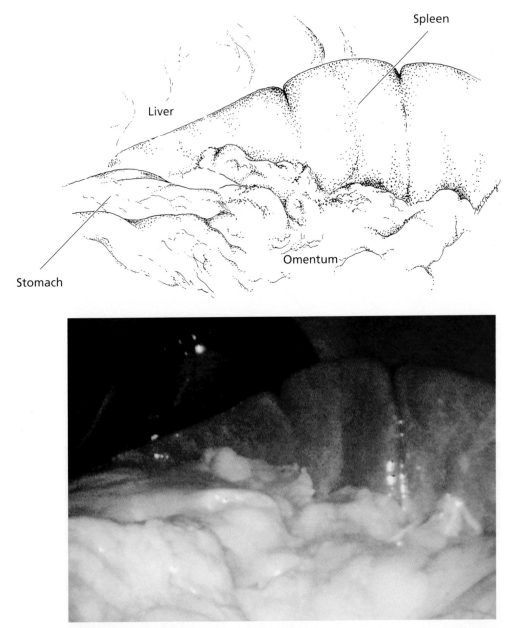

Fig. 2-2. Left upper quadrant. The diaphragm, segments II and III of the liver, stomach, greater omentum, and an enlarged spleen are seen. Note how the greater omentum covers the transverse colon and only the supramesocolic viscera are visible.

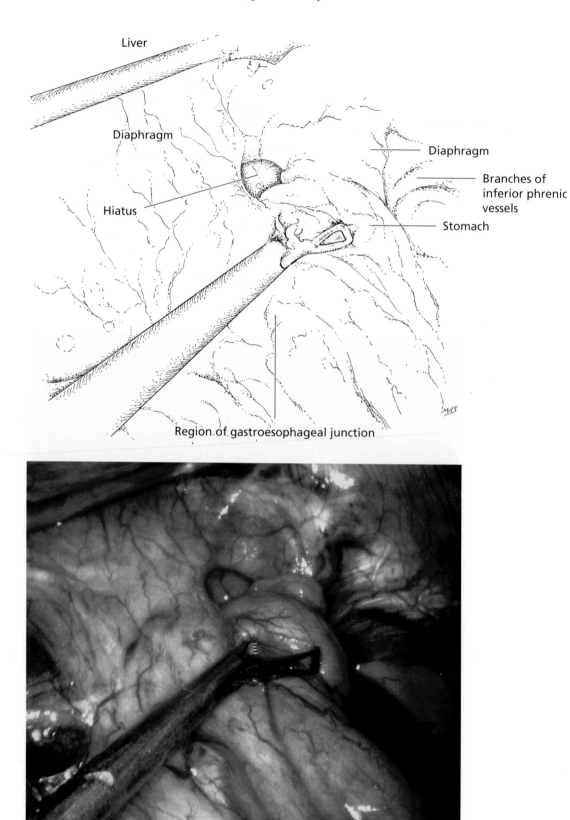

Fig. 2-3. Region of esophageal hiatus. The liver has been elevated to display the gastroesophageal junction and esophageal hiatus. A paraesophageal hernia is being reduced.

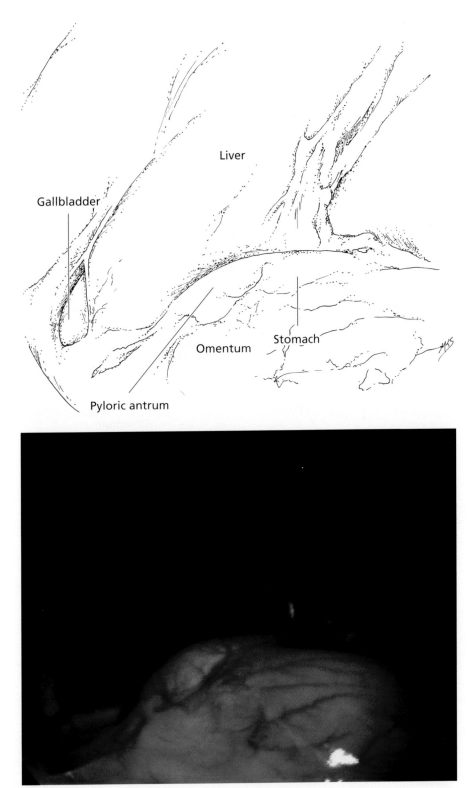

Fig. 2-4. Right upper quadrant. The liver, gallbladder, and greater omentum covering the transverse colon are noted.

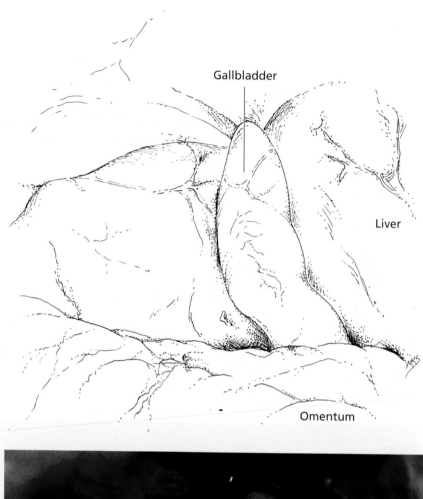

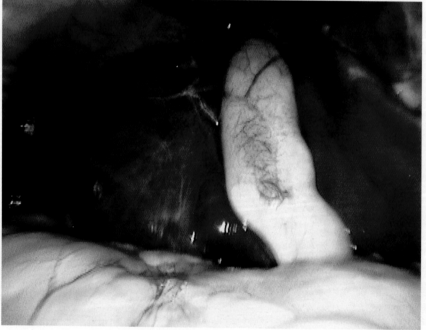

Fig. 2-5. Subhepatic space. The subhepatic space has been opened by elevating the gallbladder before laparoscopic cholecystectomy (less traumatic methods of displaying this region are discussed in Chapter 5). The gallbladder, pylorus, and first portion of the duodenum may be seen with gentle elevation of the liver.

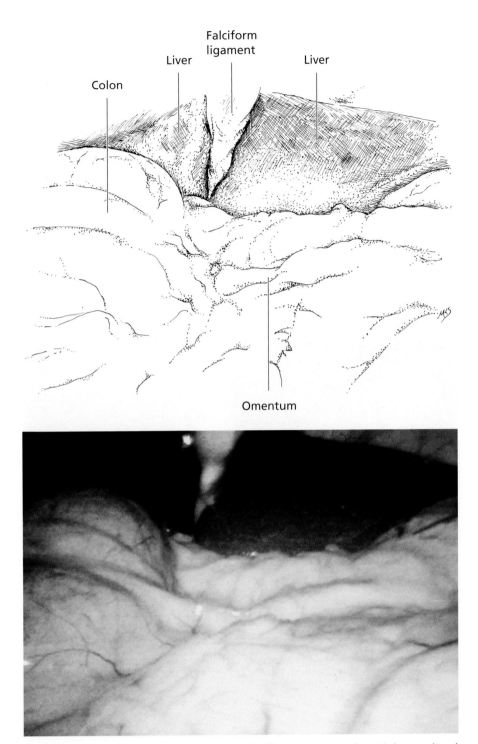

Fig. 2-6. Subhepatic space. Gentle upward traction on the ligamentum teres hepatis has produced some exposure of the distal stomach and pylorus.

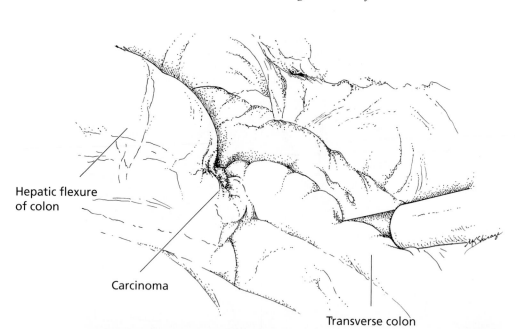

Hepatic flexure
of colon

Carcinoma

Transverse colon

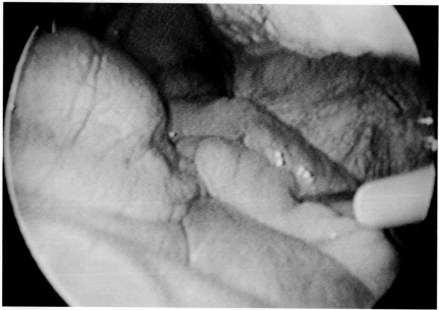

Fig. 2-7. Hepatic flexure of colon. The flexure is only partially seen. Complete visualization of the colon requires mobilization from the abdominal wall. A bulky carcinoma of the colon is barely visible.

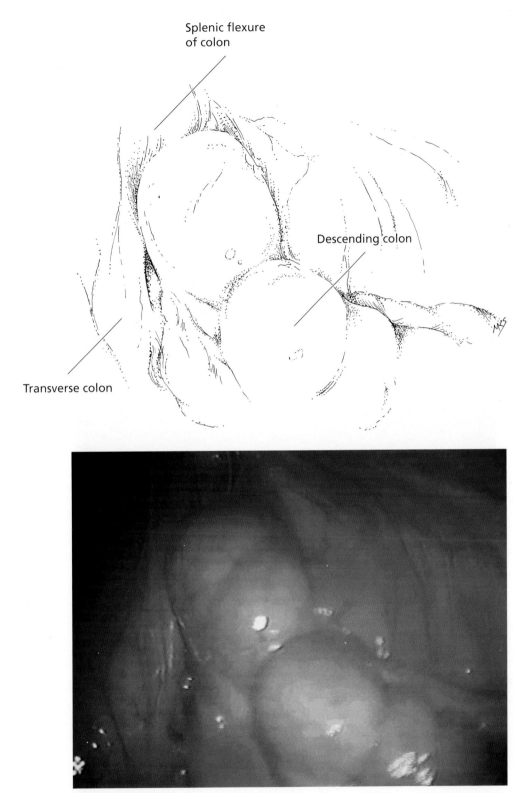

Fig. 2-8. Splenic flexure of colon. This view was obtained with the patient in the full right lateral position before laparoscopic splenectomy. A clear view of the splenic flexure is difficult to obtain with the patient supine.

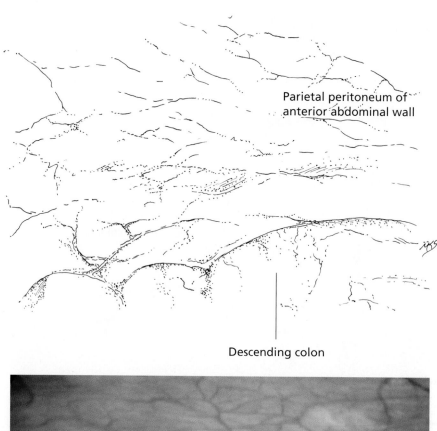

Parietal peritoneum of
anterior abdominal wall

Descending colon

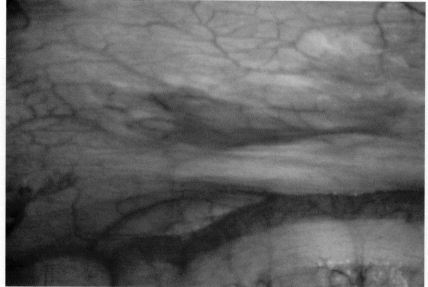

Fig. 2-9. Descending colon. The descending colon and left lateral peritoneal gutter are seen.

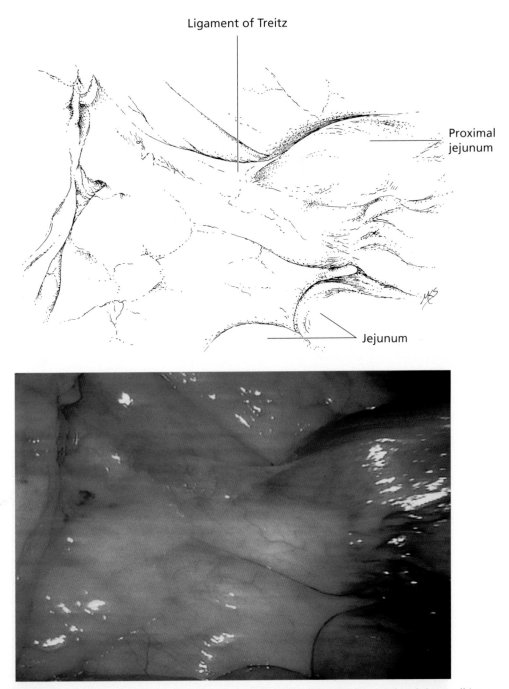

Fig. 2-10. Ligament of Treitz. With the transverse colon and greater omentum elevated and the small intestine retracted downward, the ligament of Treitz and the duodenojejunal juncture are seen.

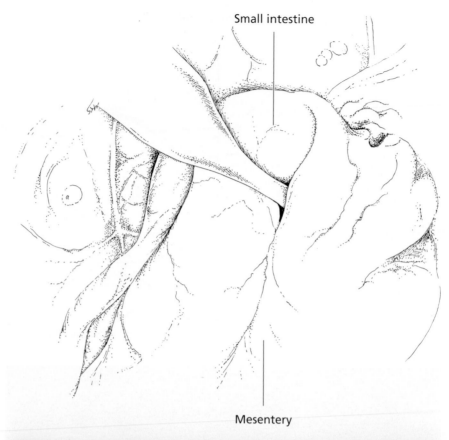

Small intestine

Mesentery

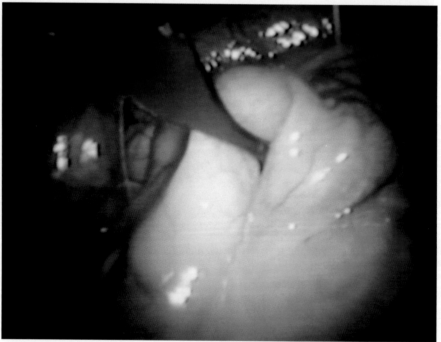

Fig. 2-11. Small intestine. A loop of jejunum has been grasped with an endoscopic Babcock clamp and will be passed to an assistant. The loop will be followed proximal and distal to inspect the entire small intestine.

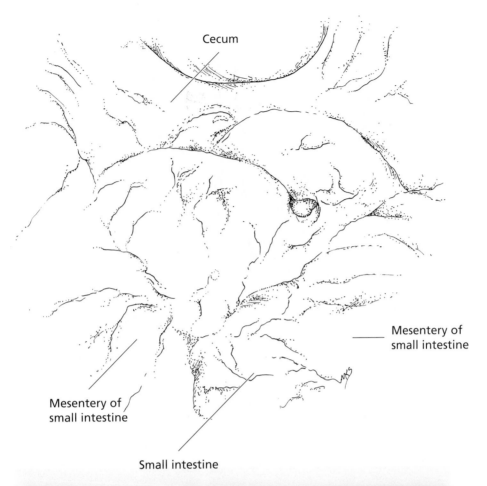

Cecum

Mesentery of
small intestine

Mesentery of
small intestine

Small intestine

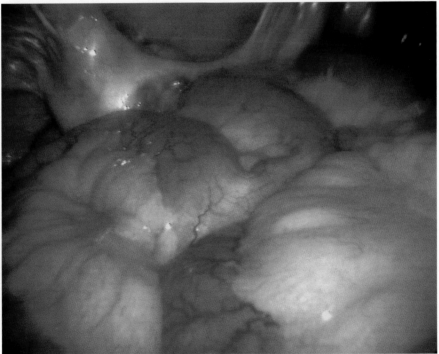

Fig. 2-12. Right lower quadrant. The cecum and distal ileum are noted.

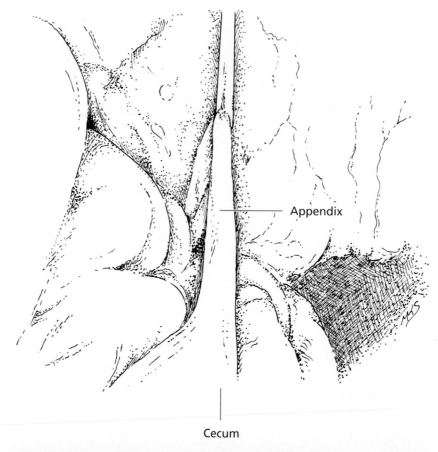

Appendix

Cecum

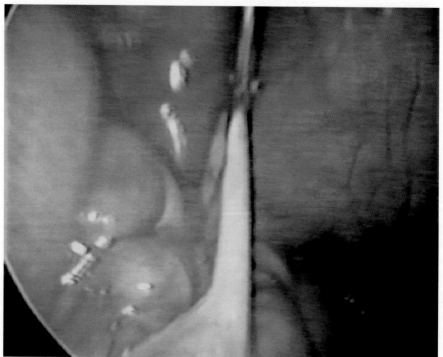

Fig. 2-13. Normal appendix and cecum. A normal appendix is displayed by traction before incidental appendectomy.

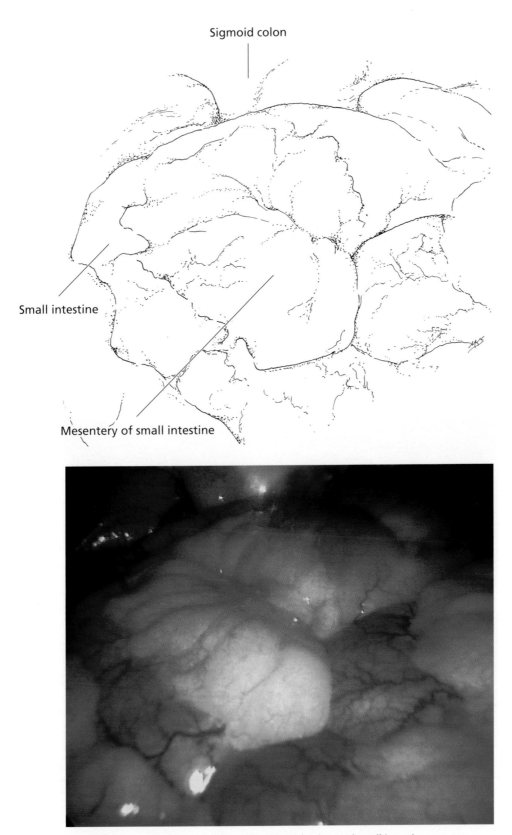

Sigmoid colon

Small intestine

Mesentery of small intestine

Fig. 2-14. Left lower quadrant. The sigmoid colon and small intestine are seen.

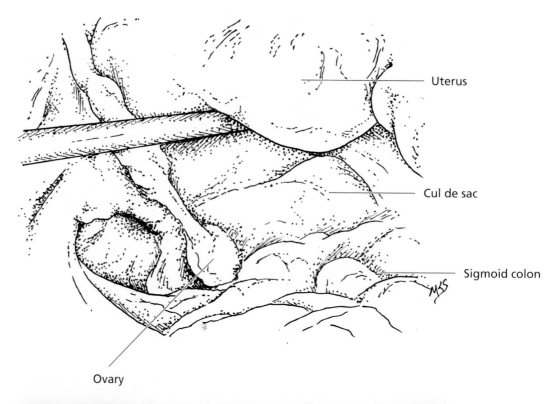

Uterus

Cul de sac

Sigmoid colon

Ovary

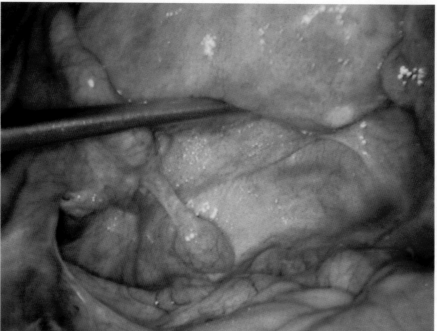

Fig. 2-15. Uterus, ovary, and fallopian tube. The adnexal structures are displayed by gentle elevation of the uteroovarian ligaments and fallopian tubes. The cul de sac is seen. A steep Trendelenburg position has allowed bowel loops and omentum to be swept out of the pelvis.

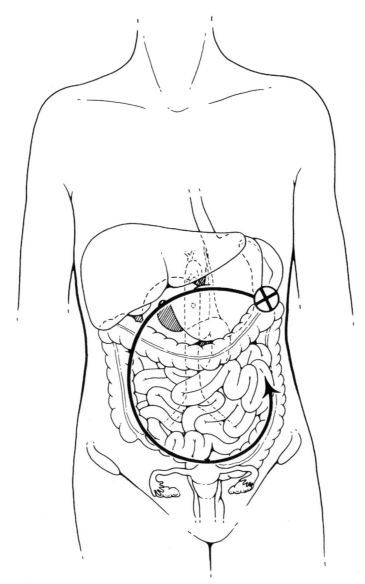

Fig. 2-16. Scheme for systematic exploratory laparoscopy. In this illustration, the greater omentum has been removed for clarity. The transverse colon is the dividing line between supremesocolic and inframesocolic compartments. A systematic approach to abdominal exploration begins with the supramesocolic compartment. The patient should be in the reverse Trendelenburg position. Inspection begins in the left upper quadrant and then progresses to the right upper quadrant. The colon, small intestine, and pelvic viscera are then inspected. A combination of steep Trendelenburg position and tilting the table from side to side will facilitate thorough exploration. The greater omentum must be elevated to expose the small intestine and the remainder of the colon. (From Scott-Conner CEH, Dawson DL. *Operative Anatomy*. Philadelphia: JB Lippincott, 1993:280, with permission.)

3

DIAPHRAGM, HIATUS, AND ESOPHAGUS

INITIAL LAPAROSCOPIC VIEW AND PRINCIPLES OF EXPOSURE

The initial survey of the left upper quadrant demonstrates the left subphrenic space, abdominal surface of the diaphragm, diaphragmatic surface of the left lobe of the liver, stomach, greater omentum, and colon. The spleen may be visible in the extreme lateral recess. The prominent ligamentum teres hepatis with the associated falciform ligament is seen to the right of the field, forming a convenient dividing point between left and right subphrenic spaces (Figs. 3-1 to 3-3).

For procedures on the esophagus, stomach, and hiatal region, the patient is placed supine with the legs separated. The surgeon stands between the patient's legs. The reverse Trendelenburg position with the left side elevated allows gravity to assist in displacing the viscera caudad to open the left subphrenic space. An angled (30- to 45-degree) laparoscope is crucial when working high in the left upper quadrant. The hiatus is high and posterior, particularly in large patients. Placement of the laparoscope through a portal in the left epigastric region (rather than the umbilicus) brings the field closer and allows the laparoscopic surgeon to look down at the region of interest.

In contrast to open surgery, laparoscopic surgery on the hiatal region is performed with the left lobe of the liver *in situ*, and the triangular ligament is generally not divided. Division of the triangular ligament may actually hinder exposure, by allowing segments II and III of the left lobe to flop down into the field. Elevation of the left lobe of the liver is produced by passing a liver retractor from a right lateral port, slipping the retractor under the ligamentum teres hepatis and into the left subhepatic space, and then opening or expanding the retractor (see Fig. 5-6). Downward pressure on the handle of the retractor, coupled with a "toeing in" motion of the retractor (so the edge of the retractor closest to the esophageal hiatus is most firmly elevated), displays the subhepatic space and hiatal region by flattening and elevating the left lobe of the liver up into the diaphragm. The laparoscope is slipped into the space thus created to look directly at the hiatal region behind the undisturbed left lobe.

For simple procedures in the left upper quadrant, an alternative method of exposure may be used. Grasping forceps are passed from an epigastric portal and gently slid under the left lobe of the liver. The forceps are then gently swept cephalad to elevate the left lobe. In slender patients, the right crus of the diaphragm may be visible and can be grasped, providing stable positioning and holding the left lobe in an elevated position. The exposure thus obtained may be adequate for diagnostic laparoscopy or simple biopsies, allowing exposure of the region with a minimum number of instruments and portals.

In the left subhepatic space, obvious landmarks include the lesser omentum, through which the caudate lobe of the liver is generally visible, and the stomach (Fig. 3-4). The intact phrenoesophageal membrane precludes visualization of the esophagus, but Belsey's fat pad may provide a clue to its location (see Fig. 3-4; Figs. 3-5 to 3-8). Gentle traction on the stomach displays the notched medial margin of the spleen, with the attached gastrosplenic folds.

For many procedures on the esophagus, it is extremely helpful to have a flexible esophagogastroduodenoscope (EGD scope) in place in the upper abdominal esophagus at the start of the procedure, with its tip positioned just below the diaphragm. The esophagus may be identified by palpation of the EGD scope through the muscular wall or by visualization of the light through the esophageal wall (with the laparoscope light source turned down or off). Gentle deflection of the tip of the EGD scope upward elevates the esophagus, enhancing visualization and facilitating dissection, but caution must be used not to injure the esophagus.

Procedures on the spleen and tail of pancreas are facilitated by tilting the patient's left side upward (see Chapter 6). Some laparoscopic surgeons place the patient in the right lateral position to maximize the effect of gravity. An angled laparoscope facilitates visualization of the extreme left upper quadrant, and it may be necessary to move the viewing port closer to the left upper quadrant to minimize distance.

ANATOMY AND SPECIFIC SURGICAL PROCEDURES

Liver

The apparent "left lobe" of the liver is actually segments II and III in the Couinaud terminology. It is sometimes called the lateral segment of the left lobe of the liver (see Figs. 3-1 and 3-2). The falciform ligament divides segments II and III from segments I and IV, which are the remainder of the anatomic left lobe of the liver. Segment I, the caudate or spigelian lobe, is visible through the filamentous portion of the lesser omentum (see Fig. 3-8) and forms a useful landmark as the laparoscopic surgeon approaches the hiatus and vagal trunks. The liver is discussed and illustrated in greater detail in Chapter 5.

The left triangular ligament is a peritoneal fold attaching the diaphragmatic surface of segments II and III to the underside of the diaphragm. It is formed by two leaves of the coronary ligament of the liver that approach and fuse (see Fig. 3-7). The anterior layer of the coronary ligament forms a fold enclosing the ligamentum teres hepatis and forming the falciform ligament. The left triangular ligament must be divided to mobilize segments II and III fully for resection. The extreme leftmost edge of the triangular ligament may contain small vessels or accessory bile ducts; hence it is prudent to secure this with clips before division. Medially, the triangular ligament surrounds the hepatic veins. The distance from the left edge of the triangular ligament to the hepatic veins varies from 5 to 15 cm, and care should be taken as the medial portion of the dissection is developed. Downward traction on the liver facilitates exposure, but it may collapse the hepatic vein, predisposing it to injury. This region is unlikely to be encountered during routine laparoscopic surgery of the left upper quadrant because the standard laparoscopic approach to the hiatus does not involve mobilizing the liver (as previously mentioned). Laparoscopic resection of segments II or III or portions thereof may require such mobilization.

Diaphragm

The diaphragm attaches by muscular insertions to the xiphoid process anteriorly, the lower six costal cartilages anteriorly and laterally, and to the bodies of several lumbar vertebrae through the crura posteriorly. Each hemidiaphragm is seen to have a central tendon and an outer muscular ring. The two hemidiaphragms communicate in the midline. The central tendinous region is a fibrous aponeurosis pierced in the posterior midline by the foramen for the inferior vena cava. The esophageal hiatus, to the left and somewhat anterior, is formed by the muscular crura and is variable in configuration (see Figs. 3-5 to 3-8; Fig. 3-9).

The central tendinous portion of the diaphragm is well seen as the left subphrenic space is inspected. Centrally, the tendinous portion is contiguous to the pericardium. This portion is easily identified by the vigorous pulsations of the heart, seen through the diaphragm. Access to the pericardium, for example, for pericardial window, may be obtained here. Laterally, the pericardium comes into close proximity to the right margin of the esophageal hiatus, especially when the hiatus is enlarged and attenuated. This must be kept in mind when large hiatal hernias, such as that shown in Fig. 3-6, are repaired.

The left and right phrenic nerves leave the pericardial surfaces to run for a short distance on the thoracic surface of the diaphragm, but subsequently they pierce the diaphragm and are then visible on the abdominal surface of the left and right hemidiaphragm. The right phrenic nerve pierces the diaphragm just lateral to the inferior vena cava foramen. It divides into four trunks (sternal, anterolateral, posterolateral, and crural), which may be visible to the laparoscopist by their accompanying branches of the inferior phrenic arteries and veins. The left phrenic nerve similarly pierces the diaphragm just lateral to the left border of the heart and also divides into four identifiable trunks. Near the posterior border of the central tendon the left and right inferior phrenic arteries divide into medial and lateral branches. The medial branch curves forward to anastomose with its contralateral counterpart, thus forming an anastamotic arcade in front of the central tendon. These vessels also anastomose with the musculophrenic and pericardiacophrenic arteries. The locations of these nerves and vessels are important when incisions are made in the diaphragm or when diaphragmatic hernias are repaired. These neurovascular bundles are generally visible through the peritoneal surface overlying the diaphragm and may be seen in most of the figures accompanying this chapter. The left inferior phrenic artery courses upward from its origin, running laterally in front of the left crus of the diaphragm and then passes anterior to it. Anomalies of the left inferior phrenic artery are common and may be particularly problematic during hiatal dissection (see later).

Repair of Diaphragmatic Hernia

Mild eventration of the diaphragm is fairly common and is usually clinically insignificant. It is demonstrated laparoscopically by a normally formed but unusually high diaphragm. Hernias of the hiatal region are common (see Fig. 3-6). Other occasional sites of diaphragmatic hernias include the bilateral anteriorly located foramina of Morgagni, the posterolateral foramina of Bochdalek, and the anatomically weak central tendon or posterior attachment region prone to rupture with blunt abdominal trauma.

The foramina of Morgagni are located anteriorly and are difficult to visualize laparoscopically. An angled (45-degree) laparoscope is essential for visualization. Anatomically, these hernias represent defects in the region where the diaphragm attaches anteriorly to the xiphoid and are frequently bilateral. The alternate terms "subcostosternal" or "retrosternal" emphasize this anatomic location. Hernias in this location are traditionally repaired transabdominally, and laparoscopic repair has been described.

Hernias through a posterolateral defect (Bochdalek) are usually symptomatic at birth and are increasingly diagnosed before delivery (using ultrasound). The typical location is at the posterior costal margins of the 10th and 11th ribs. On rare occasions, a small right-sided defect is asymptomatic into adulthood and may be observed laparoscopically.

Penetrating abdominal trauma may produce diaphragmatic defects of any size and in any location, and these have been diagnosed and treated laparoscopically as well. In contrast to diaphragmatic hernias, which have well-developed sacs, acute diaphragmatic injuries allow free communication with the pleural space. Insufflation of the abdomen with carbon dioxide may produce a pneumothorax. This simple pneumothorax is easily evacuated with a catheter, if it is recognized.

Esophageal Hiatus

The esophageal hiatus is the opening between the diaphragmatic crura. This muscular tunnel is 2 to 3 cm long. The esophagus angles slightly to the left and anteriorly as it passes through the hiatus to reach the abdomen. Only the vagus nerves and esophagus pass through this hiatus; it is not traversed by any major vessels or lymphatic trunks. In approximately half the population, muscle fibers from the right crus of the diaphragm form both the right and left margins of the hiatus; in essence, the fibers of the right crus divide and surround the esophagus in a slinglike fashion (see Figs. 3-8 and 3-9; Figs. 3-10 to 3-15). In the remaining cases, fibers of the left crus contribute to the left margin in a variable fashion.

Posterior to the esophagus, the two crura fuse to form a fibrous and muscular structure termed the median arcuate ligament. In a common variant, a band of muscle fibers, the band of Low, passes from the left crus to the right of the hiatus. The median arcuate ligament varies considerably in thickness and strength. It usually crosses over the aorta just cephalad to the origin of the celiac axis. The aorta and celiac axis are generally not visualized during the course of hiatal dissection.

The anterior margin of the hiatus is reinforced by a localized thickening of the central tendon, the transverse ligament. In patients with large hiatal hernias, the anterior margin is markedly attenuated, the transverse ligament is absent, and the diaphragmatic surface of the pericardium forms the medial border of the hiatus, creating the risk of inadvertent entry into the pericardium if sutures are placed deeply in an anterior hiatal approximation, as previously noted (see Fig. 3-6).

The medial or right margin of the hiatus is innervated by the right phrenic nerve, the left by the left phrenic nerve. Although the phrenic nerve branches that innervate this region are not seen during laparoscopic surgery, the accompanying vessels are easily visualized.

The phrenoesophageal ligament (see Figs. 3-10 and 3-11) is a membranous fusion of layers of endoabdominal fascia that closes the gap between hiatus and esophagus, thus separating the retroperitoneum from the mediastinum. Although it may contain a few muscle fibers, this structure is more membranous than ligamentous, particularly in patients with hiatal hernias. It covers the anterior muscular border of the hiatus and proximal few centimeters of abdominal esophagus. On the right, the lesser sac extends to the hiatus (see Figs. 3-12 and 3-13) behind the gastrohepatic omentum. The gastrohepatic omentum ascends and fuses with the phrenoesophageal ligament on the undersurface of the diaphragm, separating the lesser sac from the general peritoneal cavity. Posteriorly, the hiatus is partially occluded by thin, fibroareaolar tissue that may contain a few muscle fibers. Although this plane is easily developed by blunt dissection, this phase of the laparoscopic dissection is generally performed last, after adequate mobilization and definition of both hiatal margins and the anterior and lateral borders of the esophagus.

Hiatal Hernia Repair

The laparoscopic surgeon generally approaches the hiatus from the right side first, because the right margin of the hiatus is closest to the umbilically placed laparoscope. The right margin of the hiatus is exposed by dividing a portion of the lesser omentum and the phrenoesophageal ligament (see Fig. 3-12). Vascular structures in the lesser omentum must be identified and either protected or clipped and divided. If this dissection is begun high, near the hiatal margin, vessels are less likely to be encountered. The junction of the crus and perigastric fat is generally identifiable. Through this opening, the posterior mediastinum is entered.

The lesser omentum is conveniently divided into the thickened hepatoduodenal ligament and the larger, sheetlike gastrohepatic ligament. The hepatoduodenal ligament, containing the common bile duct, hepatic artery, and portal vein, is well to the right of the field of view. The laparoscope must be angled to the right of the midline to visualize these structures (see Chapter 5). The gastrohepatic ligament, which connects the lesser curvature of the stomach with the fissure for the ligamentum venosum, is encountered during the dissection around the hiatus.

Much of the gastrohepatic ligament overlying the caudate lobe is transparent, and it is tempting to begin division of this structure down low, through this avascular region. However, as the dissection proceeds toward the hiatus, the hepatic branch of the vagus nerve and several large vessels may be encountered. Therefore, a more efficient approach is to begin the dissection high, next to the hiatus. The largest vessels in the lesser omentum are the left gastric artery and its branches and the associated left gastric vein. The left gastric artery comes from posterior to enter the lesser omentum, where it abruptly turns caudad as it passes within the leaves of the lesser omentum (see Fig. 3-5). It typically gives off one or two small branches that pass cephalad to supply the esophagus (discussed subsequently) before dividing into anterior and posterior branches that supply the stomach. In 12% to 20% of anatomically normal individuals, the left gastric artery gives rise to an aberrant left hepatic artery just before dividing into its two terminal branches. This aberrant left hepatic artery courses upward near the esophagus as it passes within the lesser omentum, then crosses the caudate lobe to enter the liver at the fissure for the ligamentum venosum. This sizable vessel may be encountered by the laparoscopic surgeon close to the right crus as the dissection progresses (see Fig. 3-8). It is impossible for the laparoscopist to ascertain whether this represents an accessory hepatic artery or a replaced hepatic artery, and prudence would dictate that a sizable artery in this region be preserved. Preserving this vessel may seem difficult, but as the hiatal dissection progresses into the lower mediastinum, a substantial amount of room can be developed cephalad to this anomalous vessel (which is gradually mobilized downward) without sacrificing it (see Fig. 3-23).

Beginning at the edge of the right crus, where it is easy to delineate the muscular crura from the perigastric fat, the dissection of the hiatus proceeds from right to left. The goal is to expose the muscular hiatus fully. Keeping the dissection high, in the lower mediastinum, avoids vessels associated with the stomach. The esophagus is naturally mobilized as dissection progresses, with little actual dissection on the esophagus (see Figs. 3-14 and 3-15; Figs. 3-16 to 3-20). Both vagus nerves may be encountered and should be protected (discussed later).

Smaller vessels in the vicinity of the hiatus include the left and right inferior phrenic arteries, which supply the diaphragm. Anomalies are common, and it is not unusual to find sizable branches in this region (Figs. 3-21 and 3-22). The inferior phrenic arteries arise separately from the aorta immediately cephalad to the celiac trunk, or by a common stem from the aorta or celiac trunk. From their origin, they run upward and laterally in front of the crura. The left inferior phrenic artery passes behind the esophagus and runs forward on the left side of the hiatus in a fairly constant fashion, where it may be encountered by the laparoscopist. The right inferior phrenic artery passes behind the inferior vena cava and is not seen.

Esophagus

The length of intraabdominal esophagus varies in anatomically normal individuals. Generally after adequate mobilization, dissection, and traction on the stomach, several centimeters can be exposed. A significantly greater length can be well visualized and surgically accessed as the laparoscopic dissection continues into the lower mediastinum. The dissection of the hiatus is essentially a dissection in the posterior mediastinum. The left side of the esophagus is in close contact with the parietal pleura of the left side of the chest. Inadvertent entry into the left pleural space may occur during dissection, creating a simple pneumothorax that responds to catheter aspiration.

The esophagus and stomach look different through the laparoscope. The esophagus lacks a serosa and clearly shows the dark pink color of muscle tissue (see Fig. 3-15). The stomach, covered with serosa, is shinier and whiter. In addition, the longitudinal striations of the outer muscle layer of the esophagus are evident through the laparoscope. Belsey's fat pad is found at the region of attachment of the phrenoesophageal ligament, on the stomach, just to the left of the hiatus. It provides a useful landmark to the cardioesophageal junction and may be grasped for atraumatic retraction of the distal esophagus. It may be sufficiently bulky as to render dissection difficult. Often, a small artery, called Belsey's artery, runs transversely within the fat pad and must be controlled if the pad is excised. This fat pad must be divided to perform esophagomyotomy for achalasia.

The blood supply of the distal esophagus derives from the ascending or esophageal branches of the left gastric artery with or without a branch from the inferior phrenic artery. Both enter the esophagus beneath the phrenoesophageal membrane and anastomose with the descending esophageal branches off the thoracic aorta. Belsey's artery forms a minor collateral channel running through Belsey's fat pad and can be divided. The highest short gastric artery sometimes sends a tributary to the esophagus on the left. Finally, as previously mentioned, the left gastric artery often gives rise to a major hepatic artery branch supplying the liver (Fig. 3-23) that must be avoided and preserved.

Adequate mobilization of the stomach for fundoplication generally requires division of the short gastric vessels (Fig. 3-24), which often comprise several layers, rather than the single layer shown in open surgical texts. The short gastric vessels are illustrated and described further in Chapters 4 and 6.

Esophagomyotomy

The outer layer of the esophagus is longitudinal muscle. No peritoneum, other than the phrenoesophageal ligament, covers the esophagus. The inner circular muscle overlies a well-developed submucosa with a submucosal venous plexus. The loose areolar tissue of the submucosa provides an excellent tactile landmark during the performance of esophagomyotomy. Beneath this areolar tissue, the submucosal veins are seen overlying the white epithelial tube (commonly called mucosa, but actually squamous epithelium above the Z-line and mucosa below). During the performance of esophagomyotomy, the outer muscle layer is split longitudinally, and the inner hypertrophied circular muscle layer is divided until the epithelial tube bulges out (Figs. 3-25 and 3-26). The epithelial tube is easy to recognize by its whiteness, contrasting starkly with the pink-red circular muscle.

Vagus Nerves and Truncal Vagotomy

In the region of the cardioesophageal junction, generally two vagal trunks are identifiable (see Figs. 3-15 to 3-17). Truncal vagotomy may be performed through a laparoscopic approach, but it is rarely indicated. Generally, the vagal trunks are observed during hiatal hernia repair and are protected during dissection. The anterior vagus is seen on the surface of the esophagus. It can be sought by dissecting the phrenoesophageal ligament upward and the peritoneal covering of the cardioesophageal junction downward. The posterior vagus is seen in the depths of the dissection between the right crus and the esophagus. It is actually closer to the aorta than to the esophagus. Lying between the posterolateral wall of the esophagus and the crus, it is attached to the esophagus by loose areolar tissue (see Figs. 3-19 and 3-20). It is frequently accompanied by a small arteriole. The anatomy of the vagus nerves is further described in Chapter 4. The anterior vagus can be avoided during esophagomyotomy by making the myotomy a bit to the left of the nerve of Latarjet.

BIBLIOGRAPHY

Regional Anatomy

1. Carey JM, Hollinshead WH. An anatomic study of the esophageal hiatus. *Surg Gynecol Obstet* 1955;100:196–200.
2. Gray SW, Rowe JS, Skandalakis JE. Surgical anatomy of the gastroesophageal junction. *Am Surg* 1979;45:575–587.
3. Greig HW, Anson BJ, Coleman SJ. Inferior phrenic artery: types of origin in 850 body-halves and diaphragmatic relationship. *Q Bull NW Med School* 1951;25:345–350.
4. Listerud MB, Harkins HN. Anatomy of the esophageal hiatus: anatomic studies on 204 fresh cadavers. *Arch Surg* 1958;76:835–842.
5. Suzuki T, Nakayasu A, Kawabe K, Takeda H, Honijo I. Surgical significance of anatomic variations of the hepatic artery. *Am J Surg* 1971;122:505–512.
6. Van Damme J-PJ. Behavioral anatomy of the abdominal arteries. *Surg Clin North Am* 1993;73: 699–725.
7. Van Trigt P. Diaphragm and diaphragmatic pacing. In: Sabiston DC, Spencer FC, eds. *Surgery of the chest,* 5th ed. Philadelphia: WB Saunders, 1990;957–961.
8. Wald H, Polk HC. Anatomical variations in hiatal and upper gastric areas and their relationship to difficulties experienced in operations for reflux esophagitis. *Ann Surg* 1983;197:389–392.

Anatomy of Specific Surgical Procedures

1. Baue AE, Belsey RHR. The treatment of sliding hiatus hernia and reflux esophagitis by the Mark IV technique. *Surgery* 1967;62:396–404.

2. Collet D, Cadiere GB. Conversions and complications of laparoscopic treatment of gastroesophageal reflux disease. *Am J Surg* 1995;169:622–626.
3. Collis JL, Kelly TD, Wiley AM. Anatomy of the crura of the diaphragm and the surgery of hiatus hernia. *Thorax* 1954;9:195–198.
4. Cushieri A. Laparoscopic antireflux surgery and the repair of hiatal hernia. *World J Surg* 1993;17:40–45.
5. Fernandez-Cebrian JM, De Oteyza JP. Laparoscopic repair of hernia of foramen of Morgagni: a new case report. *J Laparoendosc Surg* 1996;6:61–64.
6. Holzman MD, Sharp KW, Ladipa JK, Eller RF, Holcomb GW III, Richards WO. Laparoscopic surgical treatment of achalasia. *Am J Surg* 1997;173:308–311.
7. Kuster GGR, Innocenti FA. Laparoscopic anatomy of the region of the esophageal hiatus. *Surg Endosc* 1997;11:883–893.
8. McKernan JB, Wolfe BM, MacFadyen BV. Laparoscopic repair of duodenal ulcer and gastro-esophageal reflux. *Surg Clin North Am* 1992;72:1153–1167.
9. Porter JM. Diagnostic laparoscopy and laparoscopic transdiaphragmatic pericardial window in a patient with an epigastric stab wound: a case report. *J Laparoendosc Surg* 1996;6:51–54.
10. Swanstrom LL, Pennings JL. Safe laparoscopic dissection of the gastroesophageal junction. *Am J Surg* 1995;169:507–511.

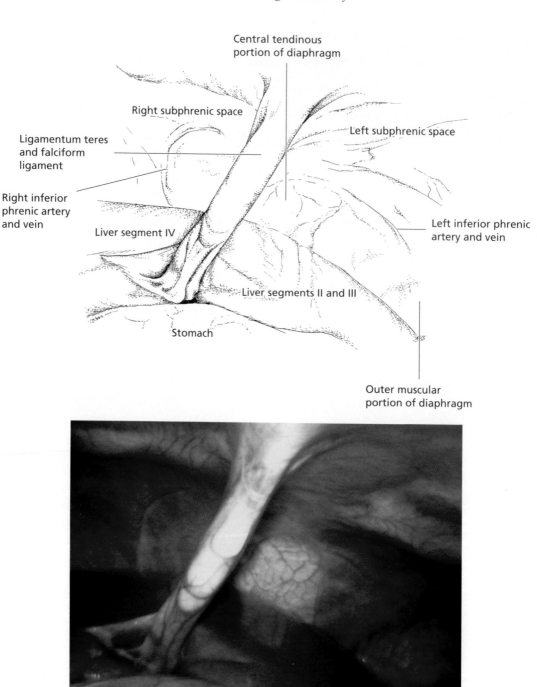

Fig. 3-1. Initial view of the left subphrenic space. The ligamentum teres hepatis and attached falciform ligament stretch across the upper foreground, dividing the subphrenic space into left and right compartments. The falciform ligament forms the external landmark for the intersegmental line between segments II and III (to the left of the falciform ligament), also termed the left lateral segment, and segments I and IV (to the right of the falciform ligament) of the left lobe of the liver. The ligamentum teres hepatis is seen to attach at the umbilical plate of the liver. Segmental anatomy of the liver and anatomy of the ligamentum teres are illustrated further and discussed in Chapter 5.

The inferior surfaces of the left and right hemidiaphragm demonstrate lateral muscular components and central tendinous portions. The portion of the left hemidiaphragm immediately adjacent to the falciform is contiguous with pericardium. This is the location through which laparoscopic pericardial window is performed. It is easily identified by visible cardiac pulsations. Branches of the left and right inferior phrenic artery (with accompanying veins) are seen arching across the inferior diaphragmatic surfaces. The left and right phrenic nerves pierce the diaphragm and run parallel to branches of the phrenic arteries.

Note the distance from the umbilically placed laparoscope to the apex of the left hemidiaphragm. The esophageal hiatus lies beneath segments II and III of the left lobe of the liver, which must be elevated to reveal it. This region is best visualized by an angled laparoscope placed through a portal closer to the left upper quadrant.

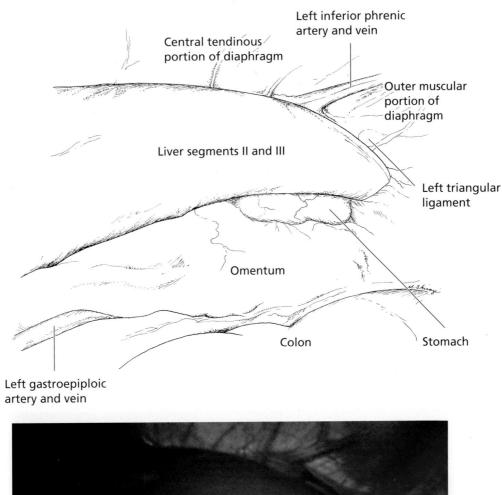

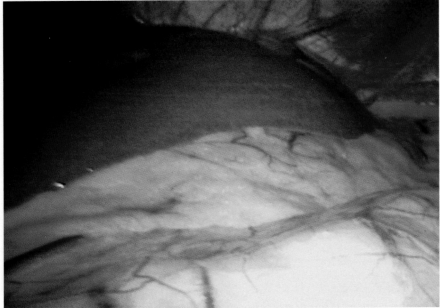

Fig. 3-2. Left upper quadrant structures *in situ*. Segment III of the left lobe of the liver is well seen. Segment II lies posterior, with no visible line of demarcation between the two segments. The triangular ligament that attaches the left lobe of the liver to the lateral abdominal wall is noted. This may contain small blood vessels or accessory bile ducts. Normally divided during open surgery in this region, the triangular ligament is left intact during the laparoscopic approach to the hiatus. The stomach, greater omentum, and colon are seen in the foreground. Branches of the left gastroepiploic artery and vein run in the omentum in the foreground. On the diaphragm, branches of the left inferior phrenic artery and vein are noted.

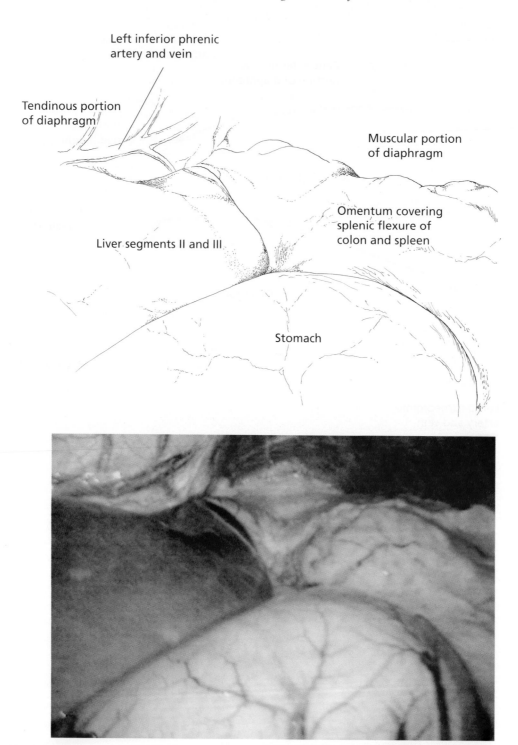

Fig. 3-3. Left upper quadrant *in situ*. In another example, the stomach is prominently seen in the foreground. Segments II and III of the left lobe of the liver obscure visualization of the proximal stomach and cardioesophageal junction. Omentum covers the splenic flexure of the colon. Branches of left inferior phrenic artery and vein are prominent on the tendinous portion of the inferior aspect of the diaphragm.

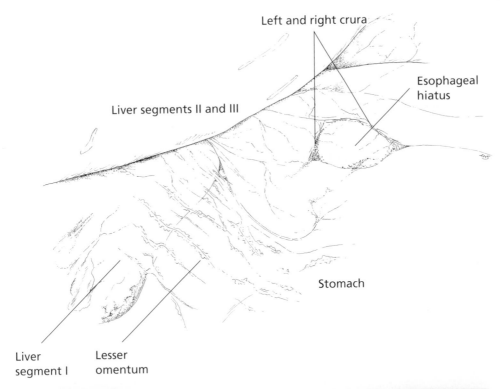

Left and right crura

Esophageal
hiatus

Liver segments II and III

Stomach

Liver
segment I

Lesser
omentum

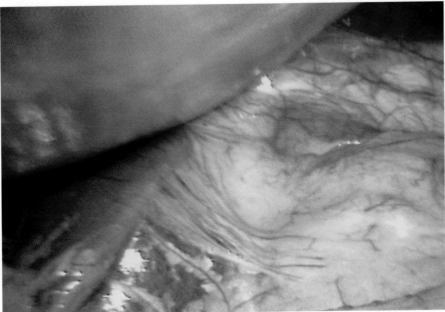

Fig. 3-4. Lesser omentum and segment I (caudate lobe) of the liver. With a retractor elevating the liver, the transparent portion of the lesser omentum is visualized. Through this transparent portion, segment I of the left lobe of the liver (the so-called caudate lobe) is visualized. The left and right diaphragmatic crura and esophageal hiatus (covered by the phrenoesophageal ligament) are glimpsed to the left. Generally, one or more sizable vessels, branches of the left gastric artery, will be found between this portion of the lesser omentum and the hiatus. These vessels run in the fatty tissue overlying the right crus of the diaphragm and between the right crus and the lesser omentum (see Fig. 3-5).

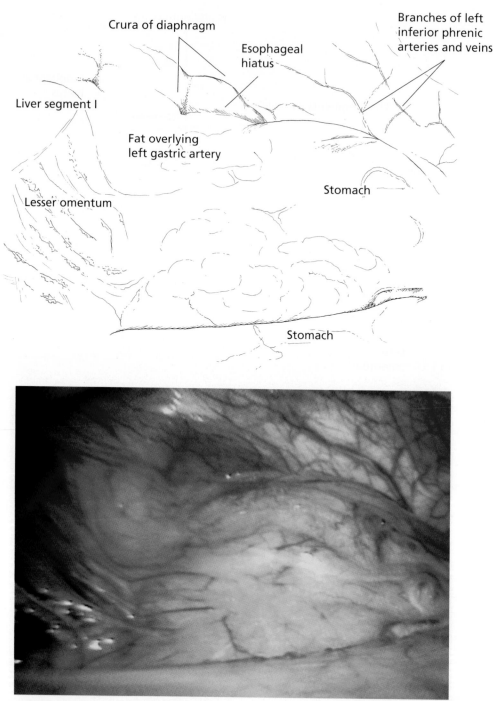

Fig. 3-5. Hiatus before dissection. The laparoscope has been moved to a closer position, and the region of the hiatus is clearly seen. The transparent portion of the lesser omentum overlying segment I of the liver lies to the right. Fatty tissue containing one or more branches of the left gastric artery lies just below the apex of the hiatus. The crura and hiatus are seen under the peritoneum. Dissection to expose the hiatus should begin on the right crus, just cephalad to the fatty tissue (which will then be swept away and left undisturbed). Branches of the left inferior phrenic artery and vein are noted.

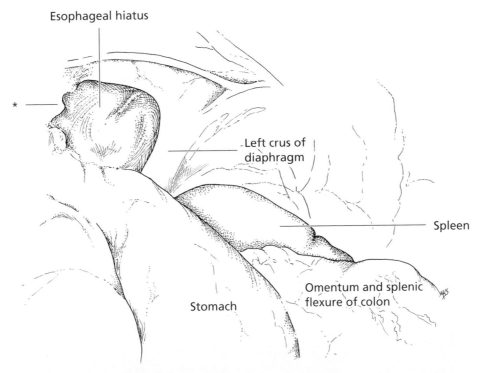

Esophageal hiatus

*

Left crus of
diaphragm

Spleen

Stomach

Omentum and splenic
flexure of colon

*Danger, may be contiguous with pericardium

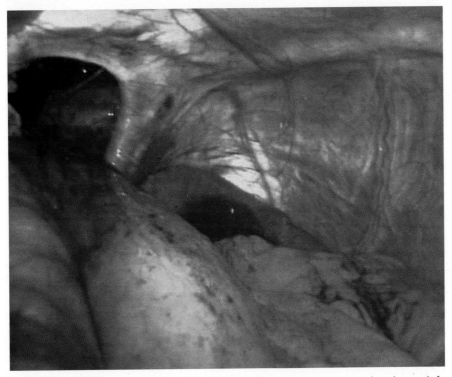

Fig. 3-6. Large hiatal hernia. In another example, elevation of the liver reveals a large defect at the esophageal hiatus with a well-developed sac going into the mediastinum. Branches of the inferior phrenic artery and vein are noted. The fairly constant left inferior phrenic artery branch that runs along the left crus is well seen. The medial aspect of this hiatus is likely to be contiguous with the pericardium above *(asterisk)*, and repair of this large defect must be undertaken with care to avoid entry into the pericardium. The notched border of the spleen, omentum overlying splenic flexure of colon, and stomach are seen in the foreground.

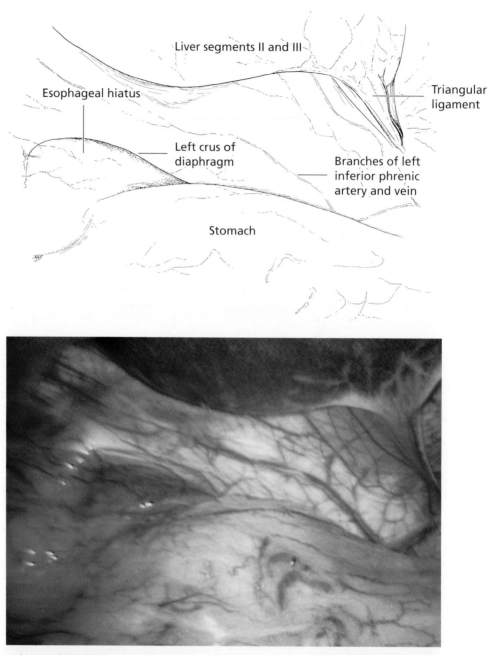

Fig. 3-7. Left crus of the diaphragm, left triangular ligament. The left crus of the diaphragm, with the left inferior phrenic artery and vein, is well seen here. The stomach lies in the foreground. Excellent exposure of the hiatus is obtained simply by elevating the liver, and the left triangular ligament is left undisturbed.

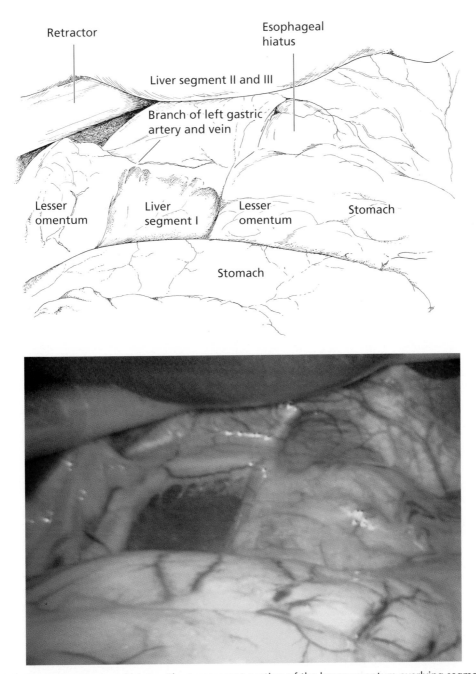

Fig. 3-8. Lesser omentum and hiatus. The transparent portion of the lesser omentum overlying segment I of the left lobe of the liver is to the left. A bridge of fatty tissue partially conceals a sizable vessel running from the left gastric artery to the liver. This is likely to be an aberrant hepatic artery. Above the vessel, the apex of the hiatus is seen. Dissection must begin above the aberrant vessel, which can then be swept down as the esophagus is mobilized.

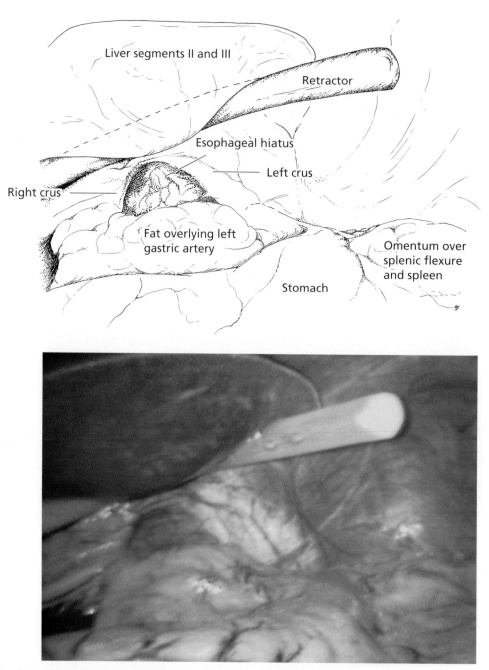

Fig. 3-9. Hiatus, with fat around the left gastric artery. In this view of the hiatus, the apex of the crura is well seen. Fat overlies the region of the left gastric artery. Dissection on the right crus allows the surgeon to enter the mediastinum and to sweep the left gastric artery and associated tissue downward. The stomach and omentum overlying the splenic flexure of the colon and spleen are noted in the foreground.

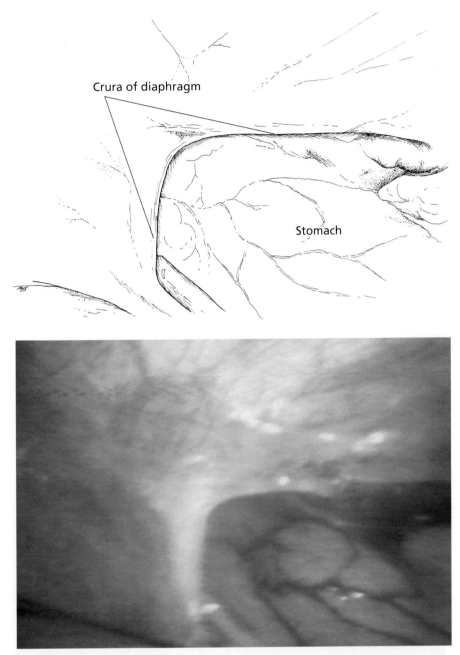

Fig. 3-10. Phrenoesophageal ligament and hiatus hernia. The phrenoesophageal ligament is seen to be infolded by a hiatus hernia. Stomach enters the hiatal opening. Esophagus lies in the mediastinum and is not seen.

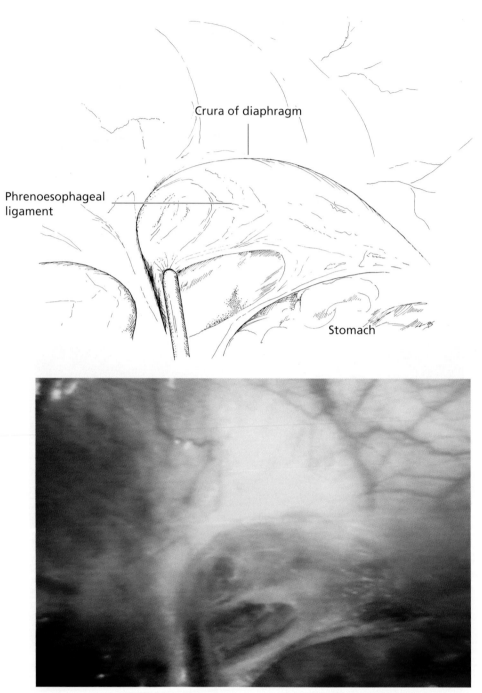

Fig. 3-11. Phrenoesophageal ligament. This view of a thin phrenoesophageal ligament demonstrates severe attenuation from a chronic sliding hiatal hernia. The esophagus and anterior vagus nerve will be found beneath the gossamer-thin phrenoesophageal ligament.

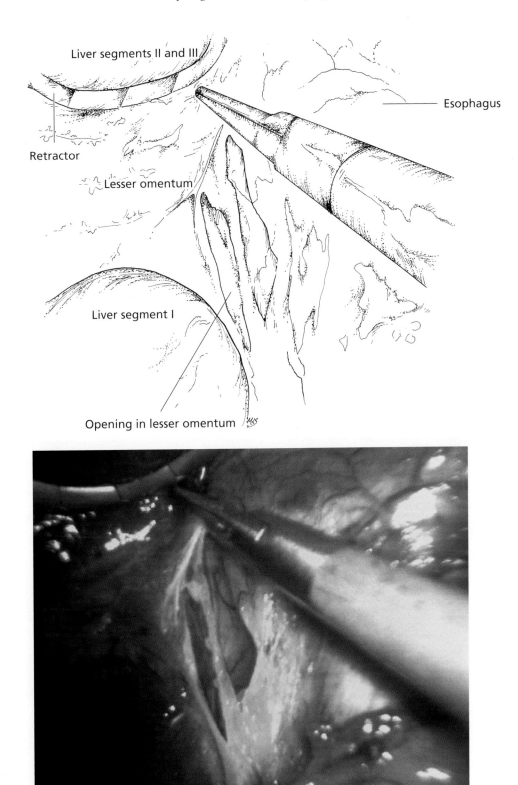

Fig. 3-12. Creating a window in the lesser sac adjacent to the right crus. Here, several slitlike defects have been created as a window is made in an avascular portion of the lesser sac overlying the right crus. The esophagus lies to the patient's left. A retractor elevating segments II and III of the liver is seen in the upper right. Segment I of the liver is noted in the right foreground.

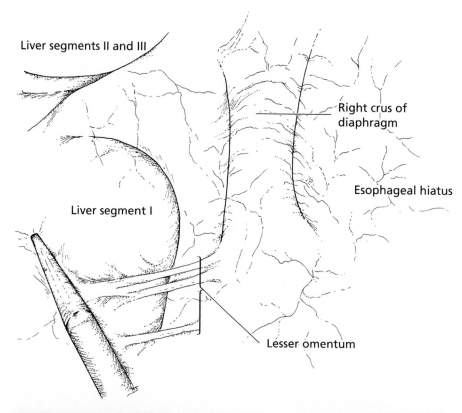

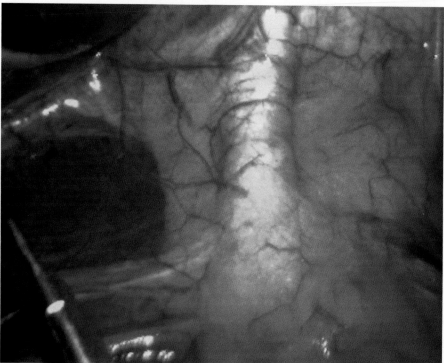

Fig. 3-13. Right crus of diaphragm and transparent portion of lesser omentum. In another dissection, the right crus of the diaphragm is noted to be covered with glistening peritoneum that is essentially continuous with the lesser omentum. Segments II and III of the liver are retracted cephalad, and segment I is clearly seen through the transparent part of the lesser omentum. The esophageal hiatus lies beyond the right crus of the diaphragm.

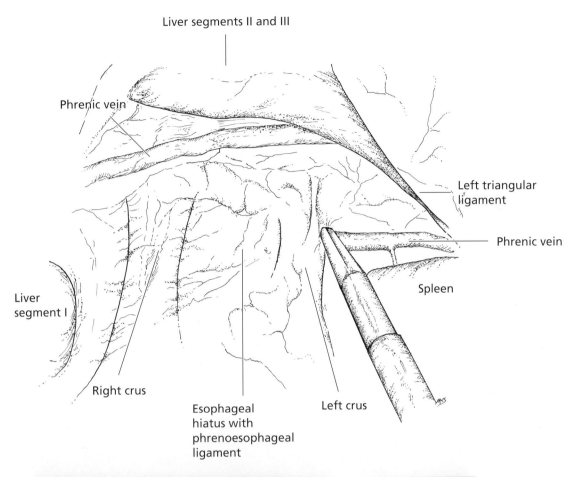

Liver segments II and III

Phrenic vein

Left triangular ligament

Phrenic vein

Spleen

Liver segment I

Right crus

Esophageal hiatus with phrenoesophageal ligament

Left crus

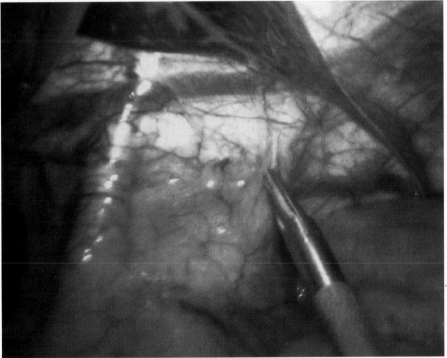

Fig. 3-14. Left and right crus of diaphragm. Both crura are seen here, with the esophageal hiatus defined between them. The apex of the hiatus is not well defined, and the two crura appear to have a more nearly parallel (rather than arch-shaped) configuration in this particular individual. Phrenic veins are seen through the peritoneal surface of the diaphragm. The triangular ligament and a portion of segments I, II, and III of the left lobe of the liver are seen. The phrenoesophageal ligament is intact. The tip of the spleen is visible.

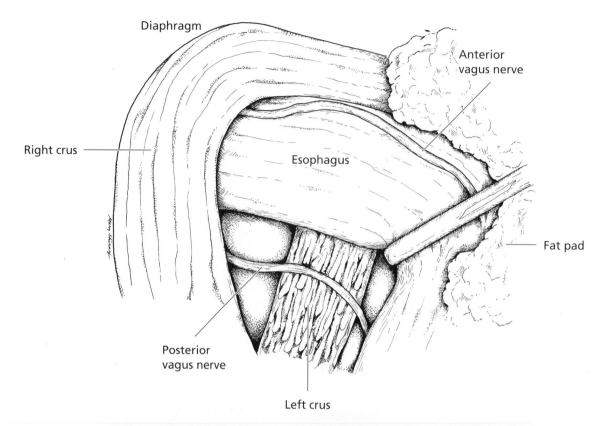

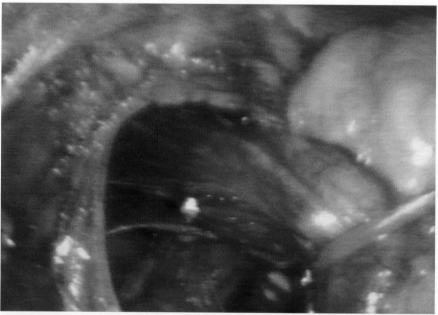

Fig. 3-15. Esophageal hiatus, esophagus, vagus nerves. The soft tissues have been dissected from the crura of the diaphragm to reveal the esophageal hiatus. The esophagus has been encircled with a Silastic loop and elevated. Two vagal fibers are seen. Belsey's fat pad is glimpsed. Note the pink-red color and longitudinal fibers of the esophagus, which contrast with the white, serosa-covered stomach. Belsey's fat pad commonly contains a small artery and vein and is a useful landmark. It can also serve as a handle for manipulating the distal esophagus without actually grasping the esophageal musculature.

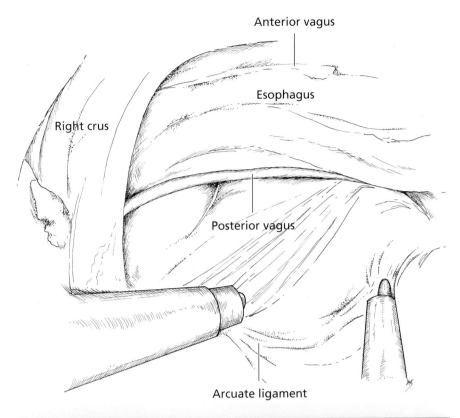

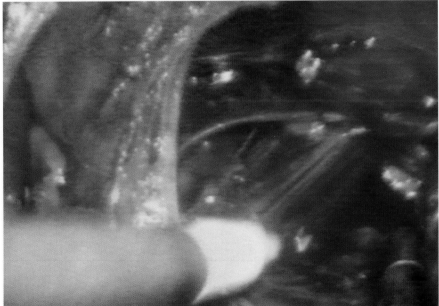

Fig. 3-16. Left and right crus of diaphragm, arcuate ligament. The left and right crus of the diaphragm converge behind the esophagus to form the arcuate ligament. Here the region behind the esophagus is being cleared. Vagal fibers corresponding to the posterior vagus and a small anterior twig of the vagus nerve are seen on the esophagus.

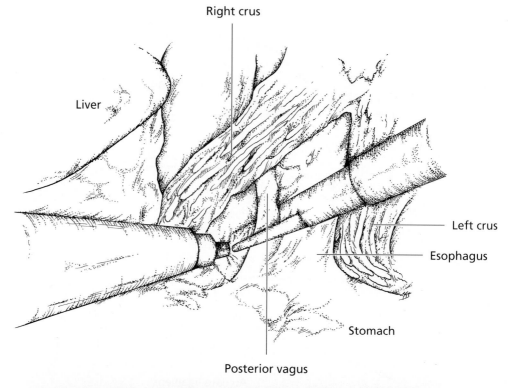

Right crus

Liver

Left crus

Esophagus

Stomach

Posterior vagus

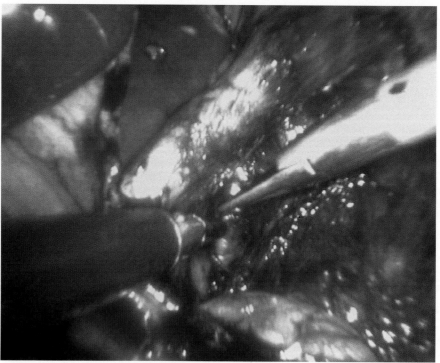

Fig. 3-17. Posterior vagus nerve on esophagus. Here a vagal fiber is being separated from the esophagus in the course of truncal vagotomy. The two crura are well defined. Liver and stomach are glimpsed.

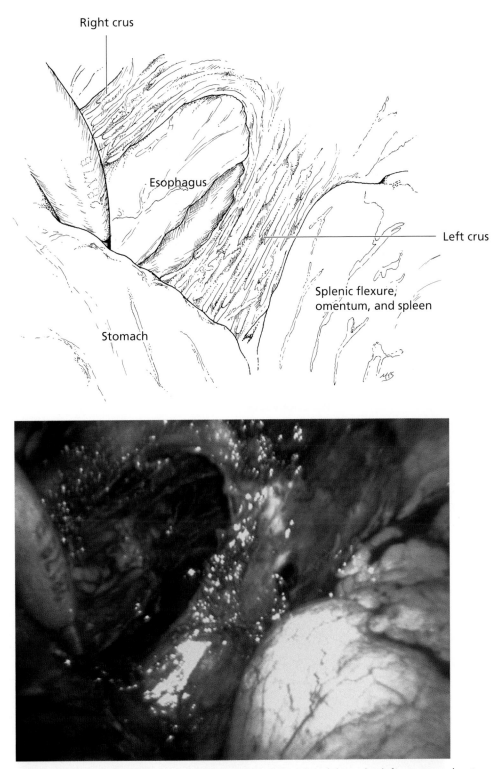

Fig. 3-18. Left crus of diaphragm. The angled laparoscope has been placed through a left upper quadrant portal, producing a more direct view of the left crus of the diaphragm. The archlike configuration of the muscular hiatus of the diaphragm is well seen. The esophagus is being retracted to the patient's right by a retractor passed to the left of the esophagus. Stomach, splenic flexure, omentum, and spleen are glimpsed in the foreground.

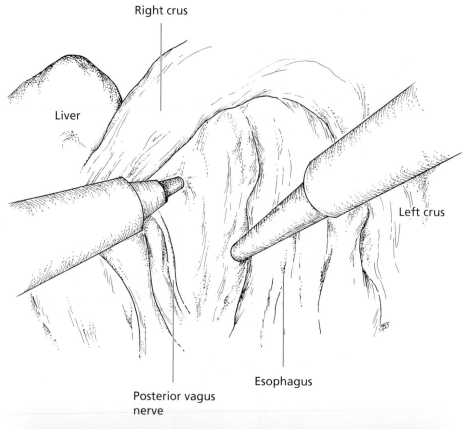

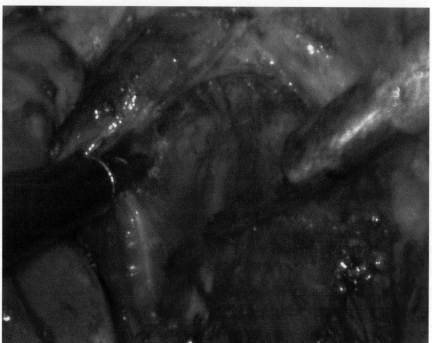

Fig. 3-19. Posterior vagus nerve. The space in the mediastinum between the posterolateral aspect of the esophagus and the right crus has been developed, and the posterior vagus nerve is shown retracted to the right. The esophagus is being gently retracted to the left. The left crus is glimpsed beyond the esophagus.

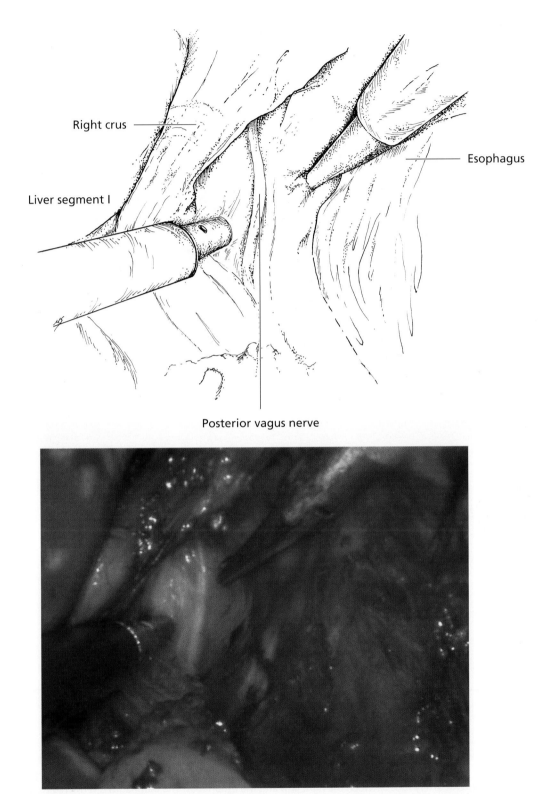

Fig. 3-20. Posterior vagus nerve. The posterior vagus nerve is shown running parallel to the esophagus. Loose areolar connective tissue between the esophagus and the vagus nerve commonly contains a small arteriole to the vagus nerve. The right crus of the diaphragm is retracted to the right, and the esophagus is being retracted to the patient's left. Segment I of the liver is seen in the foreground.

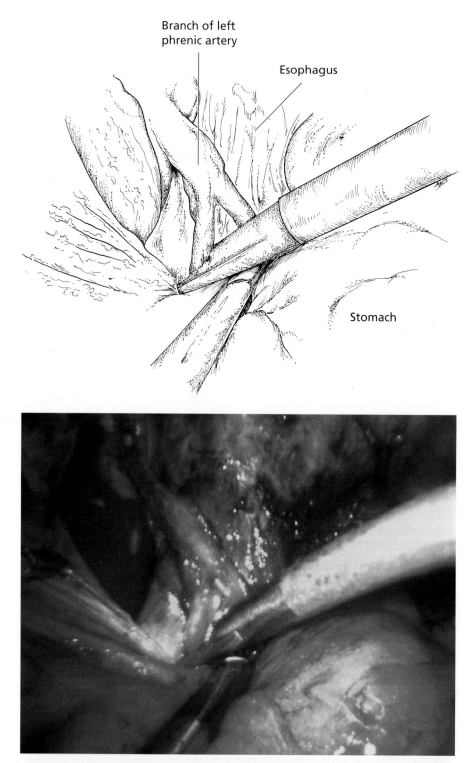

Fig. 3-21. Anomalous branch of inferior phrenic artery. A common anomaly in this area, a sizable branch of the left phrenic artery runs between the right crus and the esophagus. The esophagus is retracted to the right.

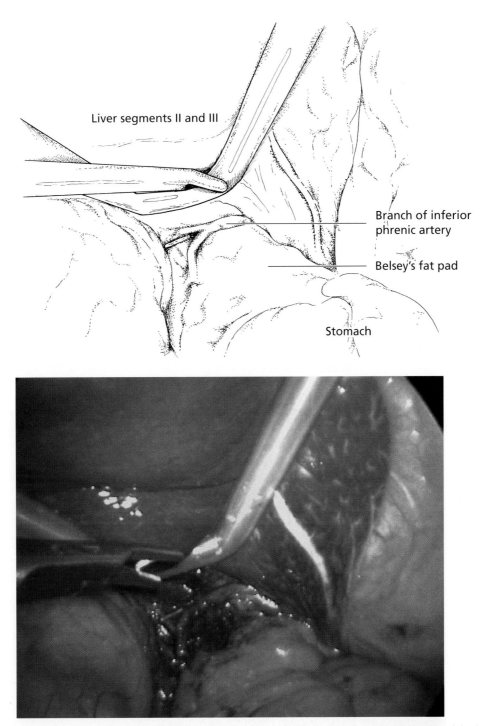

Liver segments II and III

Branch of inferior
phrenic artery

Belsey's fat pad

Stomach

Fig. 3-22. Anomalous branch of inferior phrenic artery. In another common variant, a small branch of the left inferior phrenic artery runs across the arch of the hiatus or over the phrenoesophageal ligament. Belsey's fat pad and the stomach are seen in the foreground. Segments II and III of the left lobe of the liver are being retracted upward, and the triangular ligament is noted.

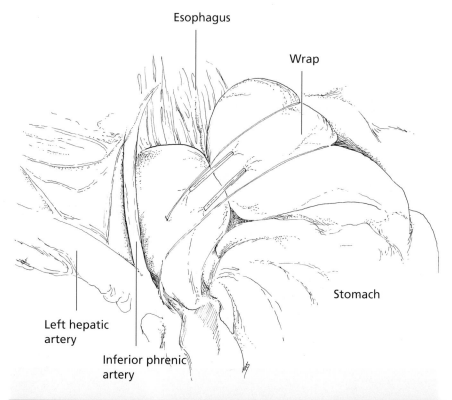

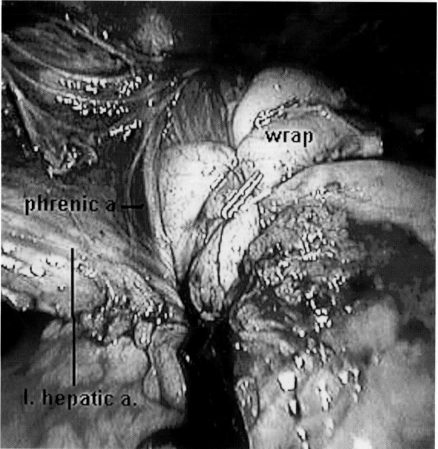

Fig. 3-23. Anomalous right hepatic artery giving rise to the inferior phrenic artery. This sizable vessel may represent a replaced right hepatic artery and has been carefully preserved. A Nissen fundoplication has been performed.

Short gastric arteries and veins

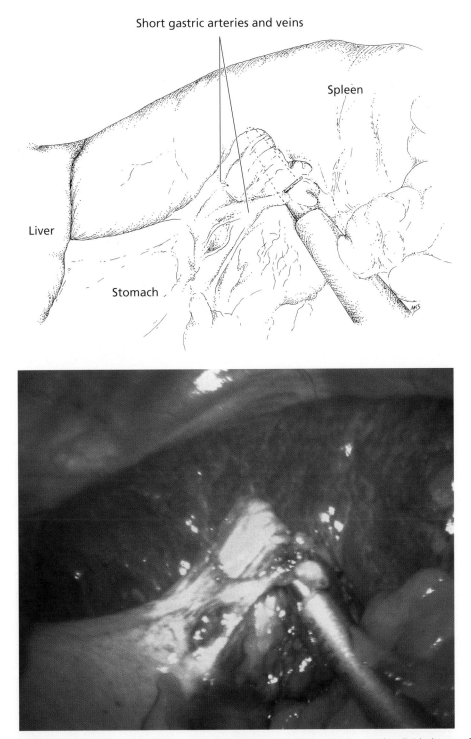

Spleen

Liver

Stomach

Fig. 3-24. Short gastric vessels. This illustrates the short gastric vessels, which must be divided to perform a floppy fundoplication. The greater curvature of the stomach is to the right, and the spleen is to the left. Segments II and III of the liver (not retracted) are seen to the right. More illustrations of the short gastric vessels are included in Chapters 4 and 6.

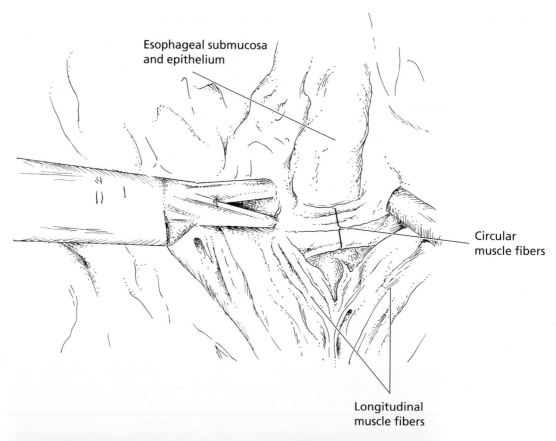

Esophageal submucosa
and epithelium

Circular
muscle fibers

Longitudinal
muscle fibers

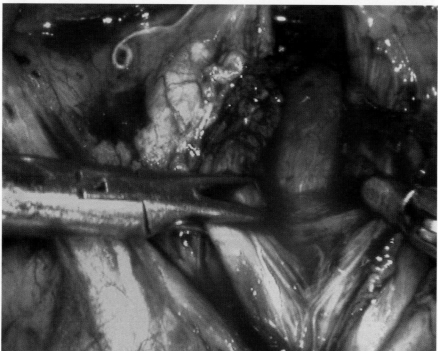

Fig. 3-25. Longitudinal muscle layer of the esophagus. This view, from the initial stage of laparoscopic esophagomyotomy, shows the longitudinal muscle layer of the distal esophagus being split to display the underlying circular muscle layer. The dissection is kept to the left of the nerve of Latarjet to avoid the anterior vagus nerve.

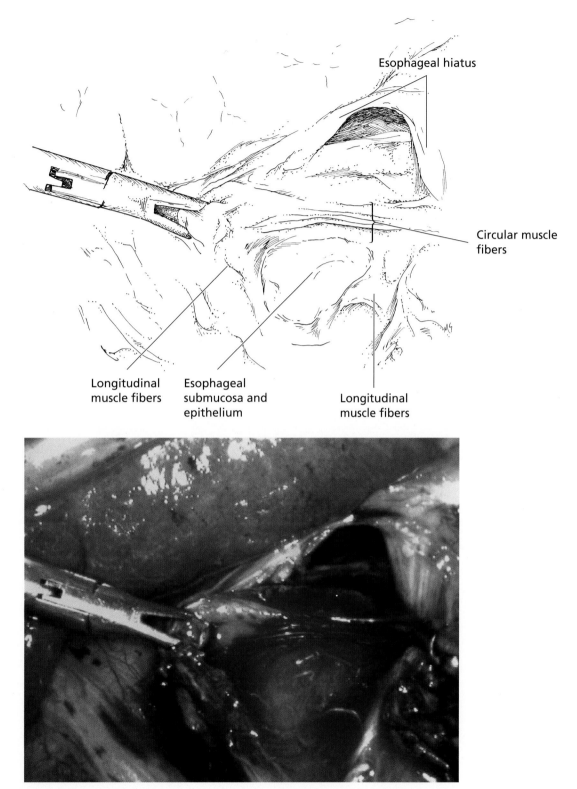

Esophageal hiatus

Circular muscle
fibers

Longitudinal
muscle fibers

Esophageal
submucosa and
epithelium

Longitudinal
muscle fibers

Fig. 3-26. Circular muscle layer and submucosa of esophagus. The circular muscle fibers are being divided to expose the submucosa, containing a rich venous plexus, and the white epithelial tube.

4

STOMACH AND DUODENUM

INITIAL LAPAROSCOPIC VIEW AND PRINCIPLES OF EXPOSURE

The stomach lies relatively close to the umbilically placed laparoscope. Effective working distance to the distal stomach and duodenum may even require placement of the laparoscope below the umbilicus. However, the proximal stomach and esophagus lie high in the left upper quadrant and may necessitate higher placement (see Chapter 3). The best solution to the problem may be to place the laparoscope through the umbilical port for the initial assessment, then move it to a port higher in the left upper quadrant for visualization of the cardioesophageal junction. A steep head-up (reverse Trendelenburg) position allows gravity to pull the abdominal viscera downward and enhances access to the upper abdomen. A 30-degree angled laparoscope facilitates visualization of structures.

The initial laparoscopic view shows the greater curvature and distal stomach, partially covered by the liver (Figs. 4-1 to 4-3). Full exposure of the anterior surface of the stomach requires retraction of the liver (Fig. 4-4; see also Chapter 3).

The posterior surface of the stomach is visible only when the lesser sac is entered. For most procedures, entry through the greater omentum with cephalad retraction of the stomach is the most direct path into the lesser sac.

The proximal duodenum is easily seen with elevation of the liver and gallbladder. Full visualization of the duodenum requires mobilization of the hepatic flexure of the right colon.

ANATOMY AND SPECIFIC SURGICAL PROCEDURES

Vagus Nerves and Laparoscopic Vagotomy

The vagus nerves descend parallel to the esophagus and form a plexus between the level of the tracheal bifurcation and the diaphragm. This plexus recombines to form two trunks, an anterior trunk and a posterior trunk (in more than 80% of cases), which pass through the hiatus. With rotation of the stomach during development, the anterior trunk comes to lie toward the left, and the posterior trunk to the right. Some individuals have more than two trunks, and additional confusion is introduced by the limited length of these two trunks, which subsequently give rise to several branches just after passing through the hiatus.

The laparoscopic approach to the vagal trunks begins by elevating the left lobe of the liver to expose the hiatus. The caudate lobe of the liver and the right crus of the diaphragm provide useful landmarks to the dissection. The dissection is begun as high as possible to avoid branches of the left gastric artery. The peritoneum overlying the right and superior margins of the hiatus, including the transparent portion of the gastrohepatic ligament, is incised. More details on this exposure and dissection are given in Chapter 3.

The posterior vagal trunk lies deep, close to the aorta, in proximity to the right crus of the diaphragm. It is only loosely adherent to the right posterolateral wall of the esophagus. The space between the right posterolateral wall of the esophagus and the right crus of the diaphragm is developed by blunt dissection in the lower mediastinum. The posterior vagus nerve is easily identified by its cylindric white structure and vertical orientation. It is a large structure when seen through the laparoscope. A small accompanying vessel derived from the left gastric artery is often noted (see Figs. 3-19 and 3-20). If the esophagus is gently rolled to the left, branches to the cardioesophageal junction may be seen.

The anterior vagus nerve lies on the esophageal surface and is exposed by dissecting the anterior peritoneal leaf caudad and the phrenoesophageal membrane cephalad (see Figs. 3-15 to 3-17). The esophagus may be gently rolled to the right, and the space between the left crus and the esophagus may be developed. As the anterior vagus nerve is retracted from the esophagus, small branches to the distal esophagus and cardia of the stomach (including a variant "criminal nerve of Grassi"; see later) may be identified.

Each of the two main vagal trunks then divides into two major divisions. The anterior vagus divides into a hepatic and an anterior gastric division. This split sometimes occurs above the diaphragm, contributing to the confusion about the number of vagal trunks at the hiatus. The hepatic division passes to the right in the lesser omentum, where the laparoscopist may divide fibers inadvertently as the space to the left of the hiatus is developed for fundoplication. It branches before entering the liver and, if seen, should be preserved. The anterior gastric division descends along the lesser curvature of the stomach and gives branches to the anterior gastric wall. A major branch of this forms the anterior nerve of Latarjet (see Fig. 4-3), which usually lies 0.5 to 1 cm from the gastric wall and gives off from 2 to 12 (average 6) branches to the stomach before terminating, inconstantly, in a "crow's foot" at the antrum of the stomach.

The posterior vagus divides into the celiac and posterior gastric divisions. The celiac is the largest of the four divisions, but it is rarely seen. It passes posteriorly, running along the left gastric artery, to the celiac plexus. It may be seen under the gastropancreatic peritoneal fold if the lesser sac is entered. If identified, it should be preserved. The posterior gastric division forms a posterior nerve of Latarjet, which passes along the lesser curvature in a manner analogous to the anterior nerve of Latarjet. The posterior nerve of Latarjet is smaller, and less constant in form, and rarely seen. The "criminal nerve of Grassi" is a small and highly variable branch (or branches) from the posterior vagus that supplies the proximal stomach. In many individuals, this small twig branches from the posterior vagus before the origin of the celiac division, in the mediastinum.

Several laparoscopic vagotomies have been developed. Truncal vagotomy is simply accomplished by identifying and dividing all vagal trunks at the level of the hiatus. Posterior truncal and anterior seromyotomy is a laparoscopic variant of the Taylor procedure that involves identification and division of the posterior trunk, followed by partial-thickness incision through the gastric wall along the lesser curvature. This divides small branches of the anterior nerve of Latarjet. Small blood vessels, branches of the left and right gastric arteries, must be secured. The seromyotomy is generally inverted with a running suture to protect against leakage and to discourage nerve regeneration. Alternatively, a formal, highly selective or parietal cell vagotomy may also be performed, in a manner completely analogous to the open procedures.

Stomach, Laparoscopic Gastrostomy or Gastrectomy

The stomach is highly variable in size and shape, quite mobile, and fixed at only two points—the cardioesophageal junction and the pylorus. The laparoscopic surgeon must rely purely on visual landmarks to determine the location of lesions or to judge the extent of resection. Some of these landmarks include the esophageal hiatus with Belsey's fat pad (see Chapter 3), which lies at the cardioesophageal junction (see Figs. 3-15 and 3-22), the crow's foot arrangement of the terminating branches of the left gastric artery and accompanying veins and nerves at the antrum, the prepyloric veins of Mayo (see Fig. 4-1), the gastrosplenic fold and short gastric vessels (Figs. 4-5 to 4-11), and the point on the greater curvature where the left gastroepiploic vessels and right gastroepiploic vessels meet (Figs. 4-12 and 4-13). The term "crow's foot" is currently used to apply to the terminal branches of the anterior nerve of Latarjet, which are preserved during conventional performance of highly selective vagotomy. The term was originally applied to the terminal branches of the left gastric artery that splay out over the antrum, and these vascular branches form the visual landmark for the distal antrum (see Fig. 4-4).

The pylorus is a muscular canal approximately 2.5 cm in length. A thin white line is occasionally visible marking its location; sometimes this is visible as a groove, marking the sulcus intermedius. The paired prepyloric veins of Mayo, when present, come from above (a branch of the right gastric vein) and below (a branch of the right gastroepiploic vein) to form a more visible landmark (see Fig. 4-1). The left and right gastroepiploic vessels meet (see Figs. 4-12 and 4-13) at a point on the greater curvature that may be used to delimit a subtotal gastric resection.

The vascular supply of the stomach are described in the following order: lesser curvature, from above downward; region of the pylorus; greater curvature from antrum to fundus. The blood supply of the lesser curvature is primarily from the left and right gastric arteries. A rich anastomotic plexus in the gastric submucosa ensures excellent blood supply despite division of one or more major vessels.

The left gastric artery is one of the three major branches of the celiac artery and is the single most important vessel supplying the stomach. It comes up from behind the stomach, initially running behind the posterior layer of the omental bursa covered with parietal peritoneum, giving off the branches to the cardia and esophagus previously mentioned, and then abruptly turning down and dividing into anterior and posterior branches that supply the lesser curvature of the stomach (Figs. 4-14 and 4-15).

The anterior branch of the left gastric artery is visible to the laparoscopist in the lesser omentum and is frequently seen during dissection for laparoscopic fundoplication (see Chapter 3). It gives off two or three smaller branches to supply the anterior lesser curvature. Each is generally accompanied by venous tributaries and branches of the anterior nerve of Latarjet (see Fig. 4-3).

The posterior branch of the left gastric artery is longer than the anterior branch and terminates by anastomosing with the right gastric artery. This vessel is hidden unless the lesser sac is entered. The left gastric ("coronary") vein receives tributaries from both surfaces of the stomach, runs upward along the lesser curvature in the lesser omentum to the esophageal hiatus where it receives several esophageal tributaries, and then turns back, down, and swings to the right to enter the lesser sac and terminate in the portal vein at the upper border of the duodenum. This region is generally not visualized by the laparoscopist.

The right gastric artery is substantially smaller and shorter than the left gastric artery. It arises from the common hepatic artery above the superior portion of the duodenum, where it may be visualized laparoscopically as it descends in the lesser omentum to the region of the pylorus, and passes from right to left to supply portions of the lesser curvature of the stomach. It may give rise to the supraduodenal artery. Veins accompany arteries in this region and are of little clinical significance, with the exception of the paired but inconstant prepyloric veins of Mayo previously mentioned (see Figs. 4-1 and 4-2; Figs. 4-16 and 4-17).

The right gastroepiploic artery, a branch of the gastroduodenal, runs along the distal greater curvature, giving branches to the antrum (see Figs. 4-12 and 4-13). There is generally a bare portion between the territory of the right gastroepiploic artery and the left gastroepiploic artery that forms a useful landmark for subtotal gastrectomy.

The left gastroepiploic artery arises from the splenic artery or one of its derivatives. It runs down along the greater curvature and sends branches to the proximal greater curvature (see Fig. 4-15). Anastomosis with the left gastroepiploic artery is through the omental arcades.

Numerous short gastric arteries supply the proximal greater curvature, region of the cardia, and sometimes the distal esophagus. These vessels run between the spleen and stomach within the gastrosplenic ligament. An avascular peritoneal fold often covers the gastrosplenic ligament (see Fig. 4-5). The number of short gastric arteries varies, but commonly, four to six are present. They arise from any vessel in the vicinity of the splenic hilum, but they often appear to be coming directly from the spleen. The lower short gastric arteries are generally longer than the upper, and the most cephalad is the shortest of all. These vessels must be divided for adequate mobilization for fundoplication (see Chapter 3) or for splenectomy (see Chapter 6). Mobilization is begun by dividing the gastrosplenic fold (if present), then making a window in the gastrosplenic ligament relatively low (close to the laparoscope; see Fig. 4-6). The dissection then progresses cephalad (see Figs. 4-7 to 4-11). By this means, the shortest and highest short gastric vessels are divided last, after adequate exposure and mobility have been obtained.

In approximately 35% of anatomically normal individuals, a posterior gastric artery arises from the splenic artery to supply the dorsal fundus. This vessel must be identified and secured if total gastrectomy is planned. For lesser procedures, it may provide an important collateral blood supply to the proximal gastric remnant, particularly if splenectomy (and hence ligation of the short gastric arteries) is required.

The lymphatic drainage of the stomach roughly parallels the venous drainage. Groups of lymph nodes along the proximal lesser curvature drain into the superior gastric lymph nodes and thence to nodes around the celiac axis. The distal lesser curvature lymphatics drain into a suprapyloric group of nodes that similarly drains into nodes around the celiac axis. The proximal greater curvature nodes drain into pancreaticoduodenal and splenic nodes, whereas distal greater curvature nodes drain into subpyloric and omental node groups. Rich anastomoses between node groups render these anatomic groupings artificial at best.

The Japanese Research Society for Gastric Cancer characterizes gastrectomies based on extent of lymphadenectomy. In this terminology, an R1 resection encompasses the stomach, omentum, and perigastric lymph nodes (those contained in the fat along the lesser and greater curvature). An R2 resection adds en bloc removal of the superior leaf of transverse mesocolon and pancreatic capsule, as well as celiac, infraduodenal, and supraduodenal lymph nodes. An R3 resection adds nodes along the aorta and esophagus, splenectomy, and resection of the tail of pancreas. The value of laparoscopic resection in gastric cancer is not yet established, but knowledge of these nodal groups and extent of resection is helpful when laparoscopic staging is performed.

Laparoscopic gastrostomy is easily performed. Minimal pneumoperitoneum is needed, and the laparoscope is primarily used to identify the anterior surface of the stomach with certainty and to guide placement of a gastrostomy tube in a manner similar to that used during percutaneous endoscopic gastrostomy. The site selected should be well away from the vessels entering the greater and lesser curvatures, with a sufficient distance above the pylorus to avoid migration of the tube. Generally, a site in the midportion of the body of the stomach is selected.

Laparoscopic gastric resection is generally performed by beginning at the pylorus and working proximally up the greater and lesser curvatures. A Penrose drain or Silastic vessel loop may be placed around the stomach to elevate it as the dissection of the gastropancreatic folds progresses. As in open gastrectomy, dissection of the greater omentum off the transverse mesocolon must be done with care to preserve the middle colic artery. The lesser sac is most easily entered to the left, where the gastropancreatic folds are less pronounced. Once the correct plane is entered, dissection can proceed proximally and distally along the greater curvature.

Duodenum, Laparoscopic Plication of Perforated Ulcer or Pyloroplasty

Lacking palpation, it may be difficult to determine where the stomach ends and the duodenum begins. The laparoscopic surgeon must rely on several visual clues to ascertain the location of the pylorus. The prepyloric veins (of Mayo) and the preduodenal arteries form useful visual landmarks that help to identify the pylorus (see Figs. 4-1, 4-16, and 4-17). The duodenum is generally pinker than the stomach. The pylorus may also be identified by a thin white line or a groove on the greater curvature termed the sulcus intermedius. Finally, an esophagogastroduodenoscope in the stomach may assist in definitive localization.

The pylorus and proximal duodenum may be visualized by simply elevating the liver. To visualize the duodenum fully, it may be necessary to mobilize the right colon. This is rarely required during laparoscopic surgery. Major current procedures on the duodenum are laparoscopic plication of perforated ulcers and laparoscopic pyloroplasty. Both involve the pylorus and proximal duodenum and can be performed with minimal dissection.

The blood supply to the pylorus and first part of the duodenum consists of the supraduodenal artery and a posterior branch of the gastroduodenal artery. The rest of the duodenum is supplied by branches of the pancreaticoduodenal arcades, which run along the anterior and posterior margins of the head of the pancreas. These are generally not seen laparoscopically. Venous drainage parallels arterial supply. Lymphatic drainage is to the pyloric and hepatic nodes (first and second part of the duodenum) and the pancreatico-duodenal and preaortic nodes (third and fourth part of the duodenum).

BIBLIOGRAPHY

Anatomy

1. Dragstedt LR, Fournier HJ, Woodward ER, Tovee EB, Harper PV. Transabdominal gastric vagotomy: a study of the anatomy and surgery of the vagus nerves at the lower portion of the esophagus. *Surg Gynecol Obstet* 1947;85:461–466.
2. Grassi G. Highly selective vagotomy with intraoperative acid secretion test of completeness of vagal secretion. *Surg Gynecol Obstet* 1975;140:259–264.
3. Gray SW, Rowe JS, Skandalakis JE. Surgical anatomy of the gastroesophageal junction. *Am Surg* 1979;45:575–587.
4. Noguchi Y, Imada T, Matsumoto A, et al. Radical surgery for gastric cancer: a review of the Japanese experience. *Cancer* 1989;64:2053–2062.
5. Skandalakis JE, Gray SW, Soria RE, Sorg JL, Rowe JS. Distribution of the vagus nerve to the stomach. *Am Surg* 1980;46:130–139.
6. Skandalakis JE, Rowe JS, Gray SW. Identification of vagal structures at the esophageal hiatus. *Surgery* 1974;75:233–237.
7. Skandalakis LJ, Donahue PE, Skandalakis JE. The vagus nerve and its vagaries. *Surg Clin North Am* 1993;73:769–784.

Laparoscopic Techniques

1. Casas AT, Gadacz TR. Laparoscopic management of peptic ulcer disease. *Surg Clin North Am* 1996;3:515–522.
2. Cuschieri A. Gastric resections. In: Scott-Conner CEH, ed. *The SAGES manual: fundamentals of laparoscopy and gastrointestinal endoscopy.* New York: Springer-Verlag, 1999:236–246.
3. Cuschieri A. Laparoscopic vagotomy: gimmick or reality? *Surg Clin North Am* 1992;72:357–367.
4. Druart ML, Van Hee R, Etienne J, Cadiere GB, Gigot JF, et al. Laparoscopic repair of perforated duodenal ulcer: a prospective multicenter clinical trial. *Surg Endosc* 1997;11:1017–1020.
5. Goh PMY, Alpont A, Mak K, Kum CK. Early international results of laparoscopic gastrectomy. *Surg Endosc* 1997;11:650–652.
6. Goh PMY. Laparoscopic Billroth II gastrectomy. *Semin Laparosc Surg* 1994;1:171–181.
7. Kitano S, Iso Y, Moriyama M, Sugimacki K. Laparoscopic assisted Billroth I gastrectomy. *Surg Laparosc Endosc* 1994;4:146–148.
8. McKernan JB, Wolfe BM, MacFadyen BV. Laparoscopic repair of duodenal ulcer and gastroesophageal reflux. *Surg Clin North Am* 1992;72:1153–1167.
9. Mouiel J, Katkhouda N. Laparoscopic vagotomy for chronic duodenal ulcer disease. *World J Surg* 1993;17:34–39.
10. Ng PCH. Laparoscopic-assisted gastrostomy in 26 patients: indications and outcome at 2 years. *J Laparoendosc Surg* 1996;6:25–28.
11. Rege RV, Merriam LT, Loehl RJ. Laparoscopic splenectomy. *Surg Clin North Am* 1996;76:459–468.
12. Salky BA, Edye M. Laparoscopic pancreatectomy. *Surg Clin North Am* 1996;76:539–545.
13. Thompson AR, Hall TJ, Anglin BA, Scott-Conner CEH. Laparoscopic plication of perforated ulcer: results of a selective approach. *South Med J* 1995;88:185–189.
14. Uyama I, Ogiwara H, Takahara T, Furuta T, Kikuchi K, Iida S. Laparoscopic minilaparotomy Billroth I gastrectomy with extraperigastric lymphadenectomy for early gastric cancer using an abdominal wall-lifting method. *J Laparoendosc Surg* 1995;5:181–187.

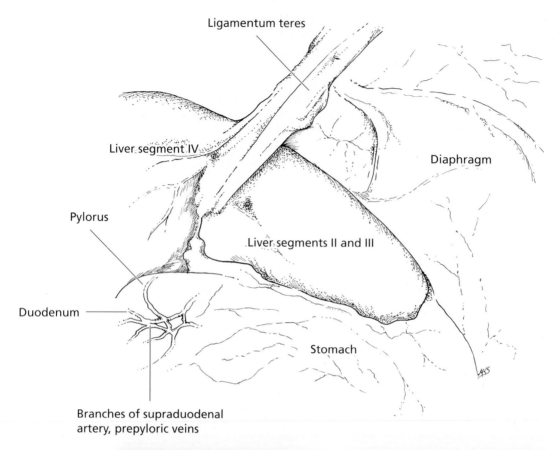

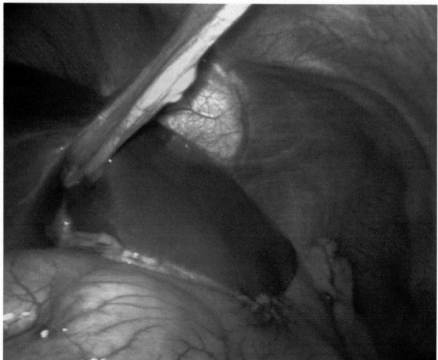

Fig. 4-1. Initial laparoscopic view of stomach and duodenum. An umbilically placed laparoscope aimed at the left upper quadrant demonstrates the prominent ligamentum teres hepatis, diaphragm, and liver. The distal stomach, duodenum, and greater omentum are seen in the foreground. Segments II and III of the liver obscure visualization of the lesser curvature of the stomach. Branches of the supraduodenal artery and prepyloric veins form a useful visual landmark to the approximate location of the pylorus.

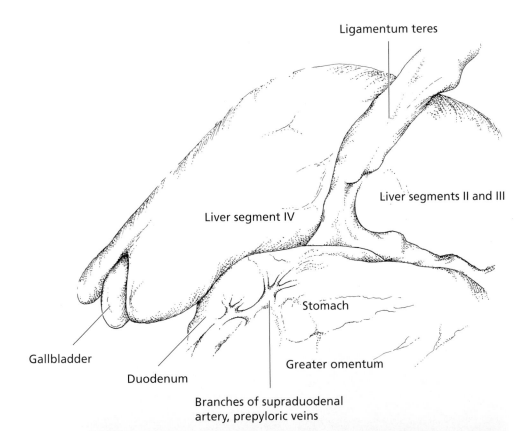

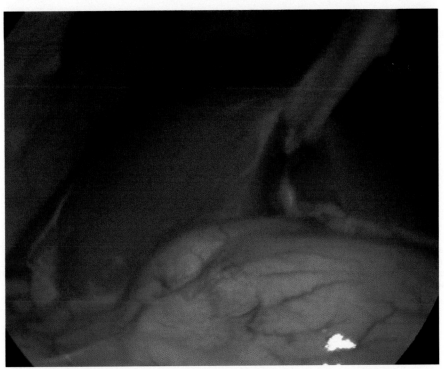

Fig. 4-2. View of upper abdomen. As the laparoscope is panned from the left upper quadrant to the midline of the upper abdomen, the relation of pylorus and duodenum to liver and gallbladder is seen. Prominent branches of the supraduodenal artery and prepyloric veins indicate the probable location of the pylorus.

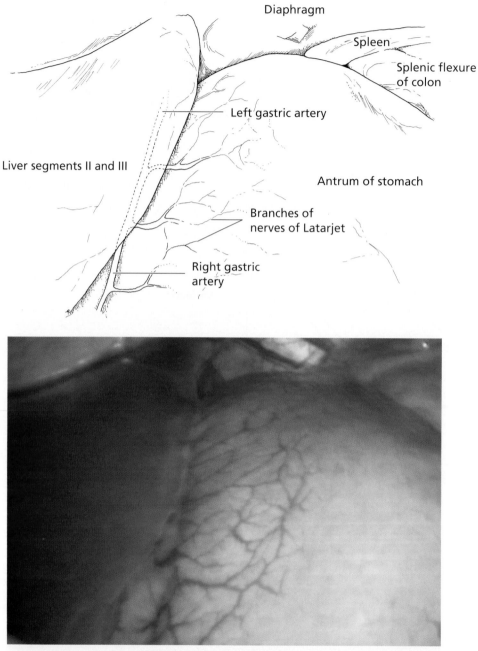

Fig. 4-3. View of gastric antrum. Segments II and III of the liver overlie part of the lesser curvature, but the vascular arcade formed by an ascending branch of the right gastric artery anastomosing along the lesser curvature with the descending branch of the left gastric artery can be seen. Accompanying nerves of Latarjet send small vagal fibers that accompany the vessels. In the background, diaphragm, spleen, and splenic flexure of colon may be glimpsed.

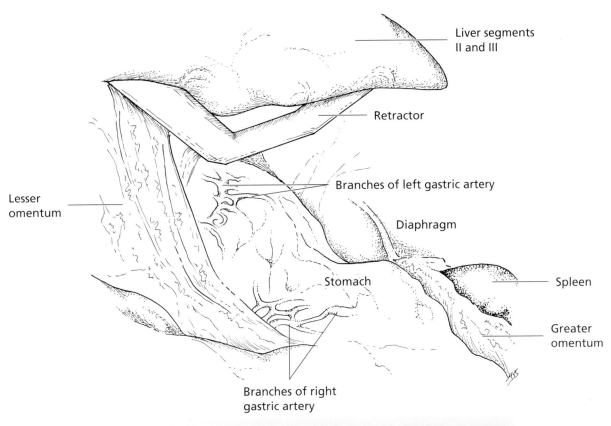

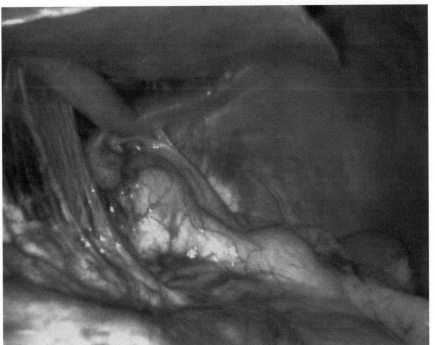

Fig. 4-4. Lesser omentum and lesser curvature of stomach. A retractor has been placed to elevate segments II and III of the liver. The transparent lesser omentum is seen draped over the liver. The stomach has been decompressed by a nasogastric tube. Branches of the left and right gastric artery (and accompanying veins and vagal fibers) are seen on the lesser curvature of the stomach. In the background, diaphragm, spleen, and greater omentum are noted.

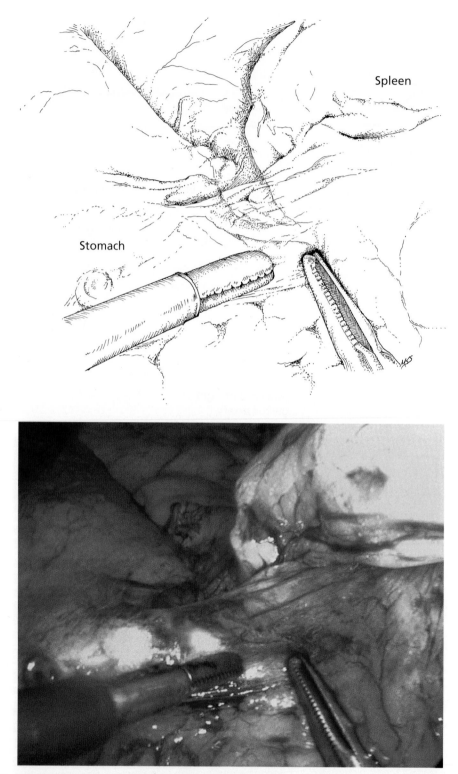

Fig. 4-5. Gastrosplenic fold. A thin veil of peritoneum covers the gastrosplenic ligament and short gastric vessels. The veil must be divided to expose the short gastric arteries (with accompanying veins) that connect stomach and spleen. Two instruments are shown providing gently downward pressure to display the peritoneal veil.

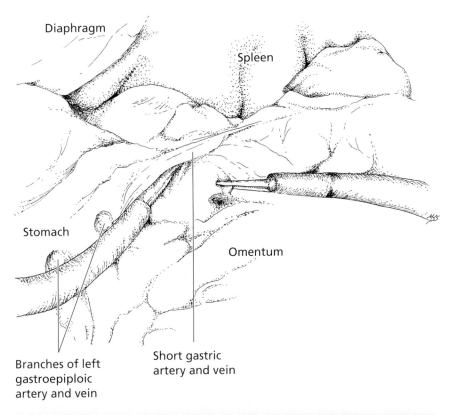

Diaphragm

Spleen

Stomach

Omentum

Branches of left
gastroepiploic
artery and vein

Short gastric
artery and vein

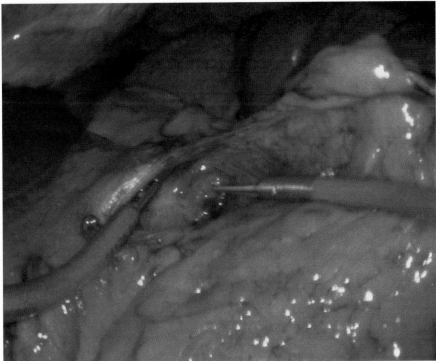

Fig. 4-6. Short gastric vessels. An opening has been made in the gastrosplenic ligament and a short gastric artery (with accompanying vein) is seen, surrounded by fatty connective tissue. The stomach, with branches of the left gastroepiploic artery and vein, and omentum are seen in the foreground. In the background, diaphragm and spleen may be noted.

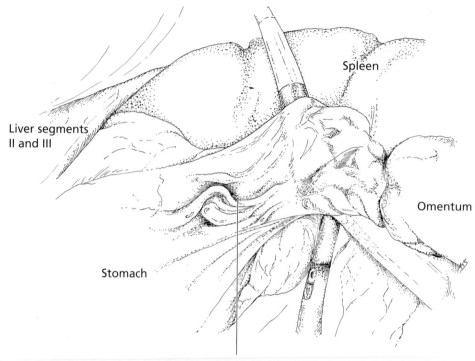

Spleen

Liver segments
II and III

Omentum

Stomach

Short gastric artery and vein

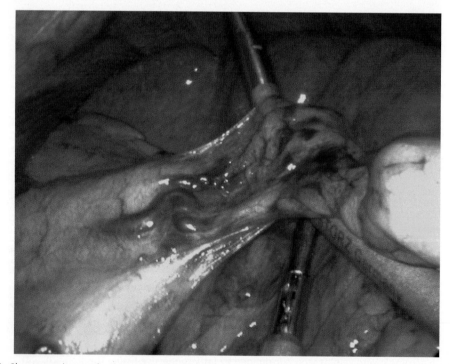

Fig. 4-7. Short gastric vessels. Fatty tissue containing short gastric vessels is shown to connect the greater curvature of the stomach with the hilar region of the spleen. Omentum overlying the splenic flexure of the colon is in the foreground. In the background, segments II and III of the liver are shown. The left triangular ligament is out of sight behind the spleen.

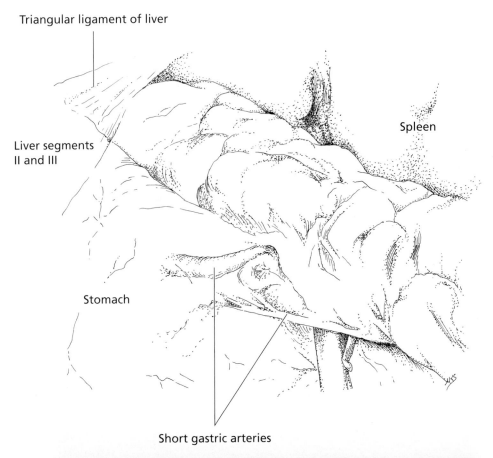

Triangular ligament of liver

Liver segments
II and III

Spleen

Stomach

Short gastric arteries

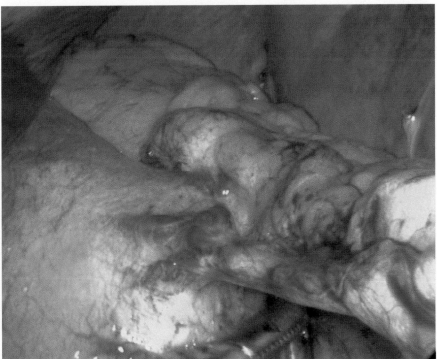

Fig. 4-8. Short gastric vessels. In this example, several short gastric vessels are seen in the gastrosplenic ligament. The triangular ligament is seen tethering segments II and III of the liver to the diaphragm.

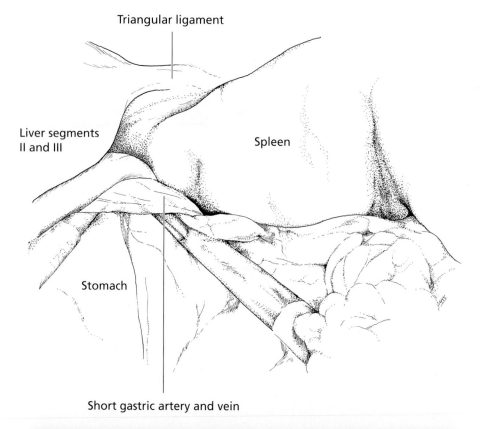

Triangular ligament

Liver segments
II and III

Spleen

Stomach

Short gastric artery and vein

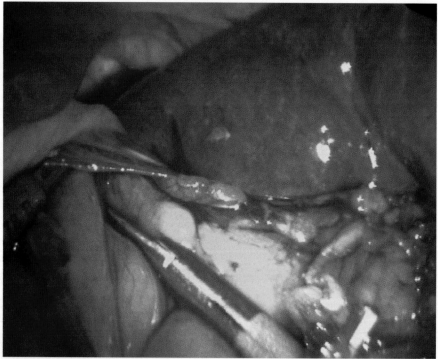

Fig. 4-9. Short gastric vessels. The stomach is being elevated by a grasper placed under the gastrosplenic ligament. As dissection progresses toward the superior pole of the spleen, the short gastric vessels tend to become shorter. Because laparoscopic dissection progresses from below upward, the most difficult part of the dissection is done last, when visualization and mobility are maximal.

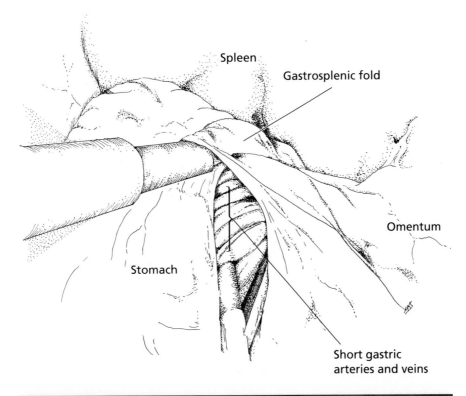

Spleen

Gastrosplenic fold

Omentum

Stomach

Short gastric
arteries and veins

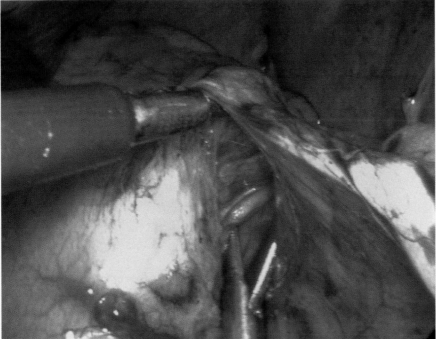

Fig. 4-10. Gastrosplenic fold and short gastric vessels. In this example, a gastrosplenic fold has been elevated to display short gastric vessels lying beneath.

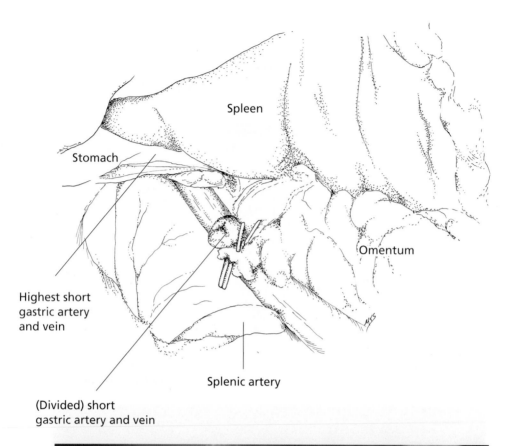

Spleen

Stomach

Omentum

Highest short
gastric artery
and vein

Splenic artery

(Divided) short
gastric artery and vein

Fig. 4-11. Short gastric vessels. All but the most cephalad short gastric artery and vein have been divided. The stomach passes almost to the capsule of the spleen.

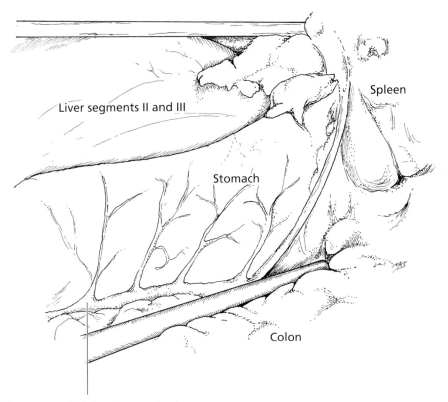

Liver segments II and III

Spleen

Stomach

Colon

Right gastroepiploic artery and vein

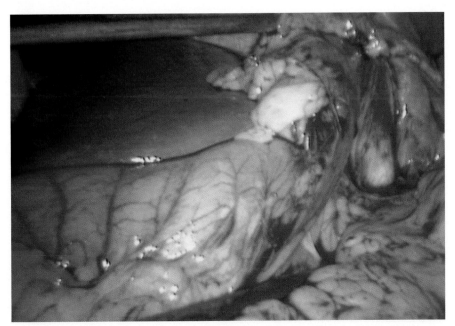

Fig. 4-12. Right gastroepiploic artery and vein. A grasper has been placed along the greater curvature and is gently pressing down on the greater omentum and transverse colon to display the vascular arcade along the greater curvature of the stomach. The right gastroepiploic artery and vein are shown sending multiple branches to the antrum and fundus of the stomach along the greater curvature. The spleen is seen in the background.

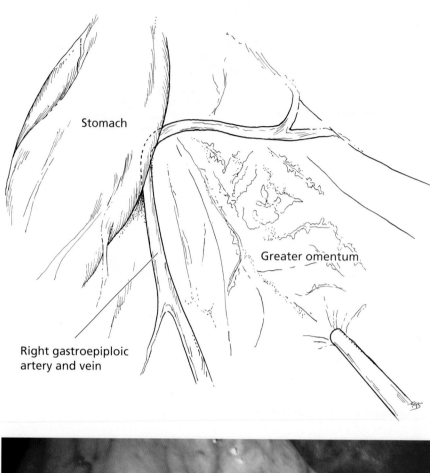

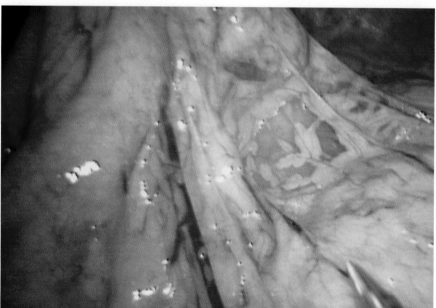

Fig. 4-13. Right gastroepiploic artery and vein. The stomach is being elevated by a grasper (out of the field of view). A second grasper pulls down gently on the greater omentum. The right gastroepiploic artery and vein are seen in the greater omentum.

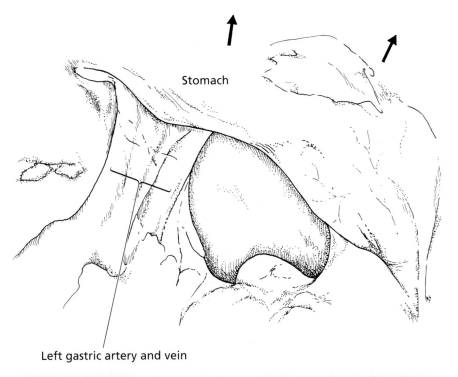

Stomach

Left gastric artery and vein

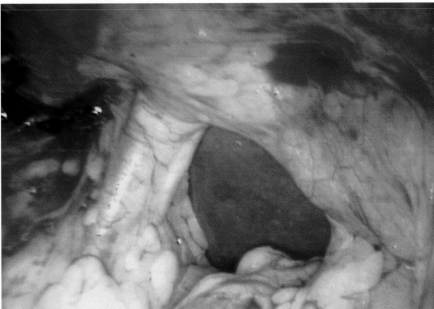

Fig. 4-14. Left gastric artery and vein. The stomach has been mobilized for resection and is being pulled toward the anterior abdominal wall (*arrows* indicate direction of pull). A prominent vascular pedicle containing the left gastric artery and vein is seen in the background.

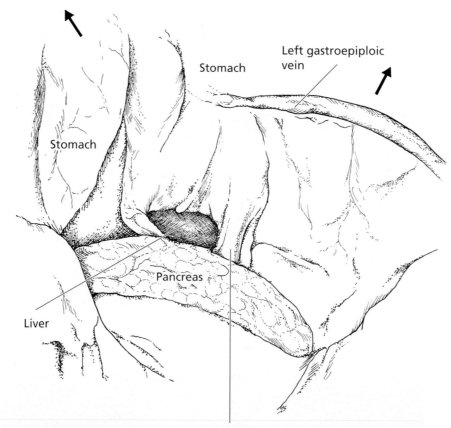

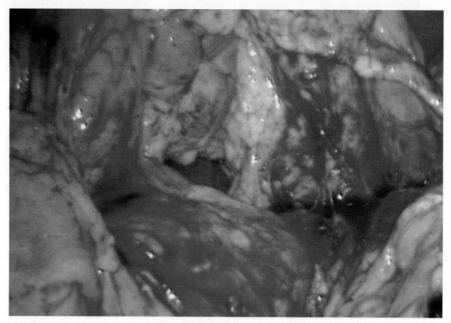

Fig. 4-15. Left gastric artery and vein, left gastroepiploic vein, pancreas. The stomach is retracted cephalad to demonstrate the left gastric artery and vein (*arrows* indicate direction of pull). On the edge of the greater curvature of the stomach, the left gastroepiploic vein and artery are noted. The pancreas is exposed in the floor of the lesser sac.

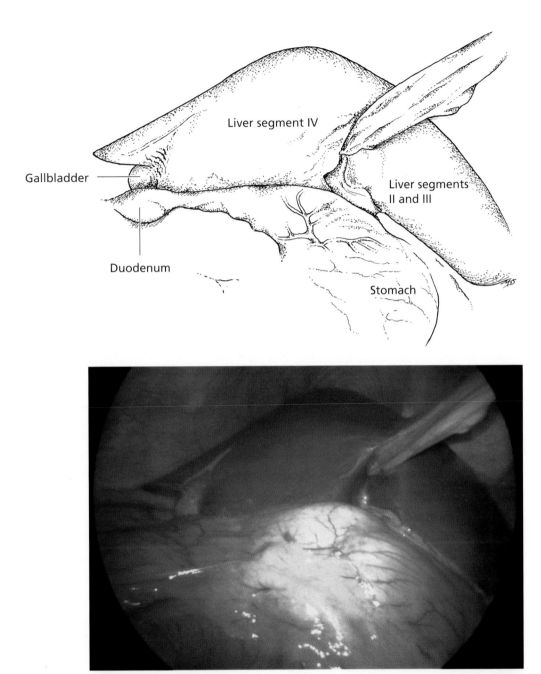

Fig. 4-16. Duodenum and gallbladder. The right upper quadrant with structures in their normal anatomic positions demonstrates the stomach, a prominent vascular pattern over the antrum, and the duodenum. In this view, it is difficult to identify the pylorus (and hence the dividing line between stomach and duodenum) with certainty.

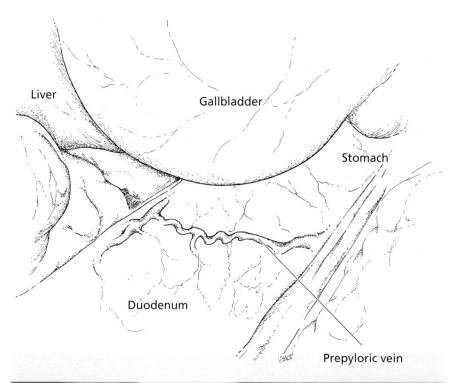

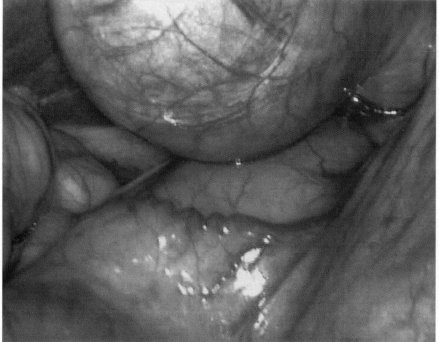

Fig. 4-17. Prepyloric veins, pylorus, duodenum. In this close-up view, the gallbladder lies over the prepyloric region. The prepyloric veins are well demonstrated and provide a useful visual landmark demarcating stomach from duodenum.

5

RIGHT UPPER QUADRANT: LIVER, GALLBLADDER, AND EXTRAHEPATIC BILIARY TRACT

INITIAL LAPAROSCOPIC VIEW AND PRINCIPLES OF EXPOSURE

The initial laparoscopic view of the right upper quadrant demonstrates primarily the sub-phrenic spaces, abdominal surface of the diaphragm, and diaphragmatic surface of the liver, but little else. The free edge of the liver nestles against stomach, duodenum, greater omentum, and hepatic flexure of the colon. The gallbladder is barely seen. The falciform ligament is a prominent dividing point between the left subphrenic space and the right subphrenic space. The ligamentum teres hepatis is seen in the free edge of the falciform. Figures 5-1 and 5-2 show a panoramic view of these structures as seen at initial explo-ration.

Exposure is enhanced by placing the patient in the reverse Trendelenburg position. Gravity pulls the viscera caudad, opening the subphrenic space even further. An angled (30- to 45-degree) laparoscope is used to inspect the surfaces of the dome of the liver, the falciform ligament, and the diaphragm.

Exposure of the subhepatic space requires elevation of the liver. The three basic tech-niques are cephalad traction on the gallbladder, falciform lift, and use of various retractors. Each is discussed in detail here. The reverse Trendelenburg position is still used, but it may be less steep, so the weight of the liver does not pull downward so strongly.

Upward traction on the gallbladder (Fig. 5-3) is the method of choice when chole-cystectomy is planned. It should be avoided under other circumstances because trauma to the gallbladder may necessitate unplanned cholecystectomy or, if unrecognized, may lead to complications. A grasper is placed on the visible portion of the gallbladder and then is pushed up over the liver. It is not uncommon for the duodenum to adhere to the region of Hartmann's pouch, and such adhesions must be carefully lysed to avoid inadvertent duodenal perforation. A second grasper, placed on Hartmann's pouch, pulls out to expose the structures of Calot's triangle and the hepatoduodenal ligament. An angled laparoscope gives the best visualization of the common duct, hepatic artery, and duodenum.

The falciform lift technique relies on upward traction on the falciform ligament. The ligamentum teres hepatis, which forms the free edge of the falciform ligament, attaches to the underside of the liver; therefore, upward traction on the ligamentum teres in particu-lar elevates the liver and makes the undersurface of the liver and structures in the subhep-atic space visible (Figs. 5-4 and 5-5). There are two ways to accomplish this traction. The least traumatic uses the shaft of an instrument passed from a lateral port. The shaft passes under and to the left of the ligament. The shaft of the instrument is then angled sharply caudad toward the undersurface of the anterior abdominal wall and diaphragm. If this ma-neuver does not produce adequate elevation, an atraumatic grasper may be used to grasp the ligamentum teres hepatis directly. The laparoscopist should place this grasper as low down, near the edge of the liver, as possible. One should take care to avoid trauma to the ligamentum teres or falciform ligament, which may bleed.

The third technique uses a laparoscopic retractor to elevate the liver (Fig. 5-6). Various such devices are available, all designed to pass through a laparoscopic port and then expand to a broad flat surface. An initial falciform lift maneuver facilitates introduction of the retractor and proper placement. Such a retractor, properly placed, provides the most stable exposure and is used for surgery on the stomach, hiatal region, or duodenum.

ANATOMY AND SPECIFIC SURGICAL PROCEDURES

Liver

The diaphragmatic surface of the liver is smooth and is covered by Glisson's capsule. The liver is partially shaped by the space it normally fills, and mamillations and fetal lobulations are sometimes seen. Most of the surface of the liver is covered with peritoneum, which forms folds at the anterior and posterior attachments of the liver to the abdominal wall and at the hepatoduodenal ligament. The anterior attachments of the liver include the ligamentum teres hepatis and the falciform ligament. Posteriorly, the left and right triangular ligaments split to form the coronary ligament, which effectively encircles the bare area of the liver. Lying extremely posterior and effectively extraperitoneal, the bare area of the liver is inaccessible to laparoscopic inspection.

The ligamentum teres hepatis stretches from the umbilicus to the umbilical plate of the liver. The falciform ligament stretches like a sail from the ligamentum teres hepatis superiorly to the undersurface of the diaphragm, inferiorly to the dome of the left lobe of the liver, and posteriorly to the inferior vena cava. It is covered with glistening parietal peritoneum. In slender individuals, it is translucent, and small vessels are easily seen. In the obese, fat is deposited in the falciform ligament as elsewhere. This thickening of the falciform ligament must be anticipated by the laparoscopist when trocars are introduced into the upper midline (see Chapter 1). The right side of the ligamentum teres is seen to be smooth and glistening. The free edge contains obliterated umbilical vessels that may remain patent or may even recanalize in portal hypertension. To the left of the falciform ligament, the diaphragmatic surface of the left lateral segment similarly assumes the shape of the space in which it is located. Posteriorly, the falciform ligament is continuous with the right and left triangular ligaments. The extreme lateral prolongation of these ligaments may be seen laparoscopically, especially on the left side (see Chapter 3).

The liver is divided into anatomic segments based on internal anatomy that is invisible to the laparoscopist. Surface landmarks include the falciform ligament and the gallbladder fossa. The older terminology is based on surface landmarks and hence may be conceptually useful to the laparoscopist (who has only the surface view to go by). Accurate description of the anatomic location of lesions is particularly important when laparoscopy is done before planned liver resection or when laparoscopic liver resection is contemplated. Thus, is it important that the laparoscopist have a mental image of the location of the major segments relative to surface landmarks. Correlation with internal (and hence segmental) anatomy is enhanced by laparoscopic ultrasound and comparison with preoperative studies such as computed tomographic portography. In the discussion that follows, the term "lobe" is used for the four visually distinct divisions of the older terminology (right lobe, left lateral lobe, quadrate lobe, and caudate lobe). The term "segment" is used for the current terminology (Couinaud) based on internal anatomy.

The portion of the liver to the left of the falciform ligament is sometimes called the left lateral lobe. It is composed of segments II (posterior) and III (anterior) (Fig. 5-7). The anatomic left lobe of the liver actually extends of the right of the falciform ligament to an imaginary line drawn through the gallbladder fossa and passing back to the inferior vena cava (Figs. 5-8 to 5-10). Elevation of the liver displays the visible landmarks for the remainder of the left lobe of the liver (Fig. 5-11). The entry of the ligamentum teres hepatis into the umbilical plate delineates the anteriorly located quadrate lobe (segment IV) and the deeper caudate lobe (segment I, or spigelian lobe). The quadrate lobe is easily visualized when the liver is elevated. The surface landmarks that delineate the quadrate lobe on the inferior aspect of the liver are the gallbladder to the right, the ligamentum teres hepatis to the left, and the umbilical plate inferiorly (Figs. 5-12 to 5-14). "Crossover structures" may be seen in the base of the falciform ligament. These are the bile duct, hepatic artery, and portal vein, which correspond to segment IV. The caudate lobe is delineated by the umbilical plate and porta hepatis superiorly and by the inferior vena cava posteriorly (not visible). To the left, the visible fissure of the liver is an extension of the ligamentum teres. To the right, the caudate lobe terminates in an edge that creates the visual impression of a separate lobe, and deep to this lies the inferior vena cava, which is generally not seen. Sometimes, the caudate lobe is visible through a transparent portion of the lesser omentum when the left lateral lobe of the liver is elevated (see Fig. 5-6) or when the gallbladder is dissected off the liver (see Fig. 5-11; Fig. 5-15). However, the caudate lobe is adequately visualized laparoscopically only with extreme elevation of the falciform ligament and left lateral lobe of the liver. It is commonly seen during laparoscopic procedures in the vicinity of the esophageal hiatus (see Chapter 3) because of the excellent exposure produced by liver retractors.

A plane through the gallbladder fossa straight back to the inferior vena cava divides the liver into its anatomic right and left lobes (see Fig. 5-13). No visible landmarks on the top of the liver can be identified. Laparoscopic ultrasound may be useful. Segments V through VIII comprise the right lobe, and there are no visible external landmarks to assist the laparoscopist (see Figs. 5-9 to 5-10). Segment V is anteromedial. Segment VI is anterolateral. Segment VIII is posteromedial, and segment VII is posterolateral.

Laparoscopic Liver Surgery

The surgical procedures performed laparoscopically currently include liver biopsy, wedge resection, and marsupialization of hepatic cysts. Major liver resections have been reported from specialized centers, but they are not commonly performed laparoscopically. Liver biopsy may be performed by several methods, depending on the location and nature of the target lesion. Biopsy needles may be used under laparoscopic guidance to obtain deep core biopsies. Biopsy forceps are used to sample lesions visible on the surface.

Laparoscopic wedge resection is reserved for small, peripherally located lesions. These minor resections are generally performed in a nonanatomic fashion, that is, without regard for the internal anatomy of the liver. If deep resection is planned, laparoscopic ultrasound is a prudent adjunct because external landmarks are difficult to interpret through the laparoscope.

Large benign cysts are easily marsupialized. Lesions on the dome of the liver may be opened with electrocautery without major concern about ductal structures. Communication with the ductal system should be excluded by aspiration.

When the cyst is on the inferior surface of the liver, the laparoscopist must use caution to avoid ductal and hilar structures that may be displaced or distorted by the mass lesion. Laparoscopic ultrasound, supplemented by cholangiography, is crucial in these cases.

Extrahepatic Biliary Tree

Gallbladder and Laparoscopic Cholecystectomy

As the gallbladder is elevated and retracted cephalad, adhesions to the omentum or duodenum may be seen. As previously mentioned, the duodenum in particular is often tented up by the traction and must be carefully mobilized. If the duodenum and transverse colon obscure visualization, a steeper reverse Trendelenburg position, greater cephalad traction on the fundus, adequate decompression of the stomach and duodenum by orogastric tube, and the use of a 30-degree laparoscope will generally overcome the difficulty. Once the gallbladder is fully mobilized and elevated, careful inspection of the surface anatomy reveals whether or not it is partially intrahepatic, on a mesentery, or possesses a phrygian cap or other odd shape. Hartmann's pouch is identified and is a valuable landmark that can be traced and seen to funnel down to a single tubular structure, the cystic duct. A redundant gallbladder infundibulum may obscure the cystic duct and hepatoduodenal ligament.

Careful placement of graspers, traction outward and upward on the fundus, and the use of the 30-degree scope improve visualization in this case (see Fig. 5-15; Figs. 5-16 and 5-17). The blue-yellow junction, in which the robin's egg blue gallbladder melds with the fat-laden yellow areolar tissue overlying Calot's triangle, is a useful laparoscopic landmark to the termination of Hartmann's pouch.

The typical angular junction of the cystic duct on the common duct (as depicted in many surgical atlases) actually occurs in a minority of patients, and the length and course of the cystic duct are highly variable. Most laparoscopic surgeons clip and divide the cystic duct high on its termination at Hartmann's pouch, rather than attempting to trace the cystic duct to its juncture with the common duct, to minimize the chances of harming the common duct (Figs. 5-18 to 5-20). Dissection down to the cystic duct–common duct junction increases the chances of traction injury to the common duct, and bleeding from the small vessels and lymphatics in the space between the cystic artery and cystic duct may obscure visualization. Control of bleeding from these small vessels may be problematic, because thermal injury to the common duct can occur. The safest way to avoid all these problems is to accept the necessity of leaving a long cystic duct remnant and to divide the cystic duct near its entrance onto the gallbladder, confirming the anatomy by the characteristic funnel shape of the infundibulum.

The boundaries of Calot's triangle are often not well seen. In particular, the common hepatic duct, which forms the medial boundary, is often not visualized or may even be tented up by extreme traction. Outward traction on the lower of the two graspers (the one placed on Hartmann's pouch) pulls the infundibulum of the gallbladder away from the liver, opening Calot's triangle, increasing the safety of dissection (see Fig. 5-17). If the first assistant pushes in or up on this grasper, the infundibulum is compressed against the hilum of the liver, Calot's triangle is narrowed, and injury to the common duct or right hepatic duct is more likely. A 30-degree laparoscope allows the surgeon to look down onto the structures of Calot's triangle directly. It may be helpful to back off and get a panoramic view with the laparoscope, looking in particular for the pulsations of the hepatic artery, which should be seen just to the left of the common duct (see Fig. 5-16).

The cystic artery is often visible under the peritoneum as it runs along the surface of the gallbladder (Fig. 5-21). Sometimes, a fatty stripe marks the location when the vessel itself cannot be seen. This important landmark helps to confirm the location of the cystic artery in its normal location arising from the hepatic artery in the hepatocystic triangle and passing up the left side of the gallbladder, a configuration that is seen in approximately 80% of individuals. Conversely, when the stripe is seen on the right side, a significant arterial branch may be anticipated (see Fig. 5-3). A posterior, or low-lying, cystic artery arising from the superior mesenteric artery or one of its branches, is seen in approximately 18% of cases, with an additional 6% having both anterior and posterior cystic arteries. This posterior cystic artery appears closer to the laparoscope than the cystic duct and may be mistaken for it. It is generally observed to be smaller than the cystic duct, to have visible pulsations when traction is relaxed, and to terminate by running onto the surface of the gallbladder, rather than by gradually funneling out to the infundibulum (Fig. 5-22).

Opening the peritoneum over Hartmann's pouch and dissecting behind the gallbladder exposes the termination of the infundibulum onto the cystic duct (see Fig. 5-20). A generous V-shaped incision, carried cephalad up the peritoneal reflections of the gallbladder on either side, allows the surgeon to dissect behind the gallbladder to create excellent visualization of the termination of the gallbladder onto the cystic duct and the cystic artery. The normally (anterior) cystic artery is seen to the left. A sizable lymph node may be seen anterior to the cystic artery in Calot's triangle and may be a useful landmark to the cystic artery, which lies deep to the lymph node (Figs. 5-23 to 5-25). It is sometimes necessary to dissect this lymph node to gain clear access to the structures of Calot's triangle. The cystic artery typically divides into superficial and deep branches and gives off a small and highly variable twig that supplies the cystic duct (see Fig. 5-25; Fig. 5-26). This tiny twig is often avulsed and bleeds as the plane between cystic duct and cystic artery is developed. Bleeding stops when the cystic duct is clipped. Usually, the laparoscopist clips and divides the cystic artery before its division into superficial and deep branches and before the origin of the twig supplying the cystic duct (see Fig. 5-23). The cystic artery and cystic duct are the only two structures that must be clipped or ligated before division.

The remainder of the dissection of the gallbladder off the gallbladder fossa is accomplished with electrocautery (Fig. 5-27). Small vessels are generally only seen at the peritoneal reflections (laterally). Accessory bile ducts are common and form a spectrum of anomalies. Any small tubular structures noted to run within the gallbladder fossa should be preserved, if possible (Fig. 5-28). These small segmental ducts, termed ducts of Luschka or subvesical ducts, drain subsegmental areas of the liver into the intraparenchymal right hepatic ductal system. Typically, these ducts run through the gallbladder fossa, where they may be injured if the dissection plane is inadvertently carried too deep. Cystohepatic ducts similarly drain variable amounts of hepatic parenchyma and typically empty into the cystic duct or right hepatic duct. These should be preserved if at all possible. Any small tubular structures passing from the liver into the gallbladder should be clipped and divided sharply (rather than cauterized) to avoid postoperative bile leakage. No sizable tubular structures should be noted. If the laparoscopist sees a tubular structure similar in size or larger than the "cystic artery" and "cystic duct" that have already been clipped and divided, anomalous anatomy or misidentification of vital structures such as the common duct or right hepatic duct may have occurred. The laparoscopist should reassess the anatomy. Cholangiography is the only way to delineate ductal anatomy with certainty. The surgeon should consider conversion to open surgery if the anatomy cannot be satisfactorily elucidated.

The right hepatic artery passes close to the cystic duct in 1% of individuals, and in another 10% it has a redundancy aptly termed the "caterpillar hump" (Figs. 5-29 and 5-30). This is often seen in association with multiple small arterial twigs supplying the gallbladder rather than a well-formed cystic artery per se. Preservation of this vessel requires that the small twigs be dissected free and individually ligated.

Structures of the Hepatoduodenal Ligament, Laparoscopic Choledochotomy

As previously mentioned, the length and pattern of termination of the cystic duct onto the common duct are highly variable. Averages from 1 to 3.5 cm in length are commonly quoted. In 10% of individuals, the cystic duct is short (around 1 cm, sometimes less). This increases the risk of injury during cholecystectomy.

There are two ways to identify the common duct laparoscopically: by following the cystic duct to its juncture with the common duct or by directly visualizing the common duct in the hepatoduodenal ligament. Because laparoscopic choledochotomy is often performed in conjunction with laparoscopic cholecystectomy, following the cystic duct to its termination is a logical method for seeking the common duct. This method is also the best way to find the common duct when the areolar tissues surrounding the duct are thickened or inflamed. Cholangiography greatly increases the safety of dissection by providing a "road map" and generally precedes the dissection. Approximately 75% of anatomically normal individuals have a relatively long cystic duct with an angled termination onto the common duct. In around 15% to 17%, the cystic duct parallels the common duct for part of its terminal portion and may share a common wall with this duct. In another 8%, the cystic duct spirals around the common duct to enter after an indirect course. As the cystic duct is traced to its juncture on the common duct, the laparoscopic surgeon must be careful to keep the dissection on the anterior surface of the duct, rather than entering into the plane behind the common duct. Alternatively, the common duct may be sought directly in the hepatoduodenal ligament. An angled (30-degree) laparoscope greatly facilitates visualization of the common duct. Laparoscopic ultrasound is a useful adjunct and may assist in delineation of structures that are hidden beneath the peritoneum. Visible pulsations in the hepatic artery, which lies to the left of the common duct, are often observed.

The structures in the hepatoduodenal ligament are best visualized with an angled laparoscope. These structures are covered by a glistening film of peritoneum that must be opened before good visualization is obtained. The hepatic artery may be identified by visible pulsations. It typically lies to the left of the common duct, which may be seen as a bluish structure. The portal vein is posterior and is not generally seen or sought.

The right and left hepatic duct combine in the hilum of the liver to form the common hepatic duct in 57% to 72% of cases. Classically, the right hepatic duct has a longer extrahepatic course than the left hepatic duct. Multiple patterns of variation include direct drainage of an anomalous right hepatic duct directly into the cystic duct or a low union of the left and right hepatic duct below the entrance of the cystic duct into the right hepatic duct. These anomalies are best identified by cholangiography, but they may be suspected whenever more than two tubular structures (one running onto the surface of the gallbladder and one terminating in Hartmann's pouch) are seen after careful dissection in Calot's triangle.

The supraduodenal common duct runs in the inferior half of the right free border of the hepatoduodenal ligament. The blood supply is axial, from branches of regional arteries, typically the retroduodenal, right hepatic, cystic, or retroportal arteries. Tiny vessels are characteristically seen running parallel to the length of the duct at the 3 o'clock and 9 o'clock positions, 60% coming from below and 40% from above. The appearance of these vessels is so characteristic that when a tubular structure is seen with two parallel vessels running along it, the laparoscopist should immediately think of the common duct. Small venous tributaries commonly form a plexus over the adventitial surface of the common duct and may cause troublesome bleeding.

The right hepatic artery passes behind the common duct in approximately 85% of cases. In the remainder, an anterior crossing, usually cephalad to the cystic duct–common duct juncture, is seen. It is not rare for the right hepatic artery to bifurcate, with one branch passing anterior to and one branch passing posterior to the common duct. These variations in the hepatic artery render it vulnerable to injury during laparoscopic choledochotomy. The magnified view obtained during laparoscopy should enable the alert laparoscopic surgeon to avoid injuring this vessel, easily identified by prominent pulsations or a transverse thickening of the tissues on the anterior wall on the common duct.

BIBLIOGRAPHY

Regional Anatomy

1. Benson EA, Page RE. A practical reappraisal of the anatomy of the extrahepatic bile ducts and arteries. *Br J Surg* 1976;63:853–860.
2. Bismuth H, Chiche L. Surgical anatomy and anatomical surgery of the liver. In: Blumgart LH, ed. *Surgery of the liver and biliary tract,* 2nd ed. Edinburgh: Churchill Livingstone, 1988;1:3–9.
3. Browne EZ. Variations in origin and course of the hepatic artery and its branches. *Surgery* 1940;8:424–445.
4. Champetier J, Letoublou C, Alnaasan I, Charvin B. The cystohepatic ducts: surgical implications. *Surg Radiol Anat* 1991;13:203–211.
5. Couinaud C. *La foie: études anatomiques et chirurgicales,* vol 1. Paris: Masson, 1957.
6. Daseler EH, Anson BJ, Hambley WC, Reimann AF. The cystic artery and constituents of the hepatic pedicle: a study of 500 specimens. *Surg Gynecol Obstet* 1947;85:47–63.
7. Eisendrath DN. Anomalies of the bile ducts and blood vessels as the cause of accidents in biliary surgery. *JAMA* 1918;71:864–867.
8. Flint ER. Abnormalities of the right hepatic, cystic and gastroduodenal arteries and of the bile ducts. *Br J Surg* 1992;10:509–519.
9. Healey JE, Schroy PC. Anatomy of the biliary ducts within the human liver: analysis of the prevailing pattern of branchings and the major variations of the biliary ducts. *Arch Surg* 1953;66:599–616.
10. Johnston EV, Anston BJ. Variations in the formation and vascular relationships of the bile ducts. *Surg Gynecol Obstet* 1952;94:669–686.
11. Lichtenstein ME, Nicosia AL. The clinical significance of accessory hepatobiliary ducts. *Ann Surg* 1954;142:120–124.
12. Lindner HH, Green RB. Embryology and surgical anatomy of the extrahepatic biliary tract. *Surg Clin North Am* 1964;44:1273–1285.
13. McQuillan T, Manolas SG, Hayman JA, Kune GA. Surgical significance of the bile duct of Luschka. *Br J Surg* 1989;76:696–698.

14. Michels NA. The hepatic, cystic, and retroduodenal arteries and their relations to the biliary ducts. *Ann Surg* 1951;133:503–524.
15. Michels NA. Variational anatomy of the hepatic, cystic, and retroduodenal arteries: a statistical analysis of their origin, distribution, and relation to the biliary ducts in two hundred bodies. *Arch Surg* 1953;66:20–34.
16. Northover JMA, Terblanche J. A new look at the arterial supply of the bile duct in man and its surgical implications. *Br J Surg* 1979;66:379–384.
17. Osler GF, Dow RS. Variations and anomalies of the biliary duct system and its associated blood supply. *West J Surg* 1945;53:316–321.
18. Parke WW, Michels NA, Ghosh GM. Blood supply of the common bile duct. *Surg Gynecol Obstet* 1963;117:47–55.
19. Pollack EL, Tabrisky J. The aberrant divisional bile duct: a surgical hazard. *Surgery* 1973;73:234–239.
20. Rocko JM, Swan KG, DiGioia JM. Calot's triangle revisited. *Surg Gynecol Obstet* 1981;153:410–414.
21. Smadja C, Blumgart LH. The biliary tract and the anatomy of biliary exposure. In: Blumgart LH, ed. *Surgery of the liver and biliary tract,* 2nd ed. Edinburgh: Churchill Livingstone, 1988;1:11–12.
22. Stokes TL, Old L. Cholecystohepatic duct. *Am J Surg* 1978;135:703–705.
23. Terblanche J, Allison HE, Northover JMA. An ischemic basis for biliary strictures. *Surgery* 1983;94:52–57.

Anatomy and Technique of Specific Surgical Procedures

1. Berci G. Biliary ductal anatomy and anomalies: the role of intraoperative cholangiography during laparoscopic cholecystectomy. *Surg Clin North Am* 1992;72:1069–1072.
2. Bouillot JL, Salah S, Baccot S, Alexandre JH. Percutaneous surgery of biliary cyst: a case report. *J Laparoendosc Surg* 1992;2:101–103.
3. Cullen JJ, Scott-Conner CEH. Surgical anatomy of laparoscopic common duct exploration. In: Berci G, Cuschieri A, eds. *Bile ducts and bile duct stones.* Philadelphia: WB Saunders, 1996;20–25.
4. Davidoff A, Pappas TN, Murray EA, et al. Mechanisms of major biliary injury during laparoscopic cholecystectomy. *Ann Surg* 1992;215:196–202.
5. Donohue JH, Grant CS, Farnell MD, van Heerden JA. Laparoscopic cholecystectomy: operative technique. *Mayo Clin Proc* 1992;67:441–448.
6. Huang SM, Wu CW, Chau GY, Jwo SC, Lui WY, P'eng FK. An alternative approach of choledocholithotomy via laparoscopic choledochotomy. *Arch Surg* 1996;131:407–411.
7. Hunter JC. Avoidance of bile duct injury during laparoscopic cholecystectomy. *Am J Surg* 1991;162:71–76.
8. Jenkins MA, Ponsky JL, Lehman GA, Fanelli R, Biachi T. Treatment of bile leaks from the cystohepatic ducts after laparoscopic cholecystectomy. *Surg Endosc* 1994;8:193–196.
9. Kaneko H, Takagi S, Shiba T. Laparoscopic partial hepatectomy and left lateral segmentectomy: technique and results of a clinical series. *Surgery* 1996;120:468–475.
10. Klingler PJ, Gadenstatter M, Schmid T, Bodner E, Schwelberger HG. Treatment of hepatic cysts in the era of laparoscopic surgery. *Br J Surg* 1997;84:438–444.
11. Phillips EH, Berci G, Carroll B, Daykhovsky L, Sackier J, Paz-Partlow M. The importance of intraoperative cholangiography during laparoscopic cholecystectomy. *Am Surg* 1990;12:792–795.
12. Robinson G, Hollinshead J, Falk G, Moulton J. Technique and results of laparoscopic choledochotomy for the management of bile duct calculi. *Aust N Z J Surg* 1995;65:347–349.
13. Sackier JM, Berci G, Phillips E, et al. The role of cholangiography in laparoscopic cholecystectomy. *Arch Surg* 1990;126:1021–1031.
14. Scott-Conner CEH, Hall TJ. Variant arterial anatomy in laparoscopic cholecystomy. *Am J Surg* 1992;163:590–592.
15. Soper NJ, Flye MW, Brunt LM, et al. Diagnosis and management of biliary complications of laparoscopic cholecystectomy. *Am J Surg* 1993;165:663–669.
16. Strasberg SM, Hertl M, Soper NJ. An analysis of the problems of biliary injury during laparoscopic cholecystectomy. *J Am Coll Surg* 1995;180:101–125.
17. Watanabe Y, Sato M, Ueda S, et al. Laparoscopic hepatic resection: a new and safe procedure by abdominal wall lifting method. *Hepatogastroenterology* 1997;44:143–147.

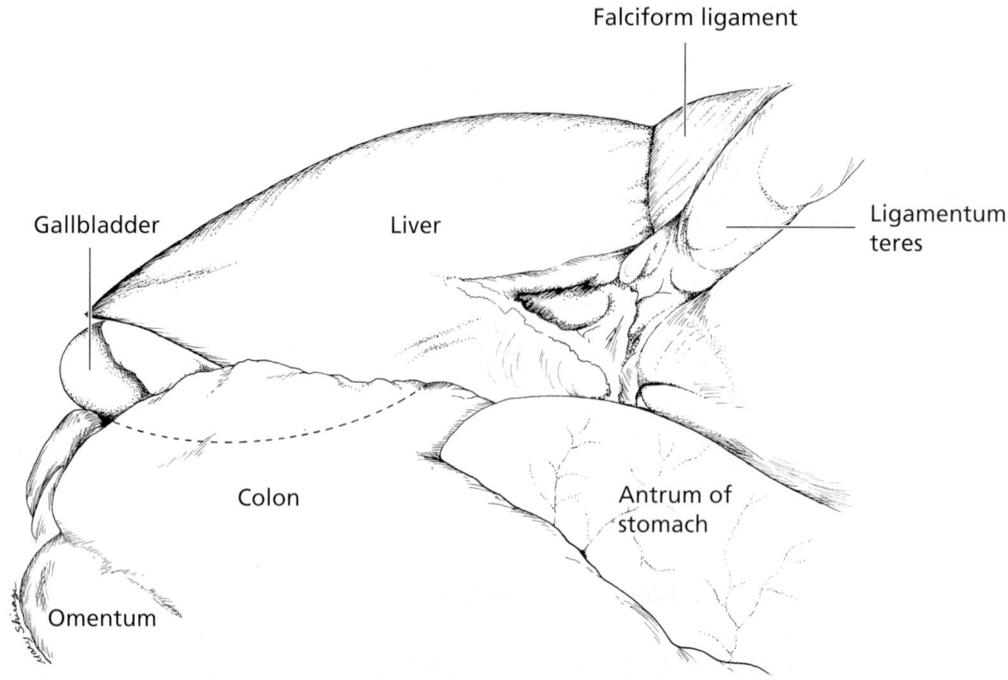

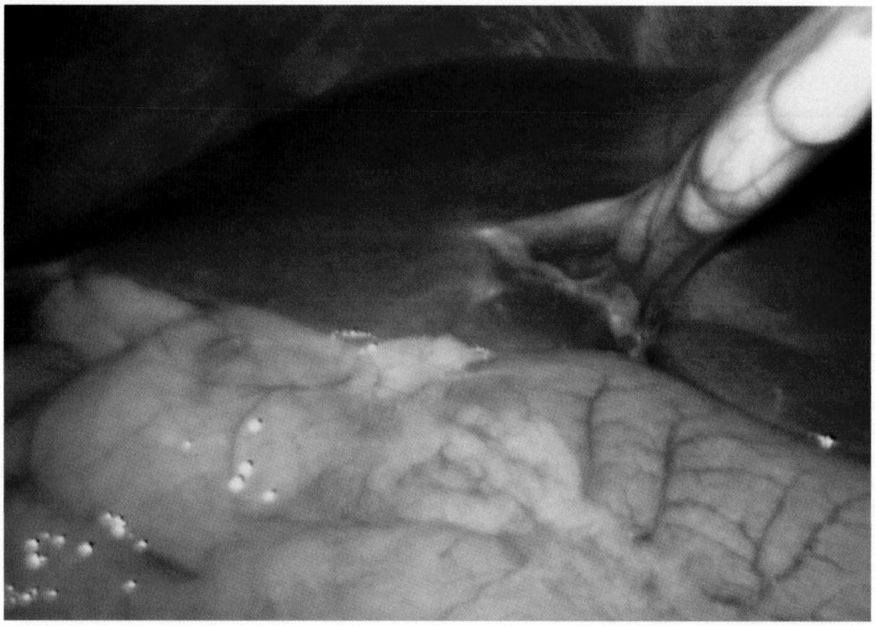

Fig. 5-1. Right upper quadrant: initial view. The ligamentum teres and falciform ligament are seen stretching across the upper foreground. The subphrenic space extends into the background, bounded by the underside of the right hemidiaphragm. The umbilical plate and segmental fissure are well seen. The liver lies against the stomach and transverse colon. The subhepatic space is closed. The antrum of the stomach is seen in the distance to the left. The hepatic flexure and transverse colon, covered by greater omentum, occupy the foreground. The gallbladder is barely seen. The *dotted line* indicates the probable location of the gallbladder fundus, hidden by omentum and colon.

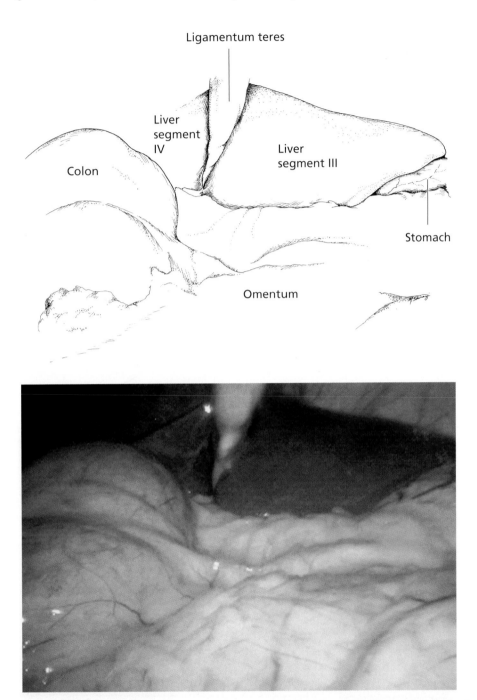

Fig. 5-2. Upper abdomen: initial view. The laparoscope is aimed directly cephalad along the midline from an umbilical portal. The ligamentum teres is seen heading directly for the umbilicus. It appears to taper as it enters the umbilical plate of the liver, as a result of foreshortening and progressively increasing distance from the laparoscope. The left lobe of the liver (primarily segment III, to the left of the ligamentum teres; and segment IV, to the right of the ligamentum teres) is seen. The transverse colon, covered by greater omentum, dominates the foreground. The stomach is barely seen in the left upper quadrant.

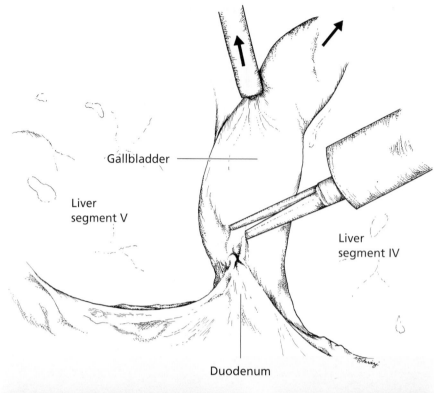

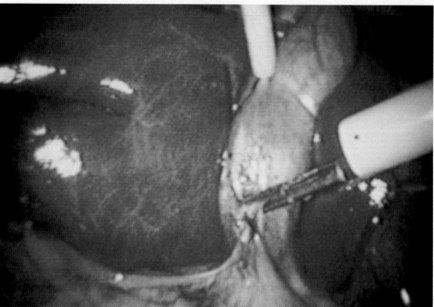

Fig. 5-3. Exposure of subhepatic space: cephalad traction on the gallbladder. Two graspers have been placed to provide traction as shown by the *arrows*. The duodenum is frequently adherent to the gallbladder, as shown here, and must be carefully dissected to avoid injury. Sharp cephalad traction on the gallbladder elevates the liver and opens the subhepatic space. This method is used to expose the subhepatic space when cholecystectomy is planned. Segments IV and V of the liver are seen.

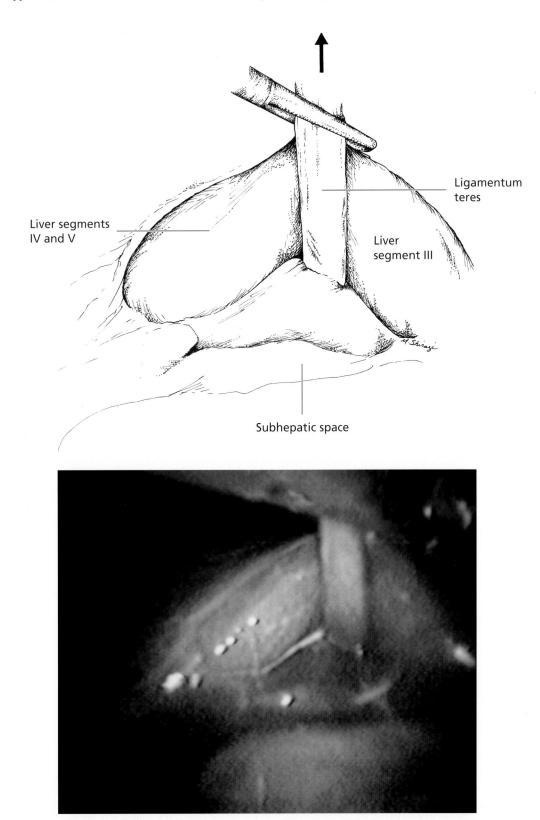

Fig. 5-4. Exposure of subhepatic space: falciform lift step 1. The falciform ligament has been grasped close to its anchor on the umbilical plate of the liver. The grasper is then angled sharply upward to produce exposure (*arrow* indicates direction of pull). Segments III and IV of the left lobe and segment V of the right lobe of the liver are seen.

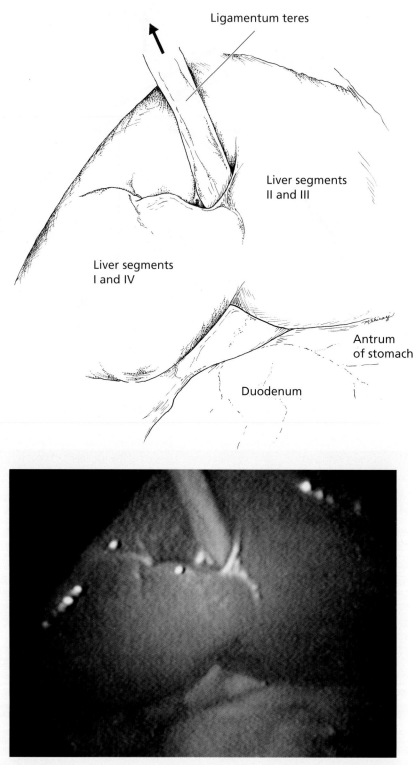

Fig. 5-5. Exposure of the subhepatic space: falciform lift step 2. Sharp upward pull on the falciform ligament is produced by upward angling of the tip of the grasper (now out of view against the anterior abdominal wall with the direction of pull indicated by the *arrow*). This maneuver opens the subhepatic space, revealing the antrum of stomach and the duodenum in the foreground. The undersurface of the left lobe of the liver, segments I through IV, is well seen. This method gives excellent exposure for procedures on the duodenum or underside of the liver. It is also a good way to expose the subhepatic space during the final inspection for hemostasis after performing laparoscopic cholecystectomy.

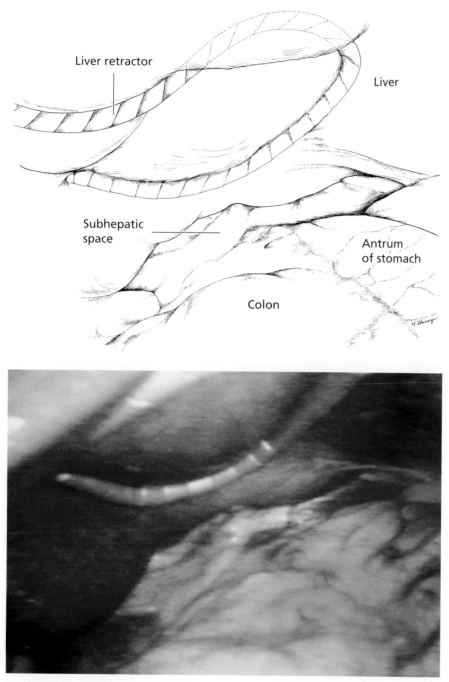

Fig. 5-6. Exposure of the subhepatic space: liver retractor. The most stable exposure of the subhepatic space is obtained by passing a retractor from a right lateral trocar site, sliding it under the left lobe of the liver, expanding it, and lifting up. Various retractors are available. The retractor shown here is a flexible metal retractor that stiffens and assumes a predetermined shape when a screw on the handle is turned. Beneath the liver, the stomach, and the lesser and greater omentum are seen. This is the method of choice for procedures on the stomach or region of the esophageal hiatus (see Chapters 3 and 4).

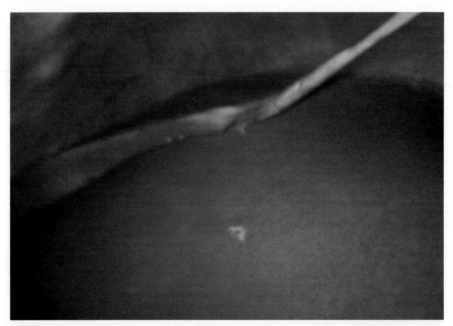

Fig. 5-7. Segments of left lobe of liver. In this view from a laparoscope placed in the left upper quadrant, segments III (anterior) and II (posterior) of the left lobe of the liver are well seen. The dividing line (indicated by *dotted line*) between segments III and II is determined by internal anatomy, and there are no external landmarks. The diaphragmatic surface of the extremely posterior segment II is best seen using an angled laparoscope placed through a left upper quadrant portal. Segments III and II comprise the portion of the liver to the left of the falciform ligament, termed the left lateral lobe in older terminology. In the distance, segment IV of the left lobe is seen beyond the falciform ligament.

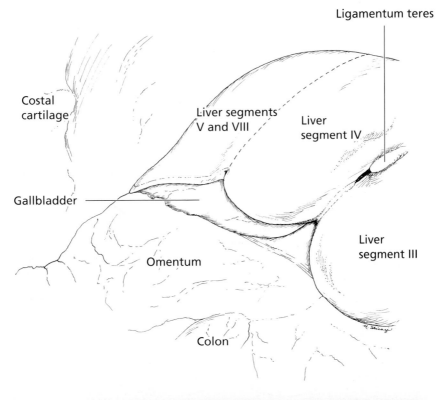

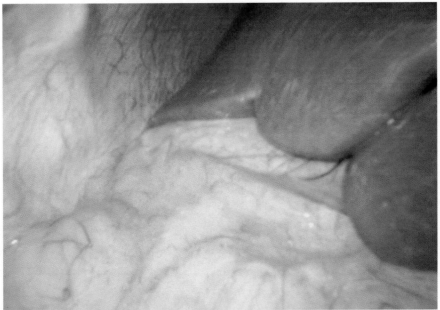

Fig. 5-8. Segments of left lobe of liver. Segments III and IV of the left lobe are seen in the foreground of this view of the diaphragmatic surface of the liver (with segments V and VIII of the right lobe in the distance). The division between left and right lobe follows an imaginary *dotted line* through the gallbladder fossa, called the interlobar fissure. In some cases, as seen here, a notch on the margin of the liver corresponds to the location of this fissure. This line forms the lateral border of segment IV. The medial border of segment IV is the intersegmental line that follows the falciform ligament. A notch is seen in the border of the liver corresponding to this line. Segment III lies medial to this line. Segment II (posterior) is not seen. The hepatic flexure and transverse colon, covered by omentum, are seen in the foreground. The gallbladder is seen extending beyond the liver's edge. A prominent costal cartilage is seen indenting the lateral abdominal wall in the background.

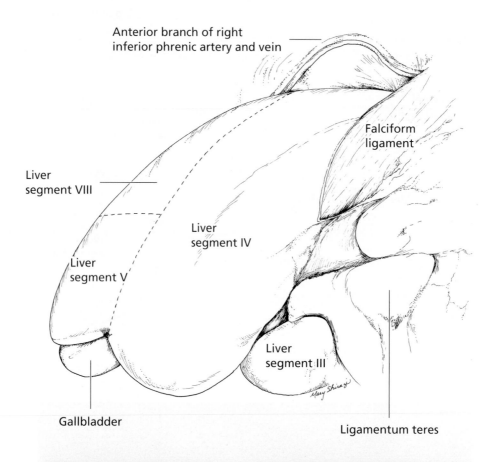

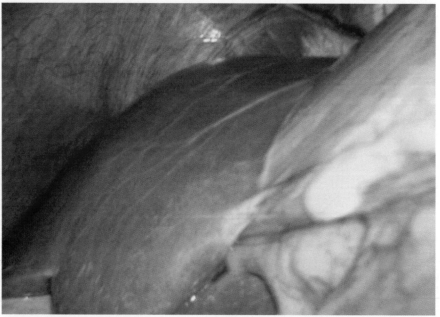

Fig. 5-9. Segments of left and right lobes of liver. The line dividing segment V (anterior) and segment VIII (posterior) of the right lobe is determined by internal anatomy. Its approximate location is indicated here *(dotted line)*. Segment IV of the left lobe is noted to occupy the territory between the interlobal line and the falciform ligament. The gallbladder is seen in the foreground to the right. To the left of the ligamentum teres and falciform ligament, the tip of the edge of segment III can be seen. The remainder of the left lobe (in the left foreground) is obscured by the falciform ligament. The anterior branch of the right inferior phrenic artery and its accompanying veins, can be seen on the undersurface of the right hemidiaphragm.

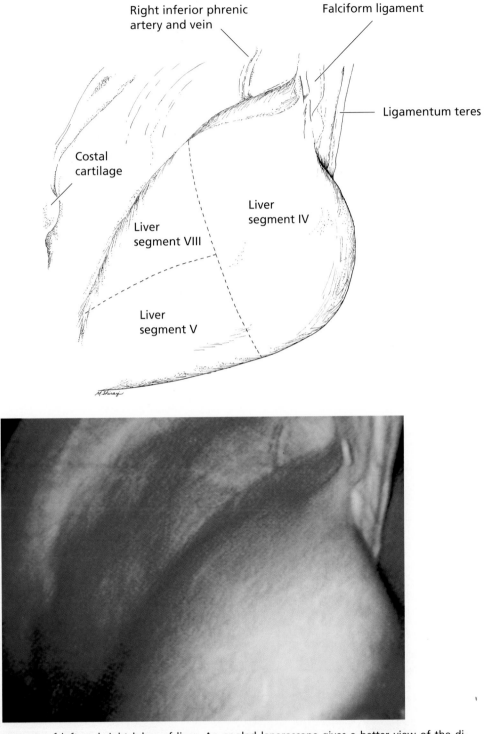

Fig. 5-10. Segments of left and right lobes of liver. An angled laparoscope gives a better view of the diaphragmatic surface of the liver. Segment IV (left lobe) extends in a bandlike fashion parallel to the falciform ligament. Segments V and VIII of the right lobe are the two segments adjacent to the interlobar fissure. In this example, the liver's edge is smooth and shows no indentation or external marking to delineate the interlobar fissure. An imaginary line through the gallbladder fossa gives its approximate location. More precise identification requires laparoscopic ultrasonography, but it is rarely needed in current clinical practice. The falciform ligament is seen extending from the liver to the anterior abdominal wall (not seen). The anterior branch of the right inferior phrenic artery and accompanying veins are seen on the inferior surface of the diaphragm.

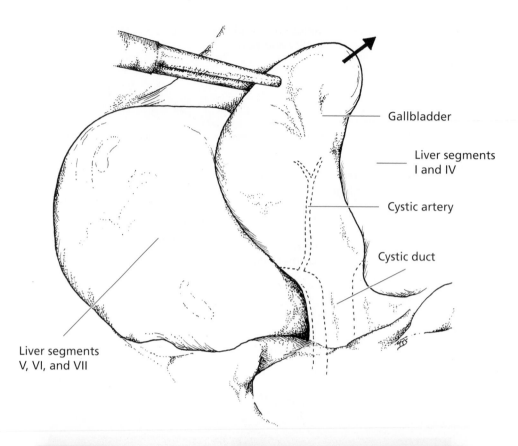

Gallbladder

Liver segments
I and IV

Cystic artery

Cystic duct

Liver segments
V, VI, and VII

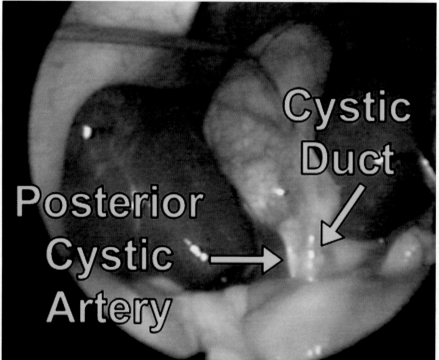

Fig. 5-11. Segments of left and right lobe. With cephalad traction on the gallbladder, segments I and IV of the left lobe and segments V, VI, and VII of the right lobe, can be seen. A posterior or low-lying cystic artery (probably originating from a right hepatic artery derived from the superior mesenteric artery) is incidentally noted. The probable course of the cystic artery and cystic duct are shown in *dotted lines* on the drawing above.

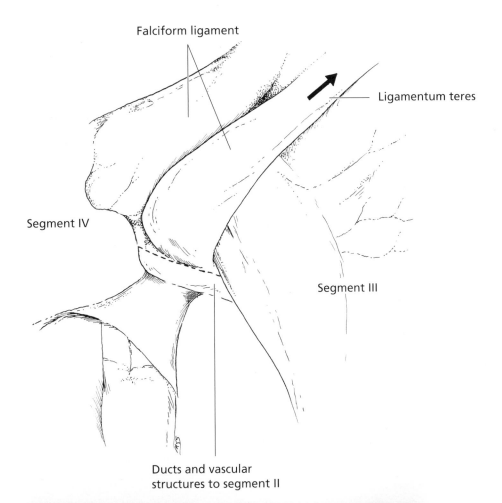

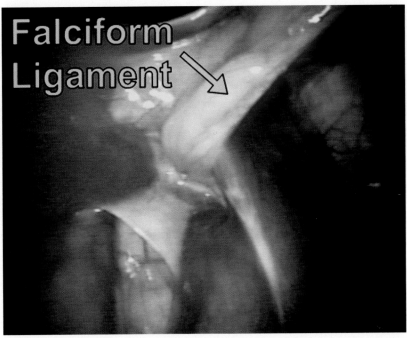

Fig. 5-12. Segments of the left lobe and crossover structures at the umbilical plate. These are bile ducts draining from and vascular structures passing to segment II of the left lobe of the liver. They are rarely seen this clearly, but they may be demonstrated by ultrasound. In difficult cases of biliary obstruction, access to the dilated biliary tree may be obtained here. Segments III and IV of the left lobe of the liver can be seen, and the falciform ligament and ligamentum teres extend to the left. The *arrow* in the drawing indicates direction of pull.

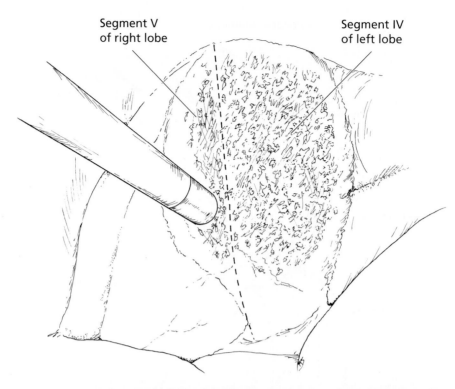

Segment V
of right lobe

Segment IV
of left lobe

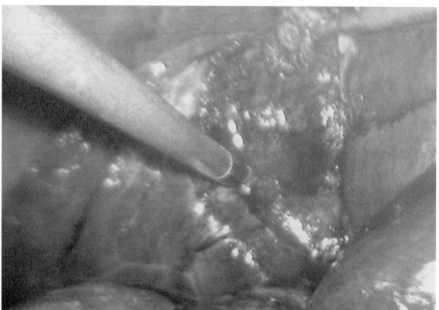

Fig. 5-13. Interlobar fissure. The interlobar fissure corresponds to an imaginary line running approximately down the gallbladder fossa (here shown as a *dotted line* in the liver bed after cholecystectomy). Segment IV of the left lobe lies medially and the right lobe lies laterally.

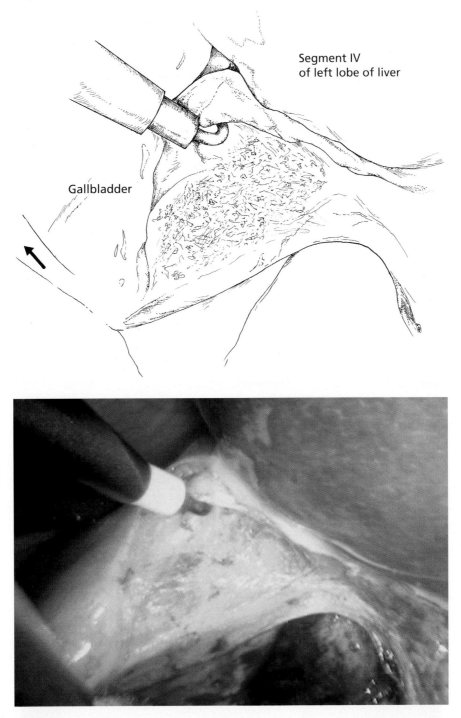

Fig. 5-14. Segment IV of the left lobe. Segment IV of the left lobe is seen as the gallbladder is removed from its bed. The *arrow* indicates direction of pull on the gallbladder.

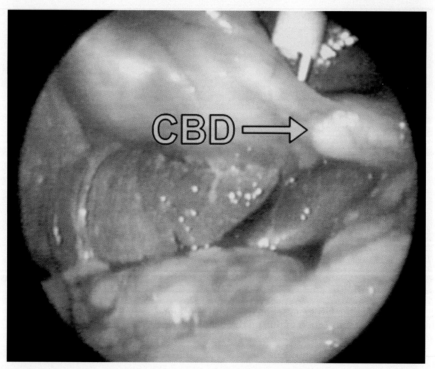

Fig. 5-15. Extrahepatic biliary tree. The subhepatic space is exposed by cephalad traction on the gallbladder. The *arrow* in the drawing indicates direction of pull. In this example, a short cystic duct appears to run directly into the common duct. As indicated by *dotted lines,* the short cystic duct terminates on the common duct. The common hepatic duct is not well seen, and the common duct might be mistaken for the cystic duct and divided. This classic error in identification of anatomy can be prevented by careful dissection and use of laparoscopic cholangiography or ultrasound to delineate anatomy. Segment I of the left lobe is seen behind the common duct. The right lobe (segment IV) lies to the right of the gallbladder.

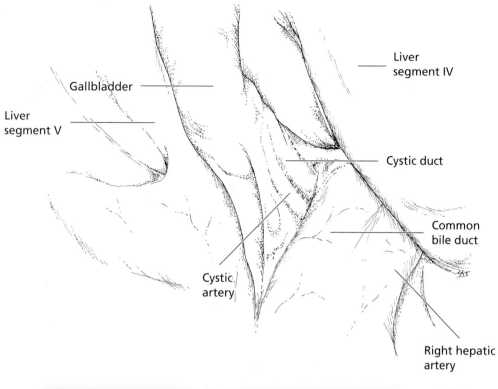

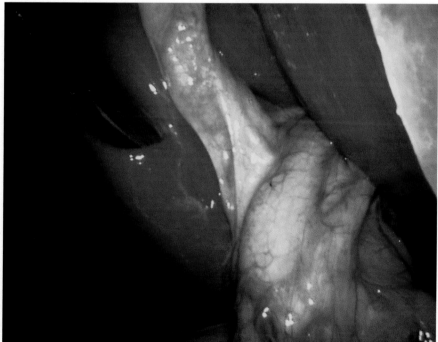

Fig. 5-16. Extrahepatic biliary tree. In the more usual situation, the common duct is seen in the foreground covered by glistening peritoneum. The right hepatic artery lies to the right and can be identified by prominent visible pulsations. A fold of peritoneum covers the cystic artery and cystic duct. The gallbladder is being elevated by cephalad traction. Calot's triangle is not well seen, because the cephalad traction on the gallbladder tends to collapse the distance between the gallbladder common hepatic duct. Segments IV and V of the liver are seen.

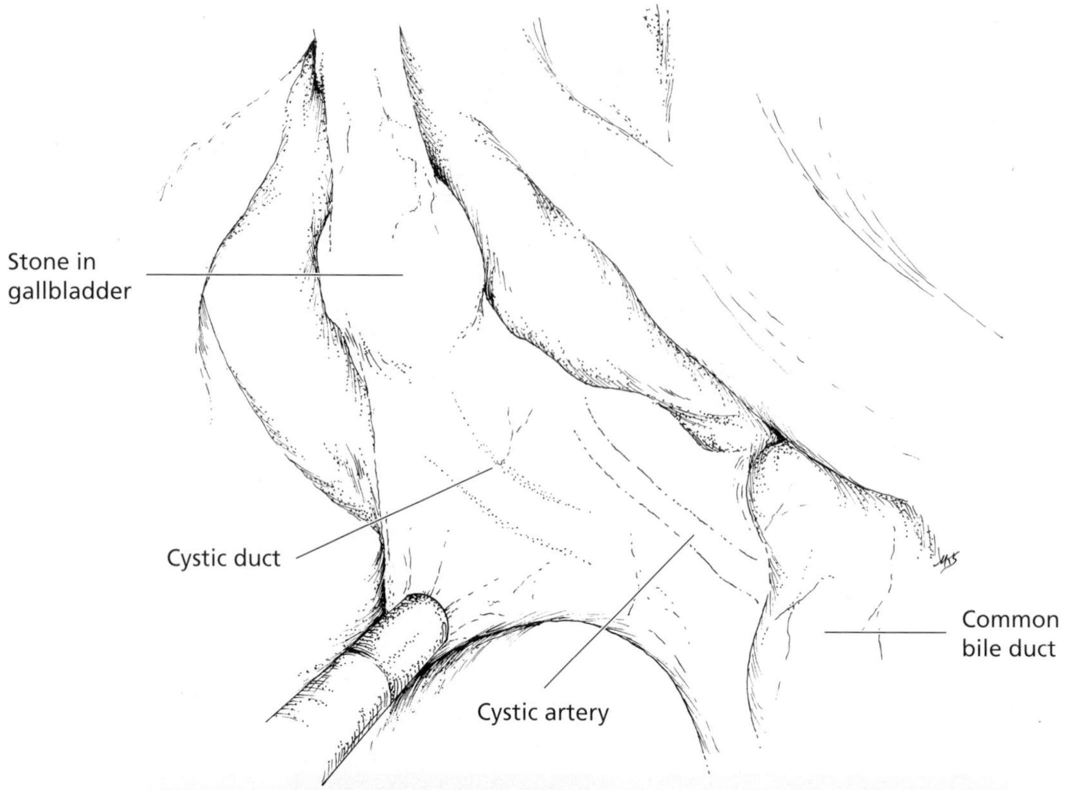

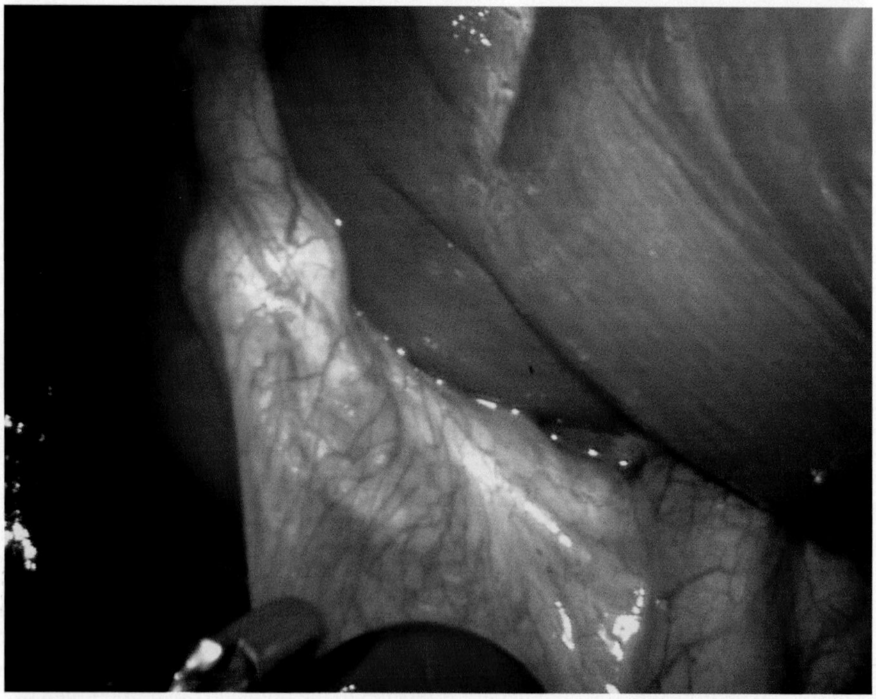

Fig. 5-17. Extrahepatic biliary tree: exposure of Calot's triangle. By placing outward traction on a grasper on Hartmann's pouch, Calot's triangle is opened, and the distance between cystic duct, cystic artery, and common duct is increased. This maneuver significantly increases the safety of dissection. Peritoneum covers all structures and must be incised to continue the dissection. A large stone is incidentally noted in Hartmann's pouch.

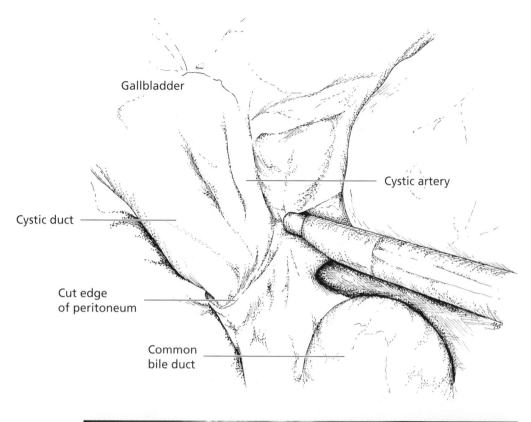

Gallbladder

Cystic artery

Cystic duct

Cut edge
of peritoneum

Common
bile duct

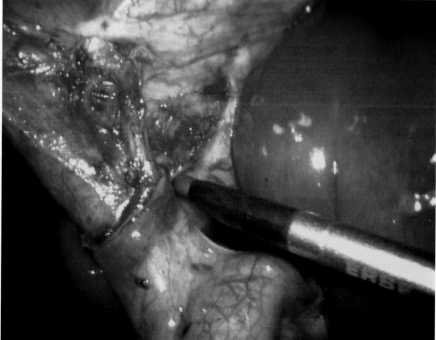

Fig. 5-18. Exposure of cystic duct and cystic artery. The peritoneum covering the cystic duct and cystic artery has been stripped away, leaving a visible cut edge at the margin of the hepatoduodenal ligament. Outward traction on Hartmann's pouch is being maintained by a grasper outside the field of view. The dissection is being performed a safe distance from the common duct, which is left covered with peritoneum and is not disturbed. In the most common anatomic situation, the cystic duct is the structure to the right and the cystic artery (usually, but not always, smaller than the cystic duct) is slightly to the left and closer to the camera. A window is being developed behind the cystic artery.

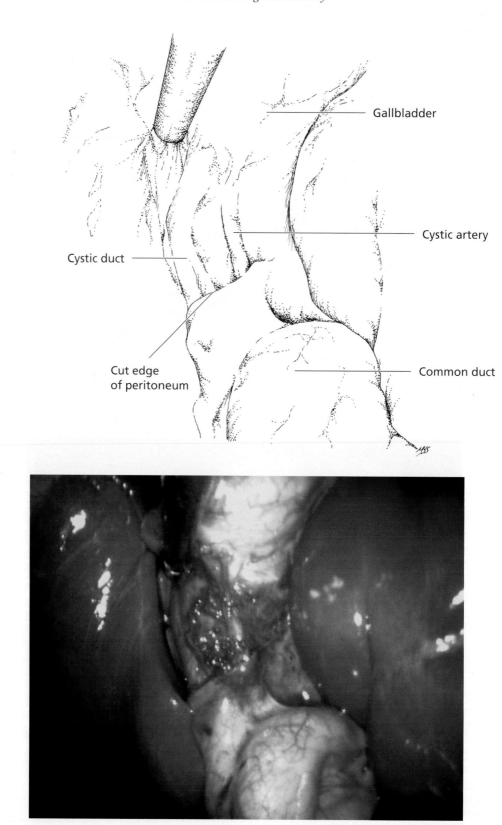

Fig. 5-19. Exposure of cystic duct and cystic artery. With the gallbladder rotated to the left, the peritoneum can be stripped from both sides of the cystic duct. Good lengths of cystic duct and cystic artery are beginning to be exposed. The common duct is seen in the foreground and is noted to be tented up from the extreme traction.

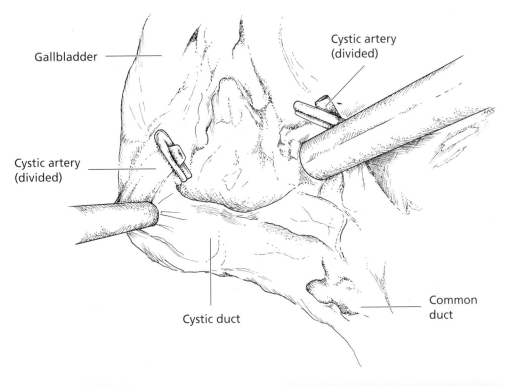

Gallbladder

Cystic artery
(divided)

Cystic artery
(divided)

Cystic duct

Common
duct

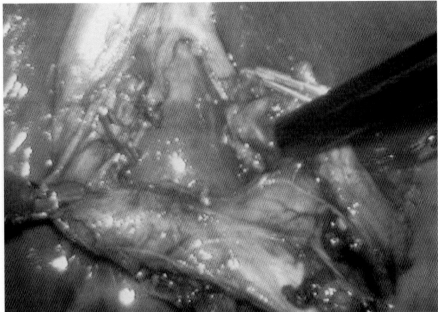

Fig. 5-20. Exposure of cystic duct and cystic artery in a patient with an extremely short, fat cystic duct. The cystic artery has been divided to enhance exposure. A large window is being created behind the gallbladder to facilitate identification of cystic duct, which can be confirmed by the way in which Hartmann's pouch funnels down to it. The cystic duct in this example is large. The common duct is tented upward. It is impossible to tell for certain that the large cystic duct is not in fact the common duct. Only careful and precise identification of all structures before clipping and division provides safety. Cholangiography (or laparoscopic ultrasound) is crucial for accurate identification of anatomy in these difficult situations.

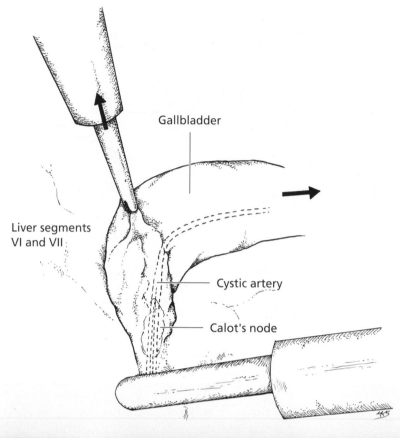

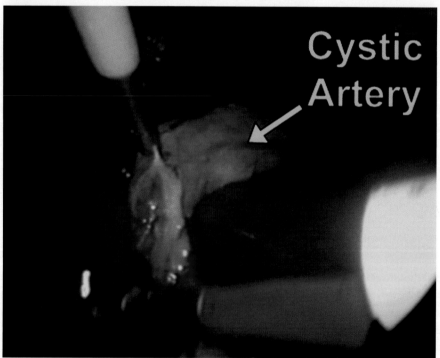

Fig. 5-21. Identification of cystic artery. A stripe under the peritoneum of the gallbladder identifies the cystic artery and may be traced down to Calot's triangle. A lymph node (Calot's node) commonly overlies the cystic artery (indicated by *dotted lines*). Both these clues are seen here. The *arrows* in the drawing indicate direction of pull.

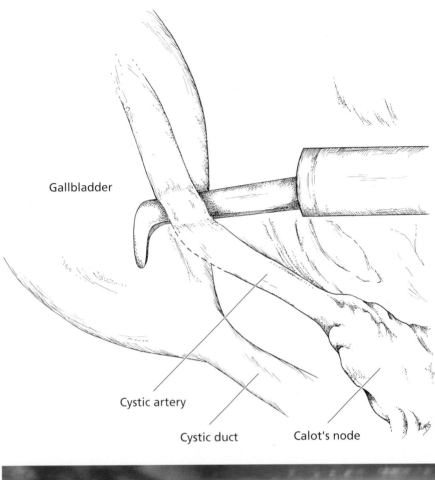

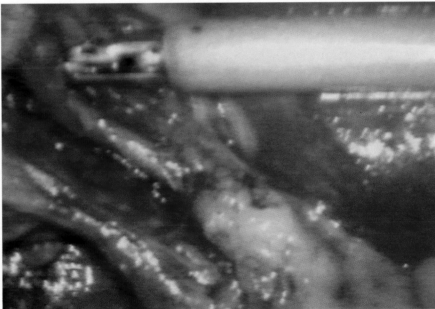

Fig. 5-22. Cystic artery. The cystic artery may be identified with confidence when it is noted to have pulsations and to terminate by running on the surface of the gallbladder. Here the cystic artery is being elevated and separated from the cystic duct. The cystic artery terminates on the gallbladder; in contrast, the cystic duct is the termination of the funnel-shaped Hartmann's pouch. Both structures will be clipped and divided close to their termination on the gallbladder.

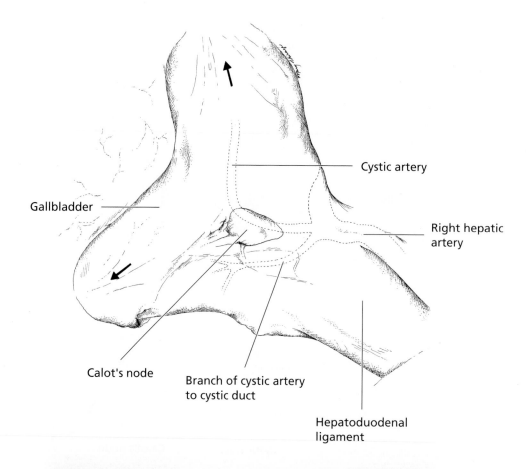

Cystic artery

Gallbladder

Right hepatic artery

Calot's node

Branch of cystic artery to cystic duct

Hepatoduodenal ligament

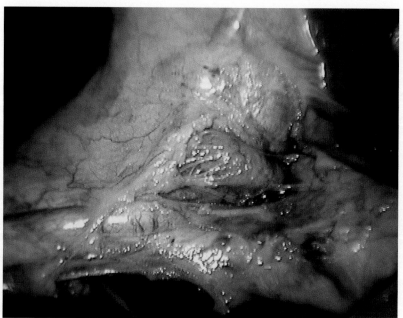

Fig. 5-23. Lymph node of Calot and branches of the cystic artery. In this example, upward traction on the gall-bladder and outward traction on Hartmann's pouch (indicated by *arrows*) have opened Calot's triangle by splaying out the gallbladder in a triangular fashion. The lymph node of Calot is shown, with the right hepatic artery and cystic artery (indicated by *dotted lines*) still covered by peritoneum. The cystic artery is seen to terminate in a stripe on the gallbladder in the background. A small branch of the cystic artery commonly supplies the cystic duct in the vicinity of Calot's triangle. Pesky bleeding may occur if this tiny branch is not identified and divided with hemostatic control. The bleeding generally ceases when the cystic artery is clipped, but it may make precise identification of crucial structures difficult. The hepatic artery runs unusually close to the gall-bladder, as indicated by *dotted lines*. It was identifiable by prominent pulsations. The hepatoduodenal ligament is seen in the foreground.

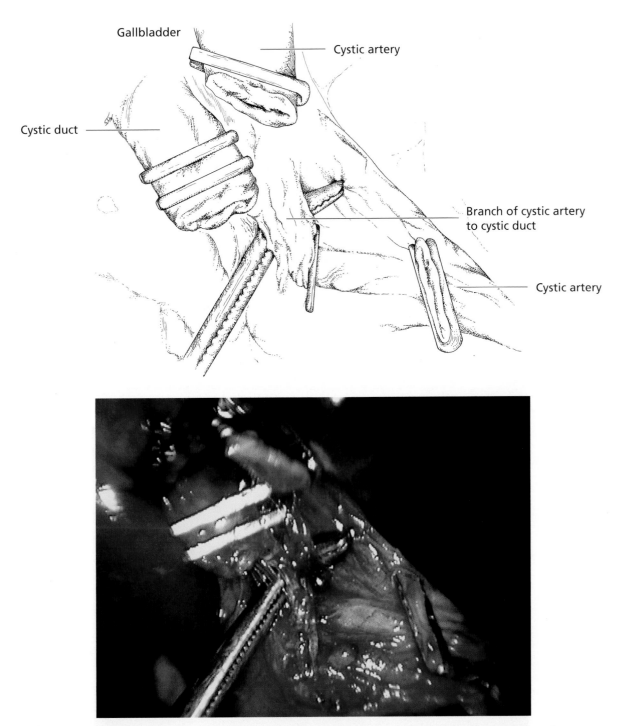

Fig. 5-24. Branch of the cystic artery to the cystic duct. In this extreme close-up view from a different dissection, the cystic artery and cystic duct have been divided. A small branch of the cystic artery is shown to run to the cystic duct. This branch must be secured to avoid bleeding.

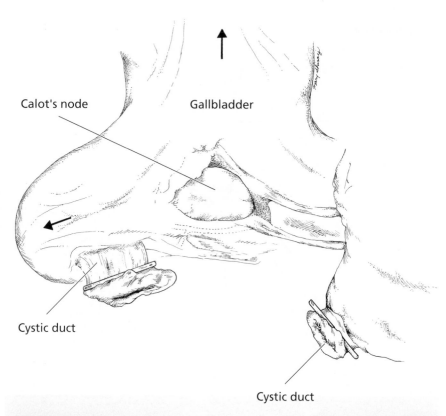

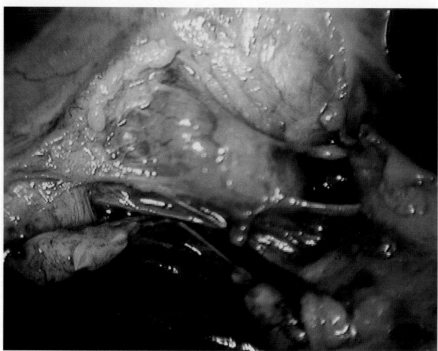

Fig. 5-25. Lymph node of Calot. The cystic duct has been divided. The *arrows* indicate direction of pull. Calot's node overlies the cystic artery, which is seen to send small branches to the node and the cystic duct. These can generally be cauterized. Small lymphatics also run in this area, but it is prudent to assume that any tubular structure is either a blood vessel or a bile duct.

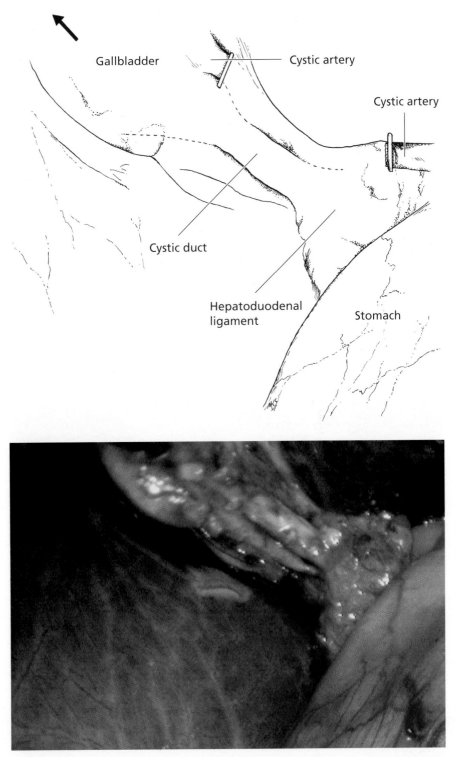

Fig. 5-26. Cystic artery and cystic duct. The *arrow* indicates direction of pull. The cystic artery (divided) runs onto the gallbladder. The cystic duct represents the termination of the funnel-shaped Hartmann's pouch *(dotted lines)*. Generally, the cystic duct is divided first. Occasionally (as shown here), it is simpler to divide the cystic artery before the cystic duct. The duodenum and stomach are seen in the foreground. The common duct is covered with peritoneum and is not well seen, but it should be assumed to be close, in the foreground (indicated as hepatoduodenal ligament).

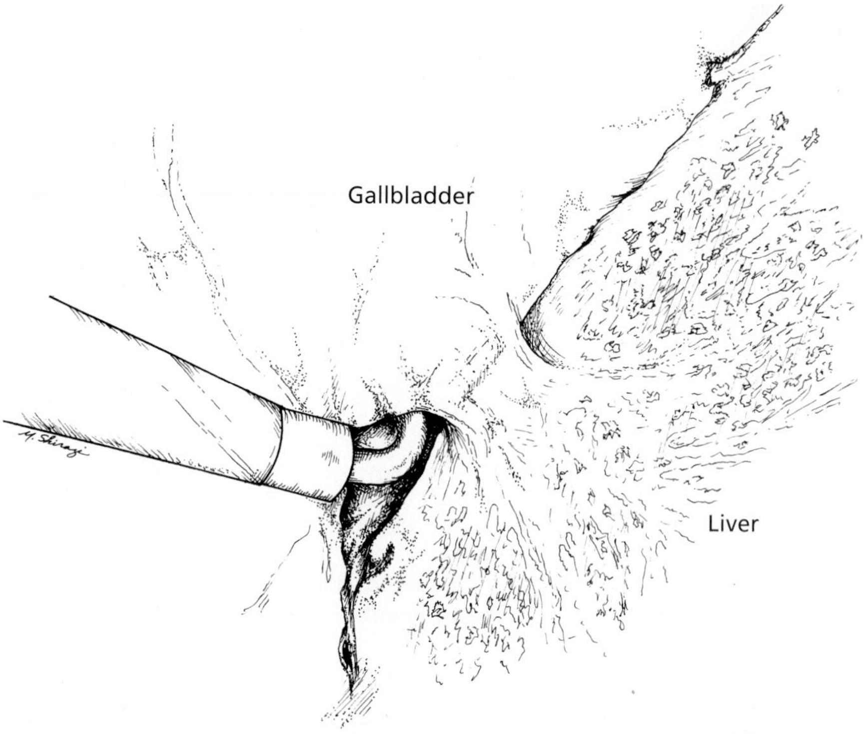

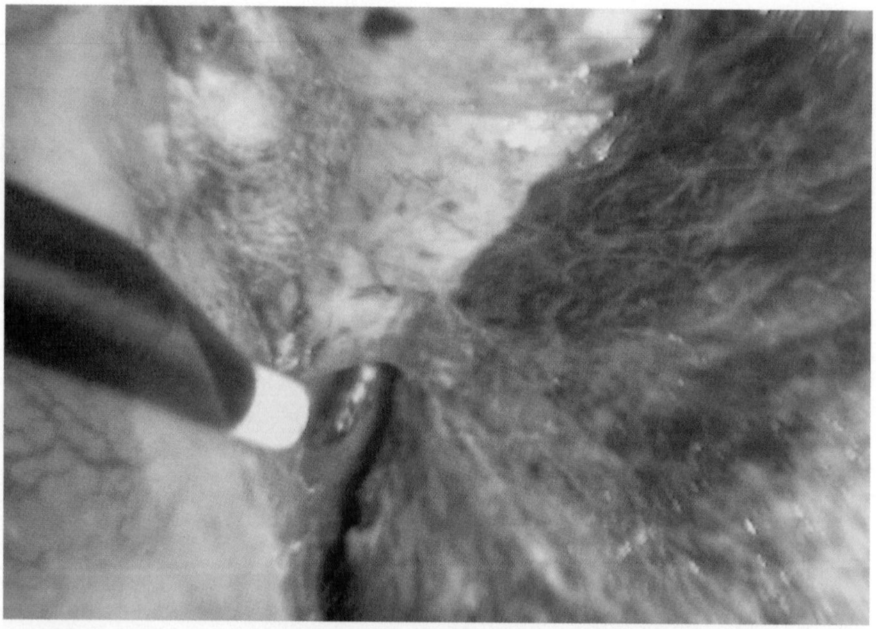

Fig. 5-27. Glisson's capsule in gallbladder fossa. As the gallbladder is removed, Glisson's capsule is left intact to avoid injuring the liver and producing bleeding. No tubular structures should be encountered during this dissection.

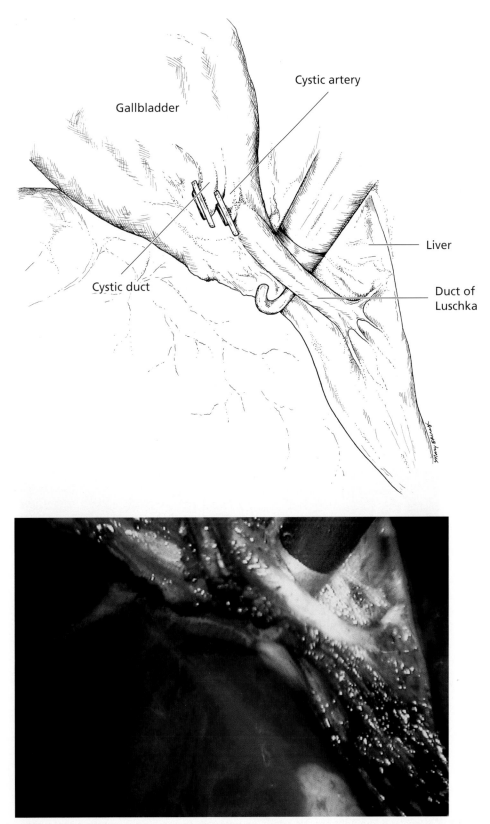

Fig. 5-28. Cholecystohepatic duct. A rare cholecystohepatic duct (sometimes termed a duct of Luschka) is seen running from the liver bed into the gallbladder. When such a tubular structure is encountered, cholangiography is advisable to avoid injury to a segmental liver duct or other anomaly. The cystic duct and cystic artery have been clipped.

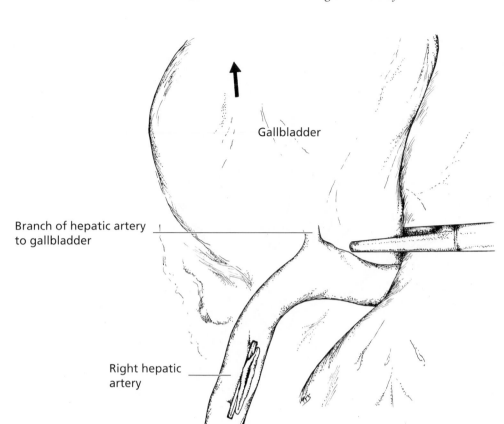

Gallbladder

Branch of hepatic artery to gallbladder

Right hepatic artery

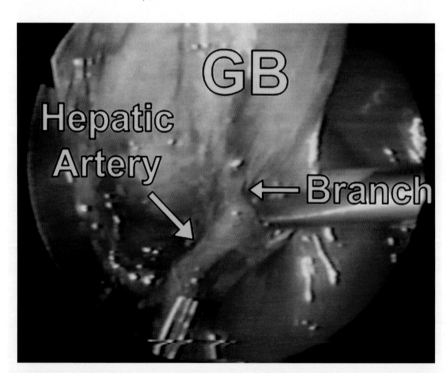

Fig. 5-29. Caterpillar hump right hepatic artery. An unusually tortuous right hepatic artery is seen closely applied to the gallbladder. Multiple small twigs, rather than a discrete cystic artery, nourish the gallbladder. This right hepatic artery is derived from the superior mesenteric artery, rather than from the celiac axis. The *arrow* in the drawing indicates direction of pull on the gallbladder.

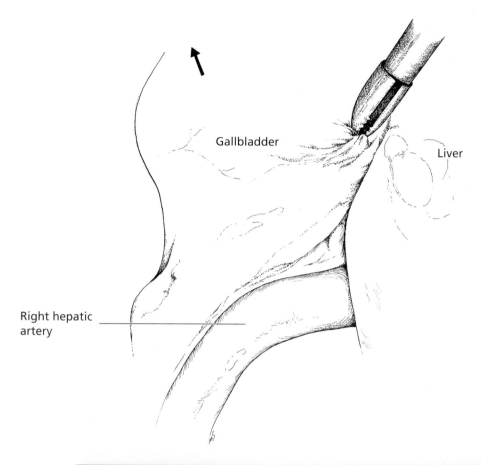

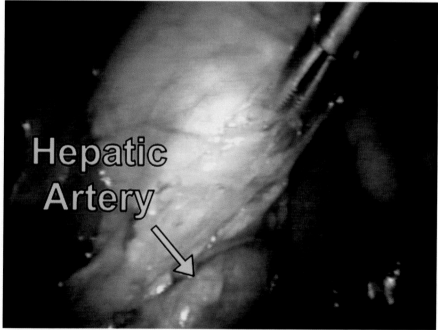

Fig. 5-30. Right hepatic artery arising from superior mesenteric artery. In this example, a right hepatic artery arising from the superior mesenteric artery or one of its branches crosses anterior to the gallbladder. Prominent pulsations make this anomaly easy to recognize. The artery should be avoided and preserved. The *arrow* in the drawing indicates direction of pull on the gallbladder.

6

SPLEEN AND PANCREAS

INITIAL LAPAROSCOPIC VIEW AND PRINCIPLES OF EXPOSURE

The initial view of the left upper quadrant reveals stomach, omentum, segments II and III of the liver, diaphragm, and perhaps the tip of the spleen (Figs. 6-1 and 6-2). The spleen is seen better if the left side of the patient is tilted upward and the table is placed in the reverse Trendelenburg position. Some laparoscopic surgeons place the patient in the right lateral position to maximize the effect of gravity.

An angled laparoscope facilitates visualization of the extreme left upper quadrant, and it may be necessary to move the viewing port closer to the left upper quadrant to minimize distance. For both spleen and pancreas, special maneuvers facilitate exposure and are discussed in the two sections that follow.

ANATOMY AND SPECIFIC SURGICAL PROCEDURES

Spleen

The normal adult spleen weighs between 125 and 175 g and measures just 8 by 15 cm. This soft, pulpy organ tends to assume the shape of the space it occupies. Thus, a convex surface abuts the diaphragm, and a concave surface, indented by stomach, colon, and kidney, faces medially.

Access to the spleen is facilitated by reverse Trendelenburg positioning, with the left side of the table tilted upward. In this position, gentle medial traction on the stomach frequently brings the anterior edge of the spleen into view. It may be necessary to elevate segments II and III of the liver for adequate visualization of the anterior margin of the spleen (see Figs. 6-1 and 6-2; Figs. 6-3 and 6-4).

Medial traction on the stomach with atraumatic grasping forceps elevates the spleen, by applying traction to the presplenic fold (if present) and gastrosplenic ligaments (see Figs. 6-3 and 6-4; Fig. 6-5). Such traction must be applied with care, because the complex and variable peritoneal folds (termed ligaments) that anchor the spleen in the left upper quadrant limit its mobility. Excess traction may cause capsular avulsion injuries at the point at which the ligament attaches to the spleen, thereby causing hemorrhage. Even minor bleeding can obscure visualization and be difficult to control during laparoscopic surgery.

The ligaments that attach the spleen may be conveniently divided into the relatively avascular attachments of the spleen to adjacent structures (splenocolic and splenophrenic ligaments) and the two major vascular pedicles (gastrosplenic, containing the short gastric vessels, and splenorenal, containing the splenic artery and vein). These are described in the order in which they are generally divided during the performance of laparoscopic splenectomy. Massive splenomegaly or portal hypertension may cause major collateral vessels in the splenophrenic and splenocolic ligaments to form; laparoscopic splenectomy is rarely performed in these situations.

The splenocolic ligament is normally divided first. This peritoneal attachment anchors the splenic flexure of the colon to the inferior pole of the spleen. It is normally avascular. The left gastroepiploic vessels may pass close to the spleen and must be avoided or controlled. The splenic flexure of the colon can be gently pushed caudad after division of this ligament. Dissection then generally progresses through sequential division of the gastrosplenic ligaments and splenic hilar vessels. The splenophrenic ligament and the peritoneal reflection to the posterior abdominal wall are farthest from the laparoscope and hence are usually divided last, in stark contrast to open splenectomy.

The gastrosplenic ligament is actually a complex and variable set of peritoneal reflections that tether the medial aspect of the spleen to the stomach and contain the short gastric vessels. These must be carefully divided to perform laparoscopic splenectomy, to mobilize the fundus of the stomach fully in hiatal hernia repair (when division of the short gastric vessels is performed), or to perform laparoscopic gastrectomy. In a significant number of cases, the gastrosplenic fold is covered by another fold, the presplenic fold, which contains relatively few vessels, with the exception of some small tributaries from the lower pole of the spleen (see Fig. 4-5; Fig. 6-6). Division of this presplenic fold proceeds easily because of the paucity of vessels. Underneath this fold lies a second, more vascular ligament, the true gastrosplenic ligament, containing the short gastric vessels (see Figs. 3-24 and 4-6 through 4-11).

There are 4 to 10 short gastric vessels—on the average 5 or 6. Division begins at a convenient point, perhaps near the middle of the group (Fig. 3-24). The lower short gastric vessels are generally longer than the upper short gastric vessels and commonly originate from the left gastroepiploic artery or directly from the interior of the spleen. The highest short gastric vessels are also the shortest, and therefore the distance between stomach and spleen is the least (giving the least distance for secure hemostasis before division). These upper short gastric arteries commonly arise from the splenic artery or a branch or from a superior polar artery. In approximately 50% of individuals, a fold of peritoneum extends from the greater curvature of the stomach to the apex of the spleen (see Fig. 4-11) and may reflect up to the posterior body wall and inferior surface of the diaphragm, blending with the splenophrenic ligament superiorly.

Complete division of the gastrosplenic ligament allows the stomach to be rotated and displaced medially, thus exposing the splenic hilum and tail of the pancreas in the splenorenal ligament. The shape of the spleen may provide a clue to the relative length of the splenic artery before branching, and the notches on the margin of the spleen (when present) may correspond to internal segments. Two general types of splenic shape have been described: a compact spleen with even borders (see Figs. 6-2 and 6-5) and an irregular form with lobulations and notched borders (see Figs. 6-3 and 6-4). The compact spleen (noted in 30% of anatomically normal individuals) corresponds to a relatively easy anatomic situation in which the hilum is narrow and the splenic artery is long and branching close to the hilum, with tributaries entering the spleen over less than one-third of the hilar area. This narrow hilar configuration renders laparoscopic splenectomy relatively easy.

In contrast, the irregular, notched, lobulated spleen (in 70% of anatomically normal individuals) predicts a shorter splenic artery with early branching (see Figs. 6-3 and 6-4). These numerous branches arise at some distance from the hilum and enter the spleen over a broad area (often exceeding three-fourths of the hilar surface and sometimes outside the hilum). Polar arteries are common. This type of configuration requires careful dissection and multiple vessels must be secured.

The usual arrangement of splenic artery and vein places the splenic artery anterior to the vein as these vessels enter the hilum, but variations, including the reverse arrangement, are possible (Figs. 6-7 to 6-12). The splenic artery, generally a branch of the celiac, is tortuous and highly variable in length, course, and number of branches. Small tributaries from the splenic artery go directly to the substance of the pancreas in the region of the pancreatic tail.

In 75% of cases, the splenic artery bifurcates into two major branches. Further branching is common and unpredictable. A superior polar artery, usually derived from the splenic artery, is generally present. Veins generally accompany the arteries. The internal anatomy is segmental, making partial splenectomy possible, and may be predicted by the pattern of hilar branches and the notches or lobulations on the surface. The tail of the pancreas enters the hilum of the spleen for a variable distance and must be assumed to be within any fat contained in the hilar region. In a significant number of individuals, the tail of the pancreas directly abuts splenic tissue in the hilum (see Figs. 6-17 and 6-18). As with open surgery, safety in laparoscopic dissection mandates dissection of hilar vessels close to the spleen.

The veins parallel the arteries in general. The splenic vein is a large vein formed by the confluence of veins draining the spleen. The left gastroepiploic vein commonly drains into an inferior terminal branch of the splenic vein. As it travels with the splenic artery, the splenic vein occasionally crosses over or under the artery. Small venous tributaries drain the body and tail of the pancreas, emptying directly into the splenic vein and tethering the splenic vein to the pancreas. After passing inferior and posterior to the pancreas and receiving the inferior mesenteric vein, the splenic vein combines with the superior mesenteric vein to form the portal vein. Veins also accompany the short gastric arteries and drain directly into the substance of the spleen.

Lymphatic drainage of the spleen is to nodes in the splenic hilum and thence to suprapancreatic and infrapancreatic nodes. These nodes may be sampled during staging procedures.

Accessory spleens occur in approximately 10% of anatomically normal individuals and in up to 30% of patients undergoing splenectomy for hematologic disorders. Of these accessory spleens, 60% are solitary; 20% of patients have two, and the remainder have more than two accessory spleens. The most common location (more than 50%) is the hilum, where the accessory spleen is likely to be confused with a splenic hilar lymph node. Other common locations include the gastrosplenic folds, other surrounding peritoneal ligaments, the greater omentum, the mesentery, or in proximity to the gonads. Most are around 1 cm in diameter, and the common hilar accessory spleens derive their blood supply from the caudal pancreatic artery. Any small, oval, or round structure noted in the vicinity of the spleen should be removed to prevent recurrence of hematologic symptoms.

Laparoscopic Splenectomy

Two different positions have been used for laparoscopic splenectomy. The first is an anterior approach with the patient supine, legs spread, and the surgeon standing between the patient's legs. The advantages of this approach are its familiarity, easy access to other quadrants of the abdomen, rapid approach to hilar structures, and ease of conversion to open laparotomy should this be required. The second approach has been termed the "hanging spleen" method. The patient is placed in the right lateral decubitus position, and the lateral attachments of the spleen are left intact. The gastrosplenic fold is divided, the hilar vessels ligated, and any polar vessels are secured. When the spleen is completely detached from its blood supply, the remaining attachments to the diaphragm and posterior abdominal wall are severed.

Pancreas

Most laparoscopic pancreatic surgery to date has been performed on the tail or body of the pancreas. A limited number of Whipple resections have been described. This chapter therefore concentrates on the laparoscopic anatomy of the body and tail. Lying in the retroperitoneum, the pancreas is hidden from view until the lesser sac is entered. The head of the pancreas nestles in the C-loop of the duodenum, with a hooklike uncinate process extending behind the superior mesenteric artery and vein. Extending to the left, the neck of the pancreas is that portion lying anterior to the superior mesenteric artery and vein. The body extends farther to the left, terminating in the tail (which commonly extends into the hilum of the spleen, as previously noted). The major pancreatic duct, the duct of Wirsung, runs the length of the pancreas and is sizable even in the tail of the pancreas.

Judging the extent of resection at the time of distal pancreatectomy is at best an empiric exercise. As a general rule, resection of the distal pancreas to a point just to the left of the portal vein corresponds to a 50% to 60% resection. Laparoscopic resection is generally performed for localized lesions that must be accurately visualized at time of resection. Meticulous hemostasis and judicious use of laparoscopic ultrasound help the laparoscopic surgeon to identify target lesions and to verify the adequacy of resection by confirming anatomic landmarks.

The pancreas derives its blood supply from both the celiac and the superior mesenteric arteries. The head of the pancreas and C-loop of duodenum are supplied by the anterior and posterior pancreaticoduodenal arcades. The blood supply of the body and tail comes primarily from the splenic artery, either directly or through a tributary, the dorsal pancreatic artery. This dorsal pancreatic artery is the first major branch of the splenic artery. Frequently, a transverse pancreatic artery parallels the splenic artery, running on the back side of the pancreas and terminating in the hilum of the spleen. Thus, several sizable vessels may run behind the tail of the pancreas and deep to it. The arterial pattern is unpredictable, and anomalies are common. The laparoscopic surgeon must proceed slowly and be aware that multiple small vessels may be found in the region between spleen and pancreas.

Venous drainage in general parallels arterial supply. Paired anterior and posterior pancreaticoduodenal venous arcades drain the head of the pancreas and the C-loop of the duodenum. The anterosuperior arcades drain into the right gastroepiploic vein; the posterosuperior arcades into the portal vein. Both anterior and posterior inferior arcades drain into the superior mesenteric vein. The splenic vein and transverse or inferior pancreatic veins (when present) form large venous channels that run behind the tail of the pancreas and receive multiple small veins directly from the pancreas. The transverse or inferior pancreatic veins either join the splenic vein in the region of the inferior mesenteric vein or drain into the inferior mesenteric vein directly.

A rich network of pancreatic lymphatics drains into five major node groups. The distal tail of the pancreas, together with the spleen, drains into splenic hilar nodes and into small nodes both inferior and superior to the tail. The body drains into superior and inferior pancreaticoduodenal nodes and into nodes just above or below the neck in the vicinity of portal or superior mesenteric vein. From there, deep lymph node groups drain into nodes to the left of the aorta and around the celiac axis. The head of the pancreas drains into anterior and posterior pancreaticoduodenal nodes.

Laparoscopic Pancreatic Surgery

Access to the pancreas for resection is obtained by entering the lesser sac, generally through an avascular region of the gastrocolic omentum (Figs. 6-13 to 6-17). A 45-degree laparoscope facilitates visualization of the pancreas by enabling the surgeon to look down at the retroperitoneum. The avascular plane along the inferior aspect of the pancreas is entered, and the pancreas is elevated (Figs. 6-18 to 6-20). The splenic artery and vein are identified, secured, and divided. Seventy-five percent of individuals have a transverse pancreatic artery that, to a variable extent, supplies the tail of the pancreas with or without twigs from the splenic artery. The transverse pancreatic and splenic arteries anastomose through the dorsal pancreatic artery. The transverse pancreatic artery may be visible or concealed within the substance of the pancreas. Transection of the pancreas with an endoscopic stapling device generally provides sufficient hemostasis to control this vessel.

Laparoscopic enucleation of islet cell tumors is performed by exposing the tumor in the lesser sac and confirming its location with endoscopic ultrasound, if necessary. Gentle dissection around the tumor is aided by the magnification provided by laparoscopy.

BIBLIOGRAPHY

Anatomic References

1. Appel MF, Bart JB. The surgical and hematologic significance of accessory spleens. *Surg Gynecol Obstet* 1976;143:191–192.
2. Baranofsky ID, Walton W, Noble JF. Occult injury to the pancreas following splenectomy. *Surgery* 1951;29:852–856.

3. Dawson DL, Molina ME, Scott-Conner CEH. Venous segmentation of the human spleen: a corrosion cast study. *Am Surg* 1986;52:253–256.

4. Garcia-Porrero JA, Lemes A. Arterial segmentation and subsegmentation in the human spleen. *Acta Anat* 1988;131:276–281.

5. Gerber AB, Lev M, Goldberg SL. The surgical anatomy of the splenic vein. *Am J Surg* 1951;82:339–341.

6. Henry AK. The removal of large spleens. *Br J Surg* 1940;107:464–469.

7. Liu DL, Xia S, Zu W, Ye Q, Gao Y, Qian J. Anatomy of vasculature of 850 spleen specimens and its application in partial splenectomy. *Surgery* 1996;119:27–33.

8. Michels NA. The variational anatomy of the spleen and the splenic artery. *Am J Anat* 1942;70:21–72.

9. Morgenstern L. The avoidable complications of splenectomy. *Surg Gynecol Obstet* 1977;145:525–528.

10. Poulin EC, Thibault C. The anatomical basis for laparoscopic splenectomy. *Can J Surg* 1993;36:484–488.

11. Skandalakis LJ, Rowe JS Jr, Gray SW, Skandalakis JE. Surgical embryology and anatomy of the pancreas. *Surg Clin North Am* 1993;73:661–697.

12. Skandalakis PN, Colborn GL, Skandalakis LJ, Richardson DD, Mitchell WE Jr, Skandalakis JE. The surgical anatomy of the spleen. *Surg Clin North Am* 1993;73:747–768.

13. Van Damme J-PJ. Behavioral anatomy of the abdominal arteries. *Surg Clin North Am* 1993;73:699–725.

14. Waizer A, Baniet J, Zin Y, Dintsman M. Clinical implications of anatomic variations of the splenic artery. *Surg Gynecol Obstet* 1989;168:57–58.

Surgical References

1. Arregui M, Barteau J, Davis CJ. Laparoscopic splenectomy: techniques and indications. *Int Surg* 1994;79:335–341.

2. Gadiere GB, Verroken R, Himpens J, et al. Operative strategy in laparoscopic splenectomy. *J Am Coll Surg* 1994;179:668–672.

3. Park A, Gagner M, Pomp A. The lateral approach to laparoscopic splenectomy. *Am J Surg* 1997;173:126–130.

4. Rege RV, Merriam LT, Loehl RJ. Laparoscopic splenectomy. *Surg Clin North Am* 1996;76:459–468.

5. Salky BA, Edye M. Laparoscopic pancreatectomy. *Surg Clin North Am* 1996;76:539–545.

6. Watson DJ, Coventry BJ, Chin T, Gill PG, Malycha P. Laparoscopic versus open splenectomy for immune thrombocytopenic purpura. *Surgery* 1997;121:18–22.

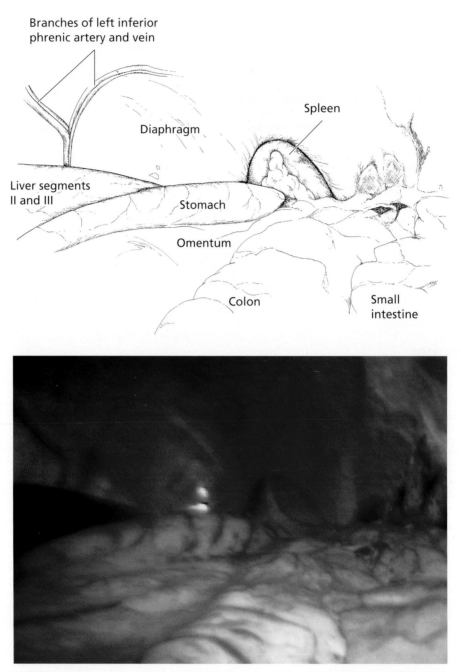

Fig. 6-1. Initial view of the spleen. This view of the left upper quadrant of a supine patient, seen from an umbilically placed laparoscope, demonstrates the omentum, colon, stomach, segments II and III of the liver, and the spleen. Fat is noted to creep up into the hilum of the spleen. Branches of the left inferior phrenic artery and vein are noted on the diaphragm. Visualization of the spleen is enhanced by placing the patient in the reverse Trendelenburg position and tilting the left side upward. Gentle medial traction on the stomach and omentum are also helpful.

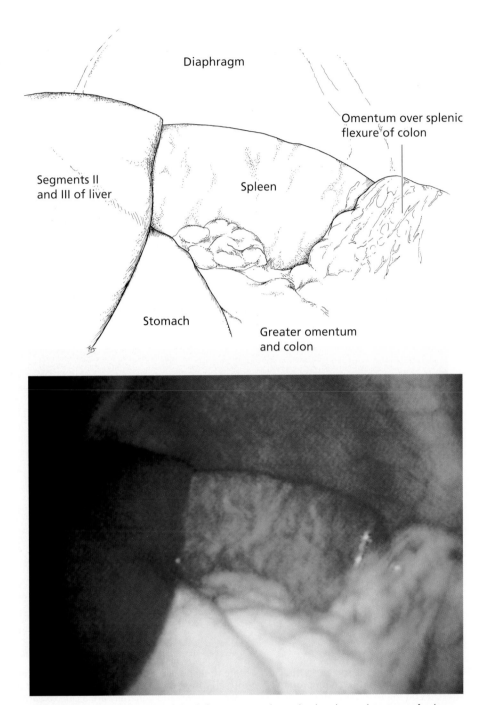

Fig. 6-2. Spleen and liver. In this view of the left upper quadrant, both color and texture of spleen are noted to be different from those of the liver. Fat is noted in the splenic hilum, as in Fig. 6-1, and the splenic flexure of the colon and omentum obscure visualization of the inferior pole of the spleen.

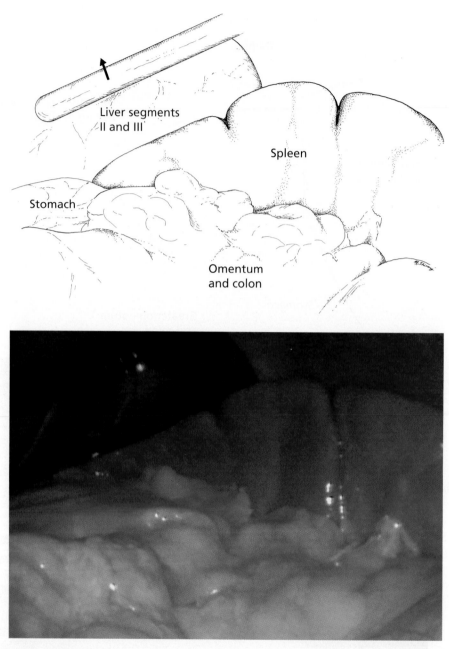

Fig. 6-3. Superior pole of the spleen. In this view, segments II and III of the liver have been reflected cephalad (*arrow* indicates direction of force on probe to produce elevation of liver) to expose the superior pole of the spleen. Notches on the anterior margin of the spleen are common and generally are a clue to early branching of the splenic artery and vein. Stomach, colon, and omentum are seen in the foreground.

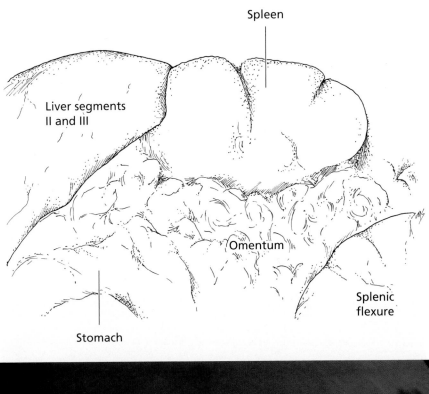

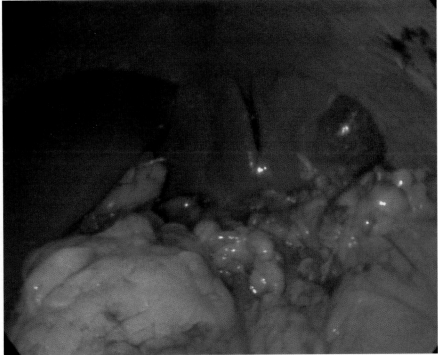

Fig. 6-4. Sharply notched splenic border. This degree of notching correlates with early branching of the splenic artery and vein and hints at the internal segmental vascular anatomy. Segments II and III of the liver, stomach, and splenic flexure of colon are seen in the foreground.

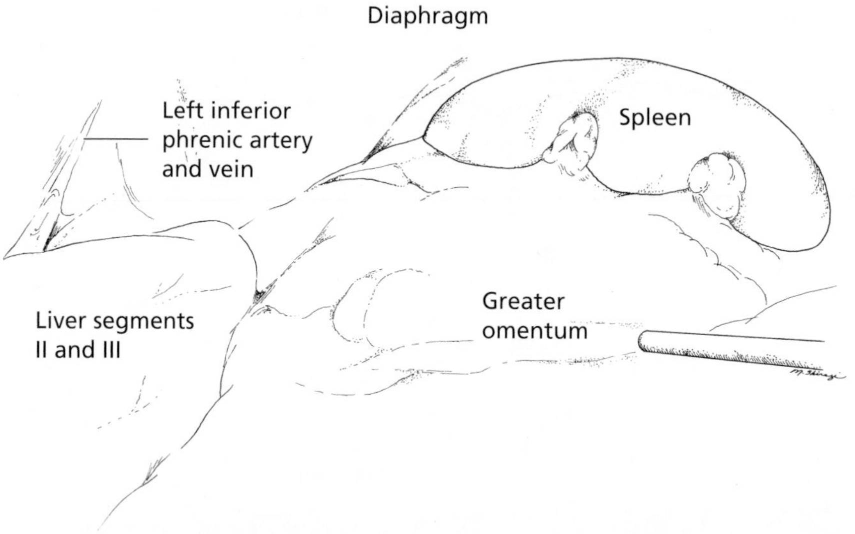

Diaphragm

Left inferior
phrenic artery
and vein

Spleen

Liver segments
II and III

Greater
omentum

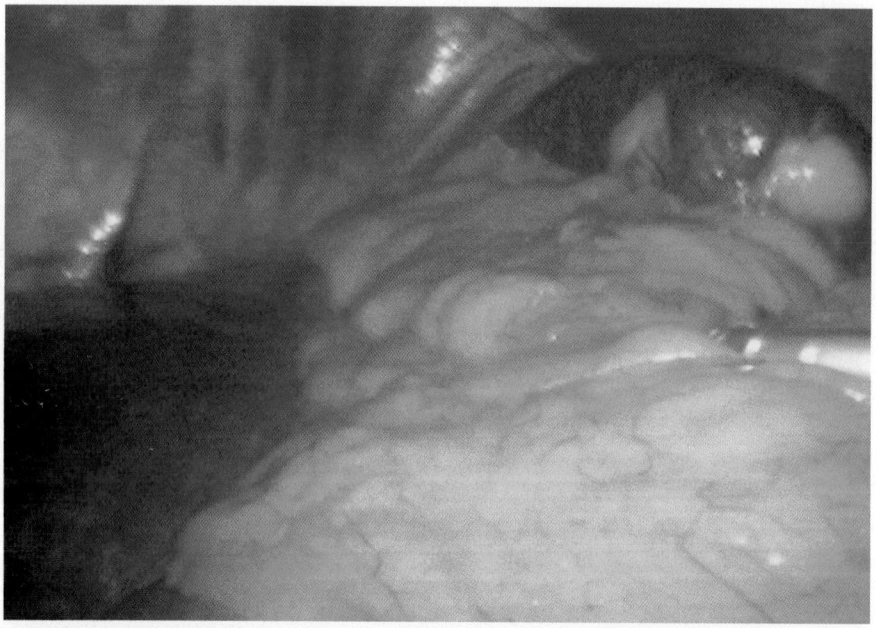

Fig. 6-5. Spleen with smooth borders. In contrast to Figs. 6-3 and 6-4, this spleen demonstrates smooth borders. This finding correlates with late division of the splenic artery and vein. Hilar fat is a clue to the location of segmental vessels. Liver and stomach are in the foreground.

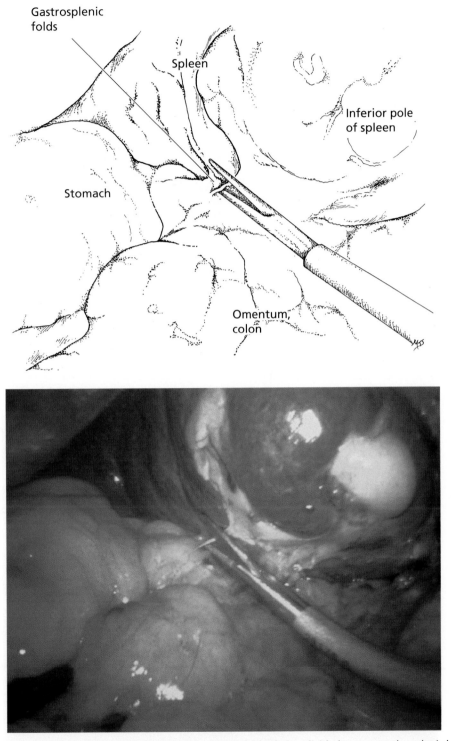

Fig. 6-6. Gastrosplenic fold. An avascular gastrosplenic fold is being divided to expose the splenic hilum.

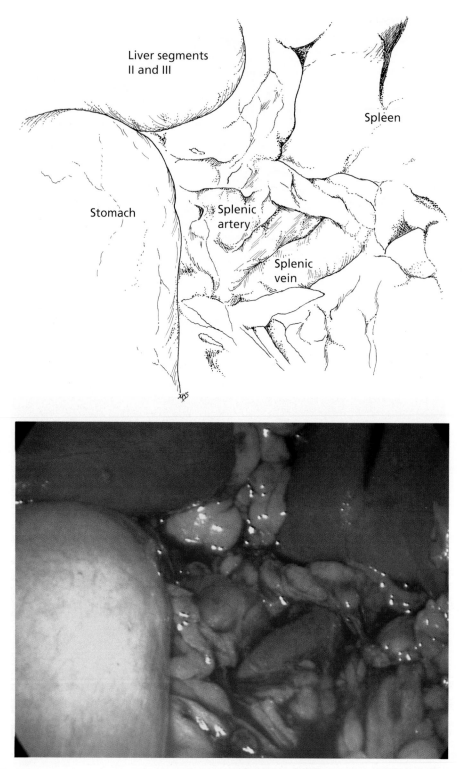

Fig. 6-7. Splenic artery and vein. Close to the splenic hilum, the splenic artery and vein have been exposed. The stomach is retracted medially. The short gastric vessels have been divided. The pancreas is not visible.

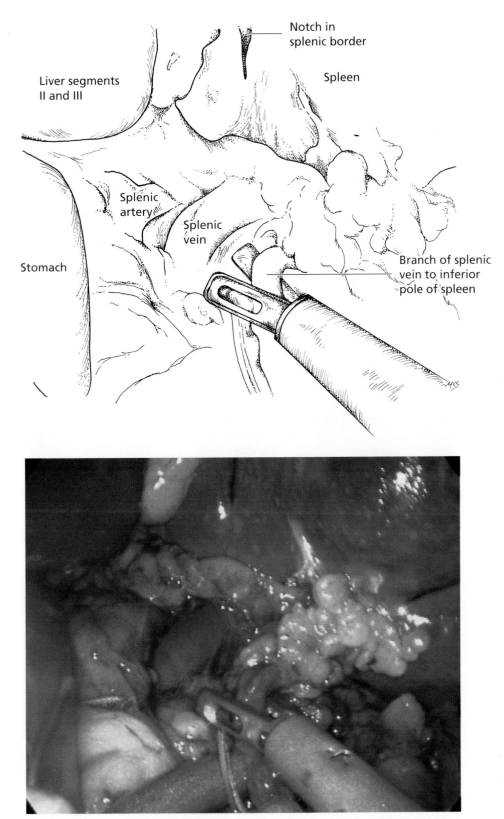

Fig. 6-8. Branch of the splenic vein. A branch of the splenic vein going to the inferior pole is being isolated. Note the notched border of the spleen, a hint to early division of the splenic vessels. The main trunks of the splenic vein and splenic artery are seen. This branch vessel appears to be running toward the left gastroepiploic vein.

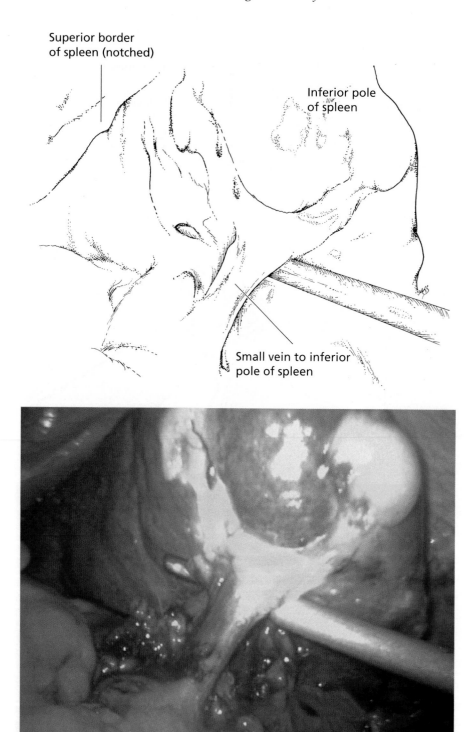

Fig. 6-9. Polar branch of the splenic vein. A significant vein, draining the inferior pole of the spleen and probably connected to the splenic or left gastroepiploic vein, is being isolated.

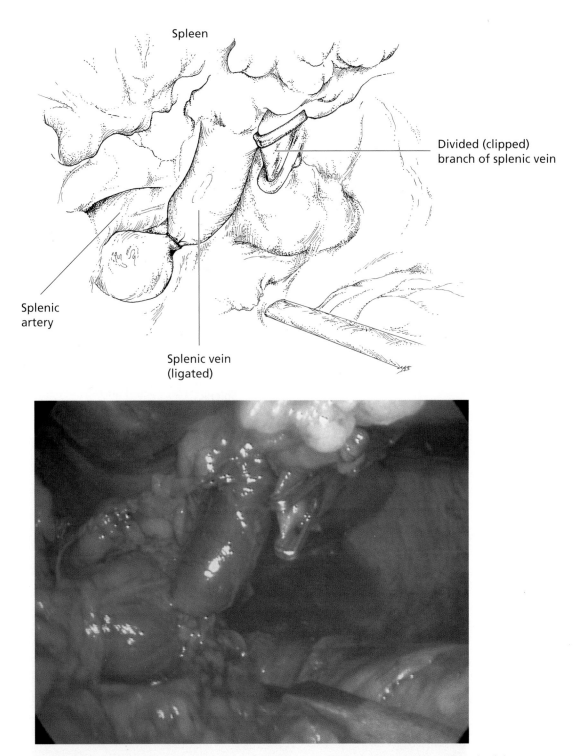

Fig. 6-10. Splenic artery and vein. The main trunk of the splenic vein has been ligated. A large branch of the splenic vein has been clipped. The splenic artery is seen cephalad, crossing anterior to the splenic vein, in the most common anatomic arrangement.

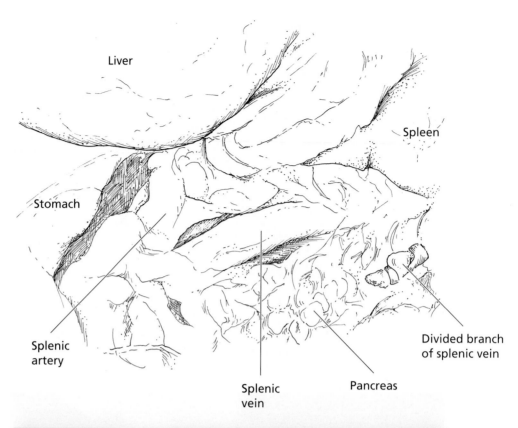

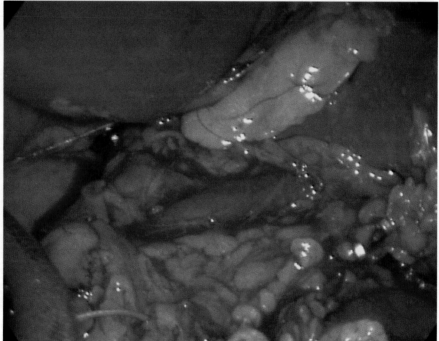

Fig. 6-11. Splenic artery and vein. An inferior polar branch of the splenic vein has been divided. Pancreatic tissue accompanies the splenic artery and splenic vein into the hilum of the spleen.

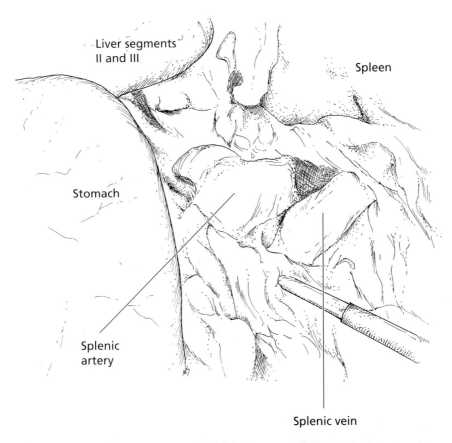

Liver segments
II and III

Spleen

Stomach

Splenic
artery

Splenic vein

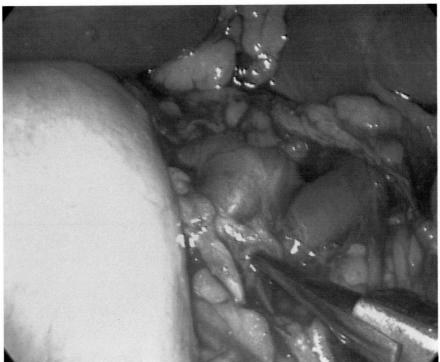

Fig. 6-12. Splenic artery and vein. In this typical example, the splenic artery is cephalad to the splenic vein in the region of the splenic hilum.

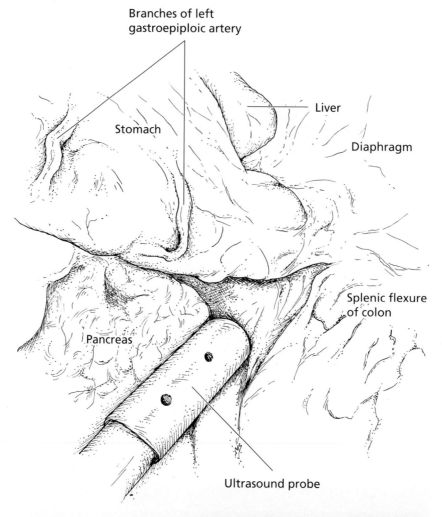

Branches of left
gastroepiploic artery

Stomach

Liver

Diaphragm

Splenic flexure
of colon

Pancreas

Ultrasound probe

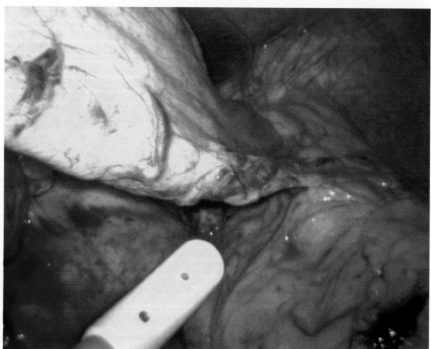

Fig. 6-13. Exposure of the pancreas in the lesser sac. The greater omentum has been opened and the lesser
sac entered. The greater curvature of the stomach with branches of the left gastroepiploic vessels is retracted
medially and cephalad. The tip of segments II and III of the liver is seen in the background. The spleen and
splenic vessels are hidden by omentum and overlying fat. The pancreas is being examined with an endoscopic
ultrasound probe.

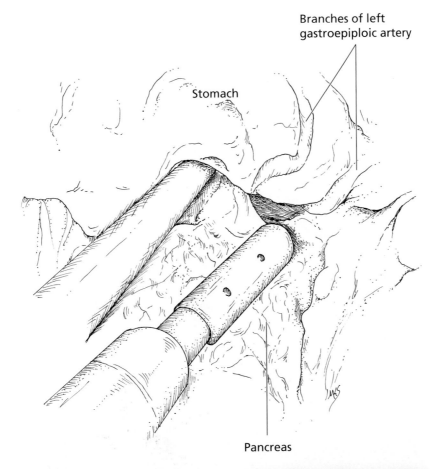

Branches of left
gastroepiploic artery

Stomach

Pancreas

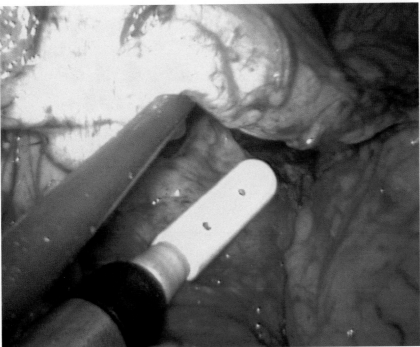

Fig. 6-14. Exposure of the pancreas and identification of vascular structures. An endoscopic ultrasound probe is being used to examine the tail of pancreas and hilum of spleen. Branches of the left gastroepiploic vessels have been divided to gain wide access to the lesser sac through the gastrocolic omentum.

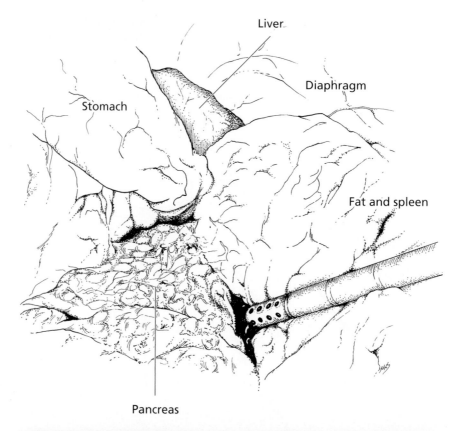

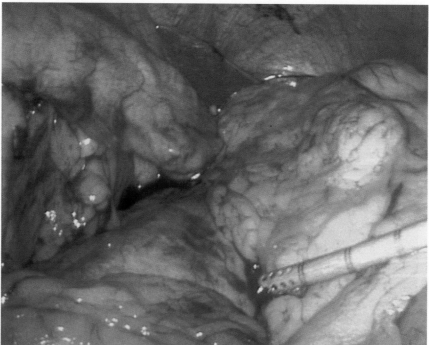

Fig. 6-15. Body of the pancreas. The stomach is reflected cephalad to expose the body of the pancreas. Segments II and III of the liver and the diaphragm are noted in the background. The spleen is obscured with fat.

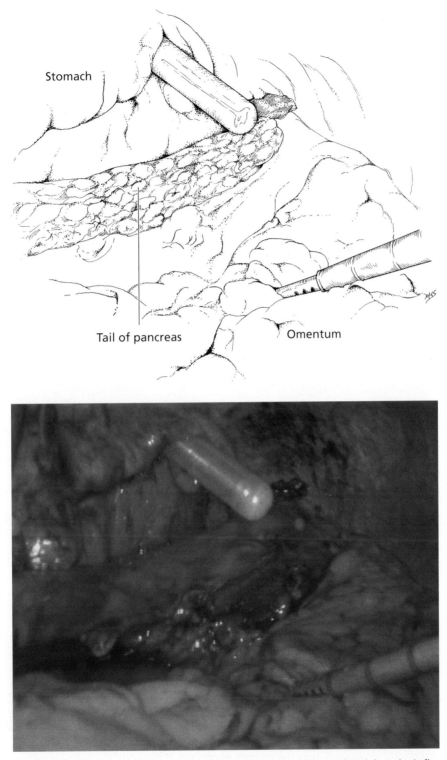

Fig. 6-16. Body and tail of the pancreas. The stomach is being reflected upward and the splenic flexure down-ward. Wide exposure has been obtained by fully opening the lesser sac through the gastrocolic omentum.

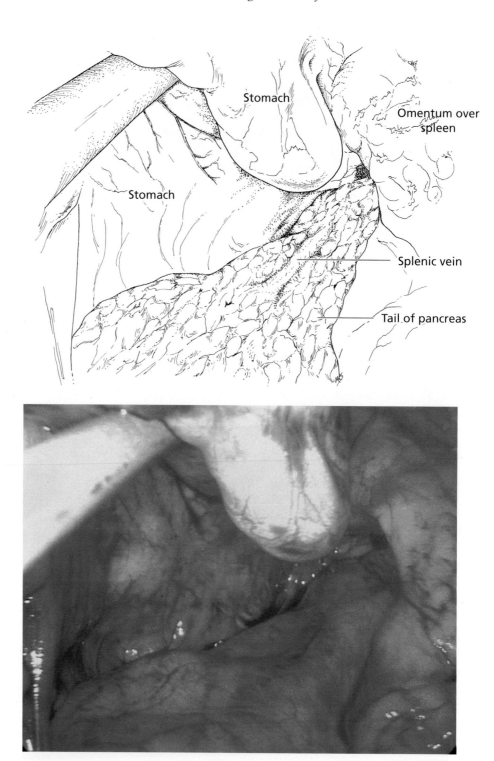

Fig. 6-17. Tail of the pancreas. The splenic vein is seen through the substance of the pancreas (anatomy confirmed by endoscopic ultrasound). Note the intimate association of the tail of the pancreas with splenic vascular structures in the vicinity of the hilum.

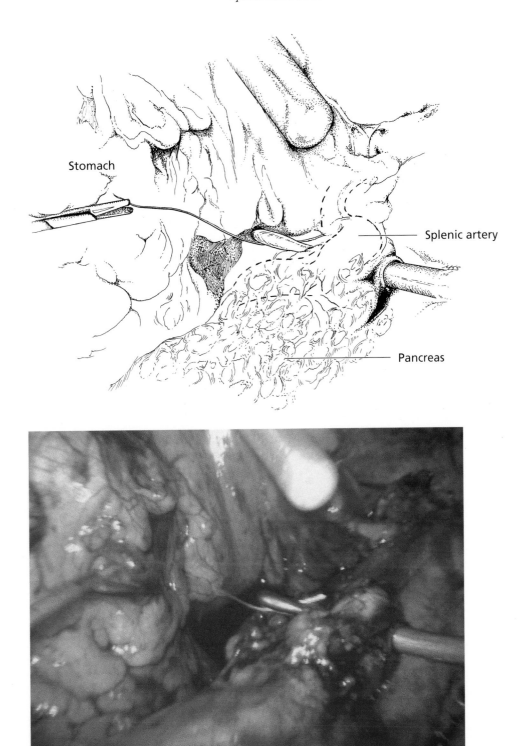

Fig. 6-18. Splenic artery and tail of the pancreas. The splenic artery is being ligated. Note proximity of the tail of the pancreas to the splenic hilum. The *dotted line* indicates the tortuous course of the splenic artery.

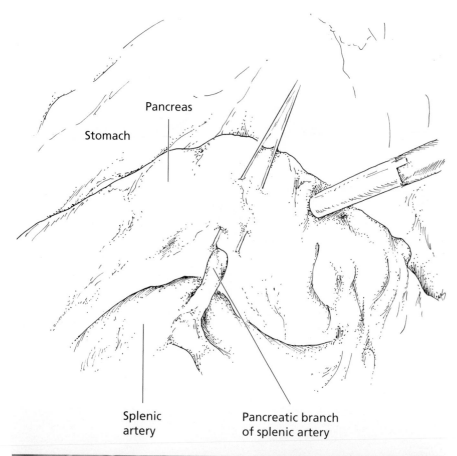

Stomach

Pancreas

Splenic
artery

Pancreatic branch
of splenic artery

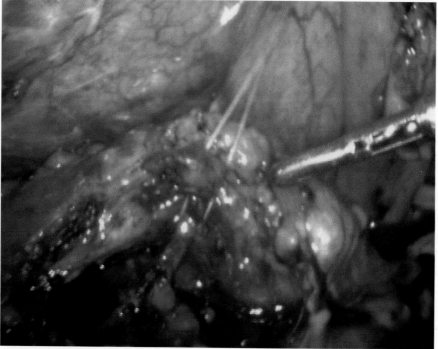

Fig. 6-19. Branch of the splenic artery to the pancreas. A small tributary of the splenic artery going directly to the pancreas is being isolated.

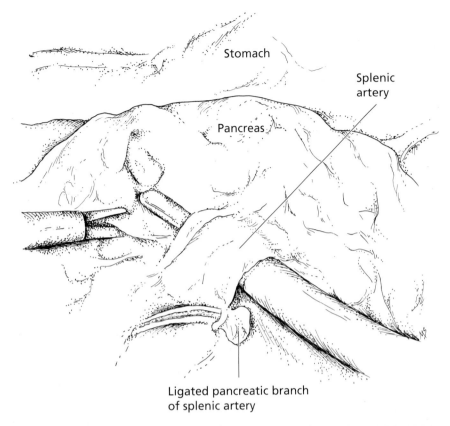

Ligated pancreatic branch
of splenic artery

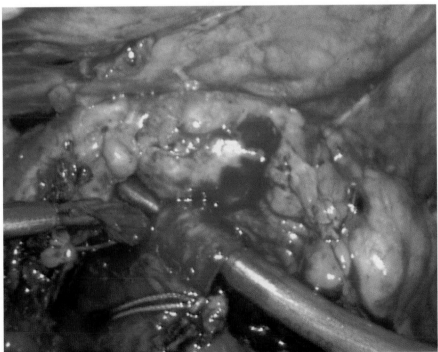

Fig. 6-20. Splenic artery, body of the pancreas. The pancreas is elevated for distal pancreatectomy. The splenic artery is being prepared for ligature. A small tributary of the splenic artery going to the pancreas has been divided.

7

SMALL INTESTINE AND APPENDIX

INITIAL LAPAROSCOPIC VIEW AND PRINCIPLES OF EXPOSURE

Because the liver occupies the right upper quadrant, the right colon occupies a relatively cramped space, and the initial view of the right lower quadrant is dominated by small intestine, omentum, and cecum. The small intestine, appendix, and Meckel's diverticulum are described in this chapter, with associated laparoscopic procedures. The cecum and right colon arc described in greater deal in Chapter 8.

ANATOMY AND SPECIFIC SURGICAL PROCEDURES

Small Intestine

The small intestine is divided into duodenum (considered in Chapter 4), and jejunum and ileum (described here). Jejunum begins at the ligament of Treitz (see Fig. 2-10) and is generally considered to comprise the proximal two-fifths of small intestine (Figs. 7-1 and 7-2). The length is generally described as around 100 cm, but this depends greatly on how the measurement is performed. The ileum is the distal three-fifths (between 100 and 150 cm). Valvulae conniventes are taller and more numerous in the jejunum than in the ileum, and the jejunum is thicker, redder, and more vascular than the ileum. The diameter of the bowel decreases as well as one progresses distally, but these differences are not of much assistance to the laparoscopic surgeon. The dividing point between jejunum and ileum is arbitrary, and the only way for the laparoscopic surgeon to differentiate proximal (jejunum) from distal (ileum) small intestine is by tracing the individual loop either to the ligament of Treitz or to the ileocecal valve (Figs. 7-3 and 7-4).

The mesentery of the small bowel serves several functions beyond simply providing blood supply and lymphatic drainage. It tethers the small intestine and provides mechanical stability, preventing internal hernias and kinking. The base of the mesentery is approximately 15 cm long and runs from a point just to the left of the midline at the ligament of Treitz diagonally down and across the right to the right lower quadrant (see Fig. 2-1). It is fan-shaped, and the broad intestinal border is approximately 6 m long. Fat is stored in the mesentery. In the mesentery of the jejunum, fat is most prominent at the base, and there may be transparent spaces between adjacent vasa recta. In the ileum, the fat becomes more pronounced and commonly encroaches on the mesenteric border of the ileum. The mesentery is longer in the midportion than in the proximal jejunum or distal ileum; it averages 20 cm in length from vertebral to intestinal borders.

The superior mesenteric artery crosses over the duodenum and provides the major blood supply of the small intestine. The superior mesenteric artery and vein can be found by elevating the transverse mesocolon and tracing the middle colic artery down to the convergence of the mesocolon and the mesentery of the small intestine. The first jejunal branches come off just after the duodenal crossing. The artery subsequently gives off multiple jejunal and ileal branches before terminating in a marginal artery that anastomoses with the ileal branch of the ileocolic artery. Veins parallel the arteries and drain into the superior mesenteric vein, which similarly crosses the duodenum.

Within the mesentery of the small intestine are multiple jejunal and ileal arcades (Figs. 7-5 and 7-6) that become more complex as one progresses distally. These arcades allow resection and the creation of long vascularized segments of ileum or jejunum for gastrointestinal reconstructive procedures. Their exact anatomy is unpredictable, and transillumination with a second laparoscope is helpful when the laparoscopic surgeon must identify the pattern of arcades in a fat-laden mesentery. The arcades terminate in end arteries termed vasa recta (see Fig. 7-6). In the most common arrangement, the vasa recta alternate supplying one side or the other of the intestine, terminating at the antimesenteric border. The antimesenteric border of the small intestine thus has the poorest blood supply and is the most susceptible to ischemia.

Lymphatic drainage of the small intestine is to nodes lying between the leaves of mesentery (Fig. 7-7). More than 200 lymph nodes within the mesentery ultimately drain into larger nodes at the root of the mesentery and superior mesenteric artery and vein.

Jejunostomy

The crucial anatomic point in laparoscopic jejunostomy, as with open jejunostomy, is accurate identification of a proximal loop of bowel (to maximize absorptive surface) that will reach the anterior abdominal wall at the site selected without tension or kinking. The only way to identify a proximal loop of bowel reliably is to trace the small intestine to the ligament of Treitz, then work distally until a suitable loop is identified. Generally, it is only necessary to pass one or two loops beyond the ligament of Treitz. Omentum must be swept aside to create a clear passage to the anterior abdominal wall. Once a suitable loop of bowel is identified, it can be anchored to the anterior abdominal wall, and a feeding tube can be passed. It may be necessary to release some of the pneumoperitoneum to allow the small intestine to reach the anterior abdominal wall without tension.

Small Bowel Resection

Laparoscopic small bowel resection is usually limited to segmental excision of a loop or two of small bowel containing an obvious abnormality. The region to be resected is identified, and the proximal and distal extents of resection are determined. Suspending the loop from the anterior abdominal wall by sutures or Silastic slings facilitates manipulation. A wedge-shaped portion of mesentery is excised. Gastrointestinal continuity may be restored either by intraperitoneal anastomosis or by exteriorizing the segment through a small incision and performing an extracorporeal anastomosis.

Meckel's Diverticulum

Meckel's diverticulum is a remnant of the persistent omphalomesenteric duct (which normally involutes between the fifth and seventh gestational weeks). It is the most common congenital anomaly of the gastrointestinal tract, found in 2% of the general population. This true diverticulum arises from the antimesenteric border of the ileum, usually within 100 cm of the ileocecal valve (Fig. 7-8). Up to 25% of pediatric patients with this anomaly have a fibrous attachment to the anterior abdominal wall, which is a potential site for volvulus. This is much less common in adults.

The blood supply comes from persistent vitelline vessels that cross the adjacent ileum to supply the diverticulum. About 50% of Meckel's diverticula examined at autopsy contain either gastric or pancreatic mucosa. The incidence of gastric mucosa is higher in symptomatic patients.

Resection of Meckel's Diverticulum

There are two ways to resect a Meckel's diverticulum. Simple excision of the diverticulum can be achieved by firing an endoscopic linear stapler across the base, taking care not to encroach on the lumen. Because the diverticulum always originates from the antimesenteric border, no mesentery (other than a small vessel to the diverticulum itself) needs to be divided.

Simple excision may not be sufficient to remove all ectopic mucosa and associated ulcerations. This is particularly significant when ectopic gastric mucosa has caused an acid-peptic ulcer to form in adjacent ileum. In this case, limited small bowel resection with restoration of continuity is performed (see earlier).

Appendix

The appendix derives from a cecal diverticulum of the fetus. During development and infancy, the cecum descends into the right lower quadrant and then enlarges. This enlargement is most pronounced on the medial aspect, and this causes the appendix to rotate posteromedially. The appendix is generally within 1.7 cm of the ileocecal junction. Its length varies from 2 to 20 cm, averaging 9 cm. The most common location in the adult is retrocecal or retrocolic (64%) and 31% lie over the pelvic brim.

To the umbilically placed laparoscope, the appendix is hidden behind the cecum (Figs. 7-9 to 7-11). The anterior taenia of the cecum leads to the appendix, and in fact the termination of the three cecal taeniae (not generally appreciated laparoscopically) reliably identifies the base. Adequate display of the appendicocecal juncture requires careful mobilization and exposure (Fig. 7-12).

A triangular mesoappendix tethers the appendix posteriorly (Figs. 7-12 and 7-13). It contains a lymph node and the appendicular artery with accompanying veins.

The appendicular artery is a branch of the ileocolic artery. It passes behind the ileum and then runs in the free edge of the mesoappendix to supply the appendix through multiple small branches (see Fig. 7-13) before terminating in a branch to the tip of the appendix. Eighty percent of individuals have two or more accessory arteries, and there may be a sizable recurrent branch of the appendicular artery that anastomoses at the base of the appendix with a branch of the posterior cecal artery.

Lymphatics from the tip and body of the appendix drain into the posterior ileocolic lymph nodes. Those from the base drain into the anterior ileocolic nodes.

Appendectomy

Laparoscopic exposure of the appendix is facilitated by gently pulling the cecum upward, toward the patient's left shoulder. The mesoappendix is farther from the umbilically placed laparoscope than the base and is generally divided last. The juncture of the base of the appendix with the cecum must be visually confirmed to avoid leaving a remnant of appendix. Generally, the cecum is seen to cone downward into the appendix when the appendix is put on traction. Convergence of the three taeniae provides another visual clue.

The appendicular artery may be secured at the base of the appendix with clips or a vascular stapler. Alternatively, small branches to the appendix may be secured individually. These branches become small enough at the point where they enter the appendix that simple electrocautery may provide adequate hemostatic control.

Exposure of the retrocecal appendix requires mobilization of the right colon. The peritoneal reflection is incised, and the cecum is gently rolled medially to bring the appendix into view (Figs. 7-14 to 7-16). Dense bands of fibrous tissue may need to be cautiously divided with electrocautery or ultrasonically activated shears.

BIBLIOGRAPHY

Anatomy

1. Backman L, Hallberg D. Small intestinal length. *Acta Chir Scand* 1974;140:57–63.
2. Jay GD III, Margulis RR, McGraw AB, Northrip RR. Meckel's diverticulum: a survey of one hundred and three cases. *Arch Surg* 1950;61:158–165.

3. Michels NA, Siddharth P, Kornblith PL, Parke WW. The variant blood supply of the small and large intestines: its import in regional resections. *J Int Coll Surg* 1963;39:127–135.
4. O'Connor CE, Reed WP. In vivo location of the human vermiform appendix. *Clin Anat* 1994;7:139–142.
5. Picken G, Ellis H, Dixon AK. The normal vermiform appendix at computed tomography: visualization and anatomical location. *Clin Anat* 1993;6:9–14.
6. Ramsden WH, Mannion RAJ, Simpkins KC, DeDombal FT. Is the appendix where you think it is and does it matter? *Clin Radiol* 1993;47:100–103.
7. Stewart JH, Storey CF. Meckel's diverticulum: a study of 141 cases. *South Med J* 1962;55:16–22.
8. VanDammer J-P, Bonte J. *Vascular anatomy in abdominal surgery.* New York: Thieme Medical Publishers, 1990:59–68, 113–125.

Laparoscopic Techniques

1. Attwood SEA, Hill AKD, Murphy PG, Thornton J, Stephens RB. A prospective randomized trial of laparoscopic versus open appendectomy. *Surgery* 1992;112:497–501.
2. Cross MJ, Snyder SK. Laparoscopic-directed small bowel resection for jejunal diverticulitis with perforation. *J Laparoendosc Surg* 1993;3:47–49.
3. Echenique M, Dominguez AS, Echenique I, Rivera V. Laparoscopic diagnosis and treatment of Meckel's diverticulum complicated by gastrointestinal bleeding. *J Laparoendosc Surg* 1993;3:145–148.
4. Kam DM, Scheeres DE. Fluorescein-assisted laparoscopy in the identification of arterial mesenteric ischemia. *Surg Endosc* 1993;7:75–78.
5. Keating J, Hill A, Schroeder D, Whittle D. Laparoscopy in the diagnosis and treatment of acute small bowel obstruction. *J Laparoendosc Surg* 1992;2:239–244.
6. Martin LC, Puente I, Sosa JL, et al. Open versus laparoscopic appendectomy: a prospective randomized comparison. *Ann Surg* 1995;222:256–262.
7. Morris JB, Mullen JL, Yu JC, Rosato EF. Laparoscopic-guided jejunostomy. *Surgery* 1992;112:96–99.
8. Nowzaradan Y, Barnes JP Jr. Current techniques in laparoscopic appendectomy. *Surg Laparosc Endosc* 1993;3:470–476.
9. Reed DN. Percutaneous peritoneoscopic jejunostomy. *Surg Gynecol Obstet* 1992;174:527–529.
10. Scott-Conner CEH, Hall TJ, Anglin BL, Muakkassa FF. Laparoscopic appendectomy: initial experience in a teaching program. *Ann Surg* 1992;215:660–668.

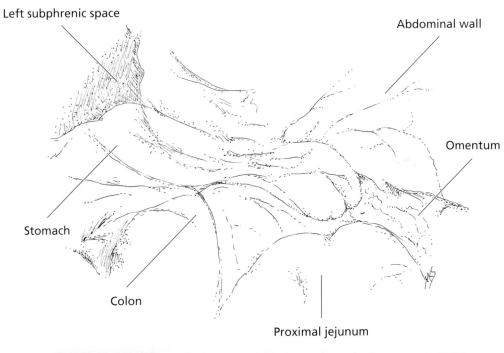

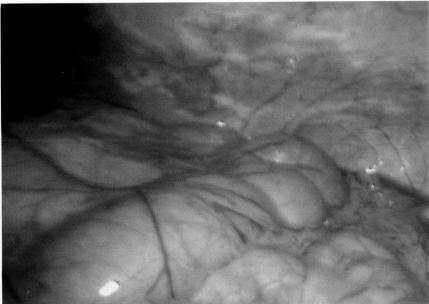

Fig. 7-1. Loops of proximal small intestine in the vicinity of the ligament of Treitz. These were displayed by reflecting the omentum cephalad (seen in background). Secure identification of jejunum versus ileum requires that an individual loop be traced proximally or distally.

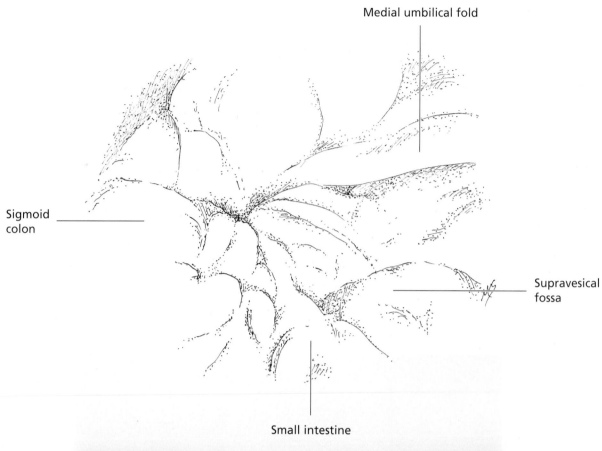

Medial umbilical fold

Sigmoid colon

Supravesical fossa

Small intestine

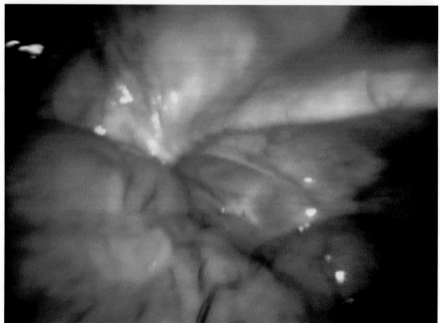

Fig. 7-2. Loops of distal small intestine in the pelvis.

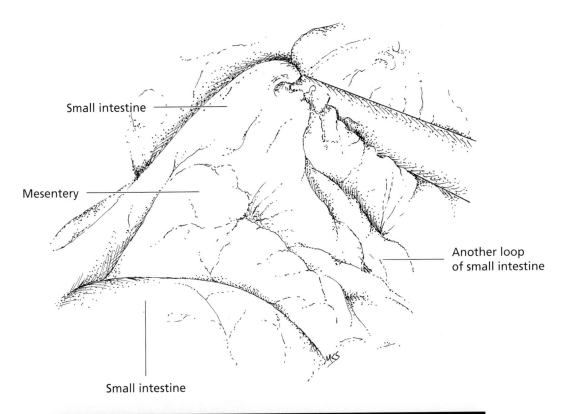

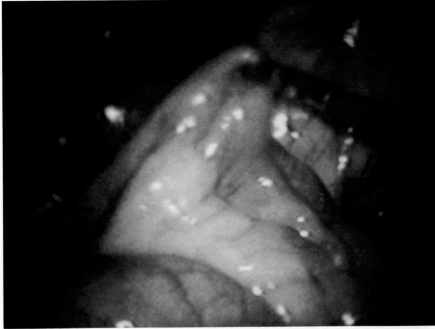

Fig. 7-3. Loop of small intestine. This loop of small bowel can be identified as jejunum or ileum only by following it proximally to the ligament of Treitz or distally to the ileocecal junction. The fatty mesentery, laden with lymph nodes, and relatively small caliber suggest that this is distal (ileum) rather than proximal (jejunum), but these differences are not reliable for laparoscopic identification.

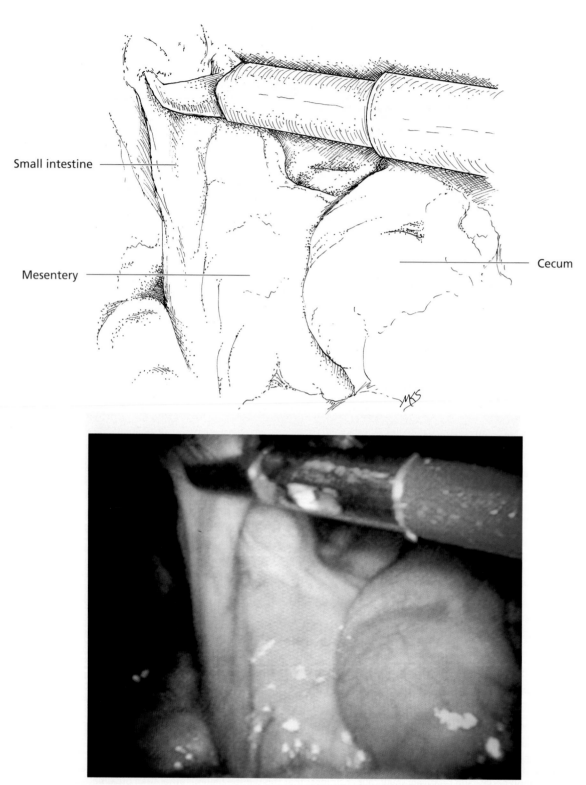

Fig. 7-4. Loop of ileum. This loop of small bowel has been traced down to the ileocecal junction and is thus identified as ileum. The fatty mesentery is laden with lymph nodes. Cecum is seen in the foreground.

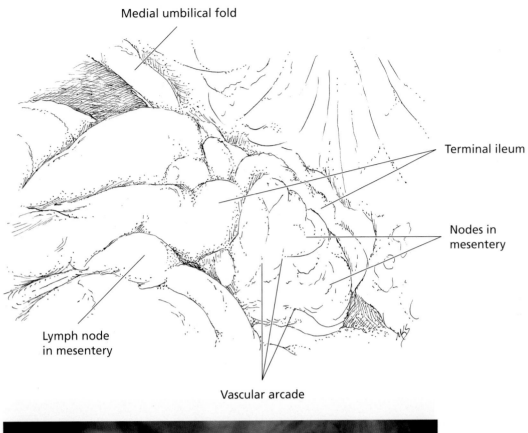

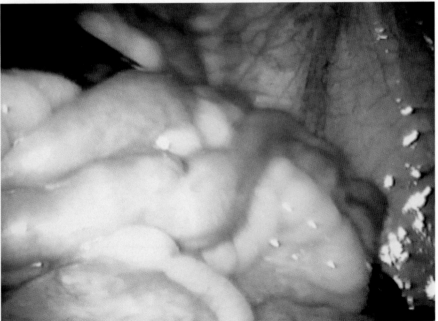

Fig. 7-5. Vascular arcade of small intestine. This loop of mid–small intestine shows the vascular arcade well. The fatty mesentery of this segment contrasts with the more filmy mesentery seen in Fig. 7-6.

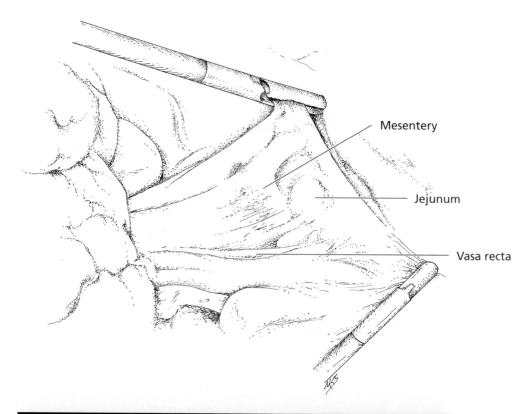

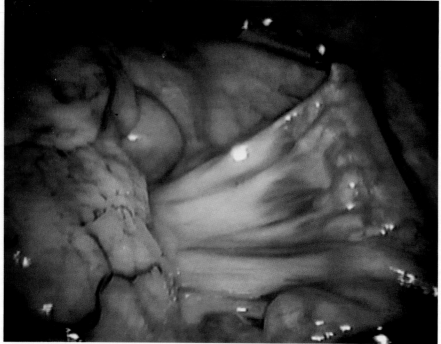

Fig. 7-6. Vasa recta of the jejunum. The terminal vasa recta of this segment of proximal jejunum are well seen. The proximal jejunum has a less fatty mesentery than the distal jejunum and ileum. These signs are useful confirmation of the level of small bowel, but only tracing the small intestine to its origin at the ligament of Treitz or to its termination onto the cecum provides definite laparoscopic identification.

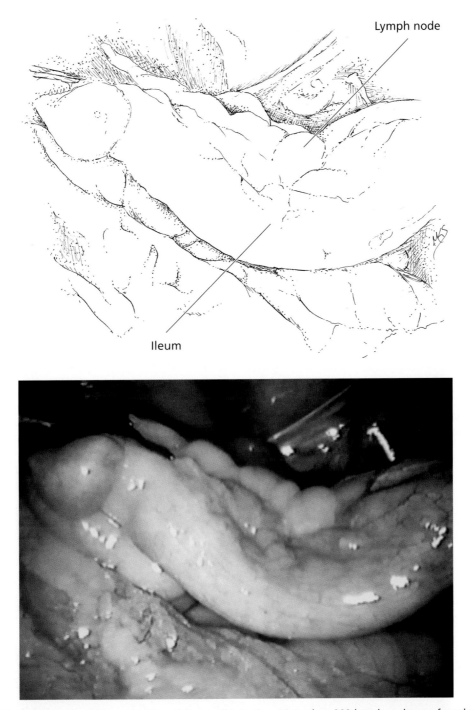

Fig. 7-7. Lymph node in the mesentery of the small intestine. More than 200 lymph nodes are found within the mesentery of the small intestine.

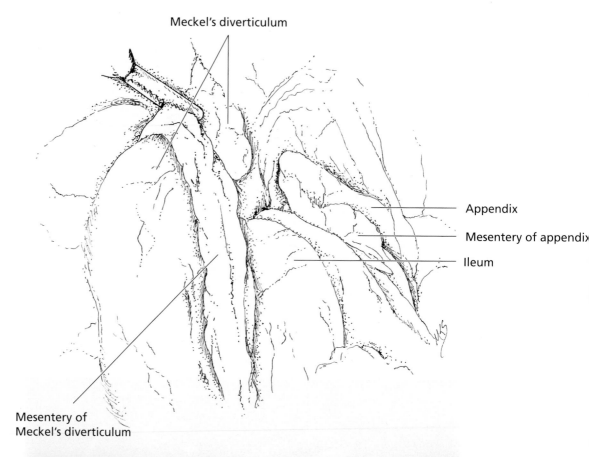

Meckel's diverticulum

Appendix

Mesentery of appendix

Ileum

Mesentery of
Meckel's diverticulum

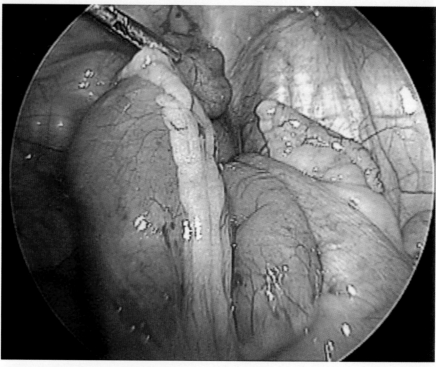

Fig. 7-8. Meckel's diverticulum. This true diverticulum arises from the antimesenteric side of the ileum, typically within 100 cm of the ileocecal valve.

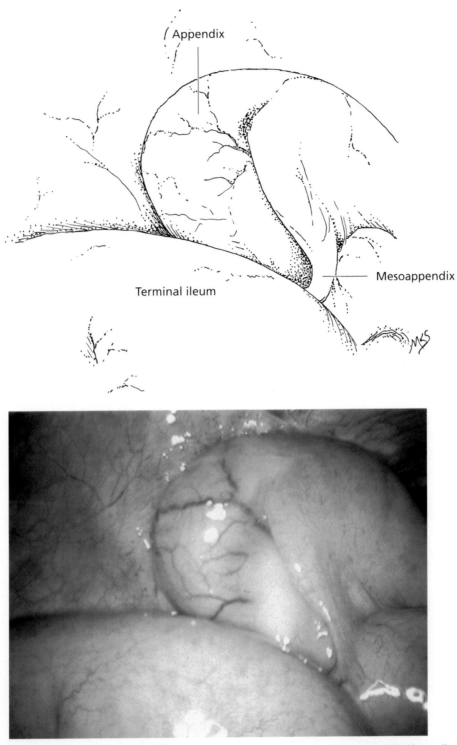

Fig. 7-9. Appendix. This inflamed and enlarged appendix is seen to curve downward by the pull of the mesoappendix. The terminal ileum is seen in the foreground. The appendix and cecum have been swept into the right upper quadrant, and the umbilically placed laparoscope is thus viewing terminal ileum, appendix, and mesoappendix from below. The cecum is not seen.

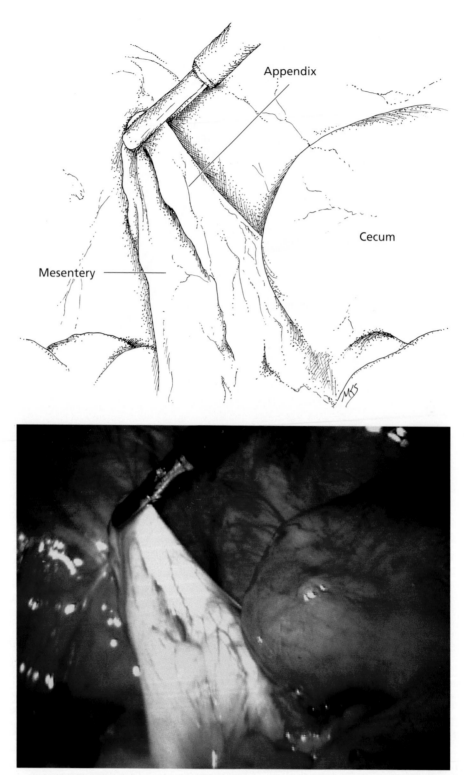

Fig. 7-10. Appendix. This inflamed appendix is being elevated to display the mesoappendix. It is tethered by peritoneal attachments. The cecum is in the foreground.

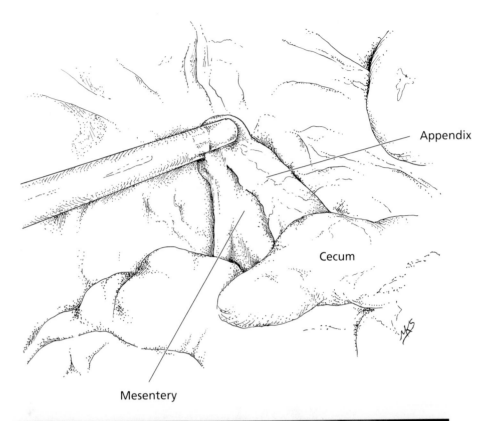

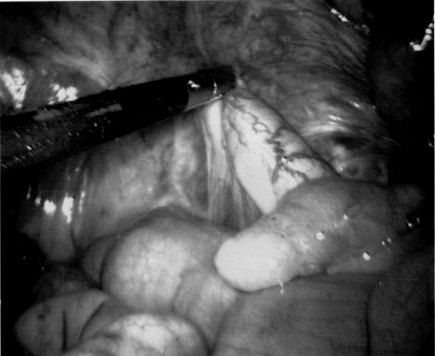

Fig. 7-11. Appendix. With additional mobilization, the appendix and mesoappendix are seen. The cecum is in the foreground. The termination of the appendix on the cecum is not identified with certainty.

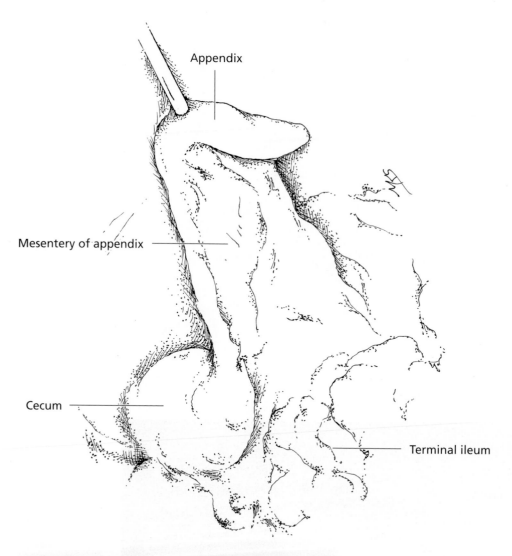

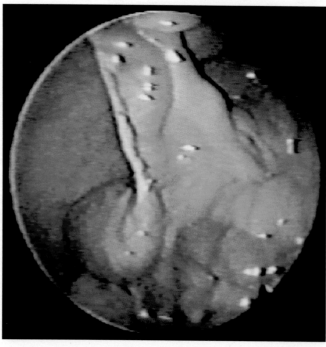

Fig. 7-12. Appendix and cecum. In this view from below, the termination of the appendix on the cecum is well displayed. The fatty mesoappendix is seen to extend like a sail, and the terminal ileum is seen in the foreground. Note how the terminal ileum is almost surrounded by its fatty mesentery.

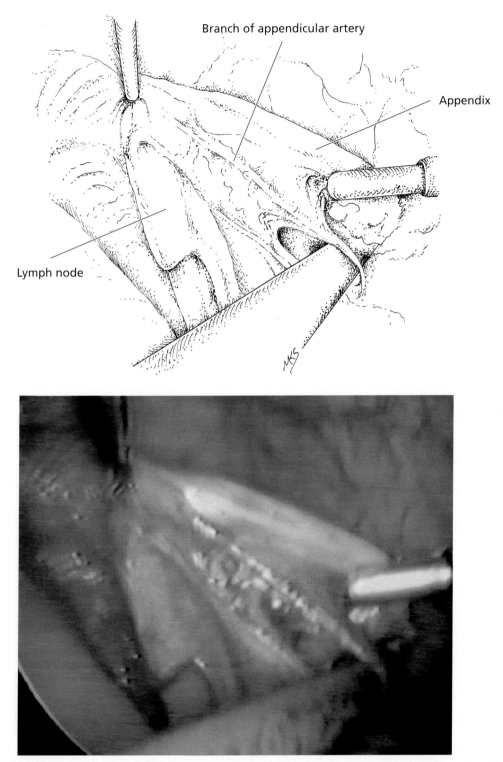

Fig. 7-13. Mesoappendix and branches of the appendicular artery. The mesoappendix contains branches of the appendicular artery. These are end arteries and may be clipped or secured with an ultrasonically activated shears. The appendix is held in tension by a pair of atraumatic graspers.

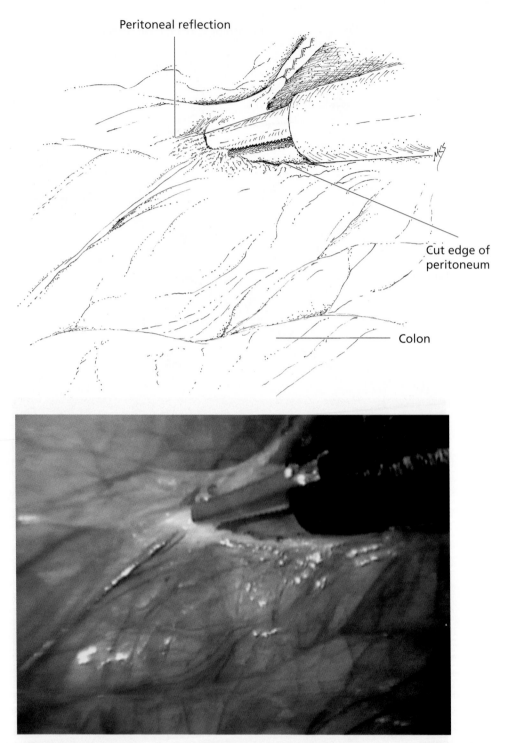

Fig. 7-14. Retrocecal appendix. When the appendix is retrocecal, the right colon must be mobilized, as shown here. An incision is made along the peritoneal reflection of the right colon, which is then retracted medially.

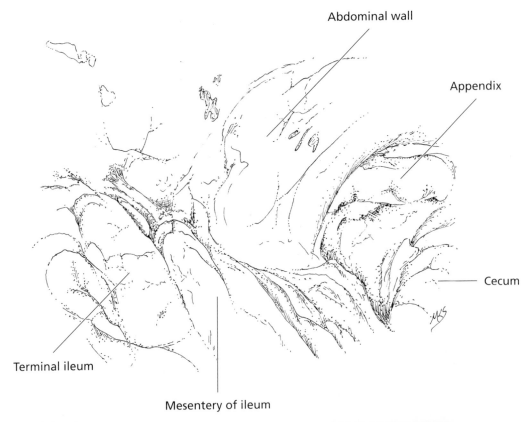

Abdominal wall

Appendix

Cecum

Terminal ileum

Mesentery of ileum

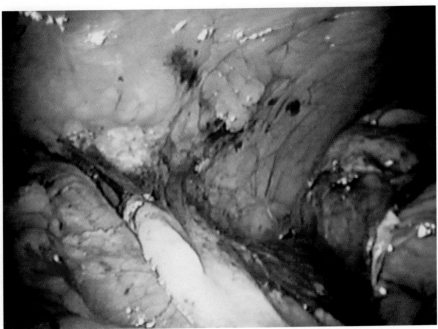

Fig. 7-15. Retrocecal appendix. Further mobilization of the right colon displays the appendix behind the cecum.

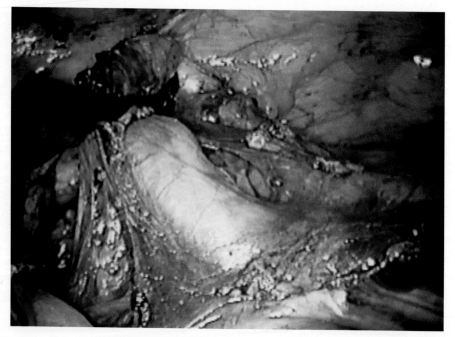

Appendix

Grasper elevating
appendix

Cecum

Mesentery of appendix

Fig. 7-16. Retrocecal appendix. Adequate dissection of the appendix from the cecum allows accurate identification of the appendiceal base and mesentery.

8

COLON AND RECTUM

INITIAL LAPAROSCOPIC VIEW AND PRINCIPLES OF EXPOSURE

An umbilical port gives the best access to all quadrants of the abdomen, usually required for laparoscopic colon surgery. An angled laparoscope may provide better visualization in the pelvis. A second laparoscope is occasionally used as a light source to transilluminate the mesentery and to identify blood vessels. As with most advanced laparoscopic procedures, it is important that the patient and monitors be placed so the surgeon can work from a variety of vantage points: from the patient's left side (for the right colon), standing between the patient's legs (for the transverse colon and flexures), and from the patient's right side (for the left colon). The operating table must be able to tilt into Trendelenburg and reverse Trendelenburg positions, as well as rotate to elevate one side or the other. This allows gravity to assist in displacement of viscera, thus improving exposure.

Seen through the laparoscope, the colon appears white and the small intestine is pink or reddish. Taeniae are often visible, and the greater omentum hangs like a fatty apron from the omental taenia of the transverse colon (see Figs. 2-2, 2-7 to 2-9, and 6-1 to 6-4). The small intestine is smaller in caliber, rounder, and more featureless than the colon, which is larger, sacculated, and distinguished by taeniae, appendices epiploicae, and the greater omentum.

ANATOMY AND SPECIFIC SURGICAL PROCEDURES

Topographic Relations

As discussed in Chapter 2, the attachment of the mesentery of the transverse colon forms the division between supramesocolic and inframesocolic viscera (see Fig. 2-1). The colon drapes like a picture frame around the inframesocolic viscera. It is conventionally divided into the right colon, transverse colon, left colon, and rectum. The right colon comprises the cecum and ascending colon. The hepatic flexure marks the juncture of the right and transverse colon. The splenic flexure is the juncture of the transverse and descending colon. Generally, the splenic flexure, descending colon, and sigmoid colon are all considered part of the left colon. The sigmoid colon terminates in the rectum, which exits the abdomen through the pelvic diaphragm.

The blood supply of the intraperitoneal colon comes from branches of the superior and inferior mesenteric arteries, which come from the medially placed aorta. Thus the mesentery of the colon lies medial to the colon itself, and the colon may be elevated along a virtually avascular fusion plane and rotated medially in preparation for resection.

Right Colon

The right colon occupies the relatively short space between the liver and the pelvis. The cecum, located in the right iliac fossa, has the largest caliber of any portion of the large intestine. Differential growth causes the cecum to rotate, placing the ileocecal junction medial to the rounded, enlarged, and protruding cecum (Figs. 8-1 to 8-3). Where the three taeniae of the cecum converge, the appendix may be seen (see Fig. 7-12). The cecum varies in mobility. In many individuals, it is completely covered with peritoneum and extremely mobile. Manipulation of the cecum and appendix may cause the laparoscopic surgeon to chase the mobile cecum into the right upper quadrant, with subsequent visual field reversal.

The peritoneal attachment of the terminal ileum and cecum often gives rise to peritoneal recesses. These are generally located medial to the cecum and above or below the terminal ileum. On rare occasions, these are the site of hernia formation.

The ascending colon is smaller in diameter than the cecum and deeper (see Fig. 8-3). This structure creates the appearance of the colon diving into the retroperitoneum in the region between the cecum and hepatic flexure. In reality, the colon is still covered with peritoneum over much of its surface, but the posterior surface and mesentery of the ascending colon above the cecum have become adherent to and have fused with the posterior abdominal wall, so peritoneum covers only the anterior surface. It averages just 15 cm in length.

The right colon lies on the fascia of the iliacus, quadratus lumborum, and psoas muscles. Several critical structures lie deep to the right colon and its mesentery. In the vicinity of the hepatic flexure, the colon overlies the right kidney (see Fig. 2-7; Fig. 8-4). The right transverse colon and right colon mesentery adhere to the duodenum. Inferiorly, the right ureter must be identified and protected (Fig. 8-5).

Transverse Colon

The transverse colon runs from the hepatic flexure to the splenic flexure. The right half is sometimes termed the right transverse colon (and is commonly resected during right hemicolectomy); the left half is frequently treated in an analogous manner. This portion of the colon averages 50 cm in length but is highly variable. It is not rare for a long, redundant transverse colon to extend into the pelvis. The greater omentum attaches to the taenia omentalis of the transverse colon, then extends downward to fold on itself and pass upward to attach to the greater curvature of the stomach. The blood supply of the greater omentum comes from the left and right gastroepiploic artery and vein (see Figs. 4-12 and 4-13), which are found in the upper leaf adjacent to and anastomosing with vessels of the greater curvature. The omentum must be elevated or pushed into the upper abdomen to reveal the transverse colon, which is adherent to its underside.

The attachment of the omentum to the transverse colon is generally avascular, and the transverse colon may be peeled off the underside of the omentum. The fusion plane between omentum and transverse colon is several millimeters from the edge of the colon where the appendices epiploicae fuse to the omentum.

The right transverse colon overlies and is normally loosely adherent to the second and third portions of the duodenum and head of pancreas. Inflammatory disease or tumor may render this adherence dense and impossible to dissect. Beyond the head of the pancreas, the transverse colon is on a mesentery (the transverse mesocolon) and is mobile. At the splenic flexure, the transverse colon ascends and becomes deep, frequently attached to the retroperitoneum and spleen. The phrenocolic ligament anchors the splenic flexure of the colon to the diaphragm, and the splenocolic ligament tethers it to the spleen (Figs. 8-6 to 8-9). Downward traction on the splenic flexure may produce a capsular avulsion injury of the spleen, resulting in troublesome bleeding. This can be avoided by dissecting in the plane between omentum and colon, pushing the omentum upward, and rolling the splenic flexure downward. The left kidney lies deep to the splenic flexure and proximal descending colon (see Fig. 8-9).

Left Colon

The splenic flexure makes an acute angle between the transverse colon and descending colon. The descending colon follows a long (approximately 25 cm), relatively straight course from the splenic flexure to the brim of the pelvis. The descending colon is attached by loose areolar tissue to the posterior abdominal wall and the fascia over the left kidney, quadratus lumborum, iliacus, and psoas major muscles.

At the brim of the pelvis, the colon becomes mobile and lies in loops forming the sigmoid colon (Figs. 8-10 to 8-12). This portion of colon averages 40 cm in length but is highly variable. The sigmoid mesocolon provides mobility to the sigmoid colon and varies considerably in length. The sigmoid colon usually lies in one or two coils in the pelvis; it overlies the bladder in the male (see Fig. 8-10) and the bladder, uterus, and adnexal structures in the female (see Fig. 8-11).

The transition to the rectum is gradual and is marked by convergence of all the taeniae to form a continuous, longitudinal outer muscle layer (see Fig. 8-11). The left ureter is the most crucial structure that must be identified and protected during dissection in this region. Other structures that cross behind the descending and sigmoid colon include the left gonadal vessels, the left external iliac artery and vein, and the lateral femoral cutaneous, femoral, and genitofemoral nerves. The right ureter is also at risk during pelvic dissection and must be identified.

Rectum

The rectum is variously defined as beginning where the taeniae converge in the distal sigmoid colon or at the level of the third sacral vertebra. The former definition is more useful to the laparoscopic surgeon, because this is a visible landmark. The upper third of the rectum is intraperitoneal (see Fig. 8-11), and its mesentery arises posteriorly. The middle third of the rectum has peritoneum only on the anterior surface, and the distal third of the rectum is completely extraperitoneal. The division between middle and distal thirds is at the peritoneal reflection (vesicorectal pouch in the male, rectouterine pouch in the female).

The levator ani muscles form the floor of the pelvis. This pelvic diaphragm is covered with endopelvic fascia, lymphatics, and fat. The rectum passes through the sling of levator muscles to terminate in the anorectal canal. Laparoscopic manipulation generally ceases at the levator ani.

In addition to the structures mentioned in the section on the sigmoid colon, surgery on the rectum involves dissection in close proximity to the seminal vesicles, ductus deferens, prostate, vagina, and bladder.

Arteries, Veins, and Lymphatic Drainage

The blood supply to the intraperitoneal colon comes from vessels derived from the superior (right colon) and inferior (left colon) mesenteric arteries. The superior mesenteric artery terminates in the ileocolic artery, which supplies the cecum, the terminal ileum, and (by way of the appendicular artery) the appendix. A highly variable right colic artery sometimes arises from the superior mesenteric artery but more commonly is derived from the ileocolic or middle colic artery to supply the ascending colon and hepatic flexure. The middle colic artery is a relatively constant vessel that arises from the superior mesenteric artery proximal to the jejunal branches just below the pancreas. It runs in the transverse mesocolon.

The inferior mesenteric artery runs in a relatively straight course from the aorta to terminate in the superior rectal branches. It gives rise to the left colic artery and the sigmoidal branches. These vessels cross the psoas major, left ureter, and left gonadal vessels. The left colic may encroach on superior mesenteric artery territory or may even derive from the superior mesenteric artery. In a rare variant, the inferior mesenteric artery arises from the superior mesenteric artery.

Each of the named vessels of the colon divides into at least two vessels that run roughly parallel to the edge of the bowel to anastomose with the counterpart from the adjacent vessel. In this manner, an anastomotic arch is formed along the edge of the bowel. These marginal arteries may become dilated and meandering when a gradual occlusion of the vessels on one side of the colon forces collateral enlargement of the remaining vessels.

The blood supply of the rectum comes from several sources. The most important are the paired superior rectal arteries (occasionally, there is just one) which are the terminal branches of the inferior mesenteric artery. These supply the proximal rectum. The middle rectal arteries derive from the internal iliac arteries, and the inferior rectal arteries (the least important) derive from the pudendal arteries. There is rich anastomotic communication among all these vessels. The mesentery of the rectum arises posteriorly in the upper third and from both sides for the lower two-thirds.

The venous drainage of the right colon closely parallels the arterial supply, to drain into the superior mesenteric vein. The left colon venous drainage diverges from the arterial supply to drain into the inferior mesenteric vein. This vein passes behind the body of the pancreas to empty into the splenic vein to the left of the aorta; hence, the venous drainage of the left colon runs into a main trunk several centimeters to the left of the main arterial trunk.

In general, lymphatic drainage of the colon parallels the arterial supply. There are four groups of lymph nodes. The epicolic nodes are tiny nodules found along the wall of the bowel and in appendices epiploicae. The paracolic nodes lie along the mesenteric border of the bowel, and the intermediate colic nodes are found along the trunks of named vessels such as the middle colic artery. Finally, terminal colic nodes cluster at the main trunks of the inferior and superior mesenteric artery and are continuous with the paraaortic nodes. The rectum drains into pararectal lymph nodes in close proximity to the bowel wall and thence into nodes along the left colic artery or to the bifurcation of the common iliac arteries.

Laparoscopic Colostomy

Laparoscopic colostomy uses laparoscopic visual control to identify a mobile loop of colon (either transverse or sigmoid) capable of reaching to the abdominal wall. The laparoscope is passed through an umbilical portal, and a suitable loop of colon is identified. A site is chosen that will allow the colon to pass through the abdominal wall without tension and that will be easy for the patient to care for and maintain. A disk of skin and fascia is excised and a trocar is passed through this disk. The colon is grasped and exteriorized. Either a simple loop or a divided loop ostomy may be formed. The laparoscopist must visualize the bowel at the conclusion of the procedure to verify position and fixation.

Laparoscopic Colon Resection (Intraperitoneal)

The role of laparoscopic colon resection is still being defined. Both segmental and anatomic resections have been described. The site of the lesion must be clearly identified either by a preoperative barium study or (preferably) by marking or tattooing the bowel wall at the time of preoperative colonoscopy.

Usually, the laparoscope is passed through an umbilical portal. Multiple trocars are used, and it may be useful to position the patient with the legs spread to facilitate access to the upper abdomen (for mobilization of the flexures).

The right colon is mobilized by incising along the peritoneal reflection (visible as the "white line of Toldt") and sweeping the bowel medially (see Figs. 7-14 through 7-16). As this dissection progresses, the hepatic flexure must be mobilized. Frequently, small veins are noted in the vicinity of the hepatic flexure; hence division of the peritoneum in this region must be done with care. As the right transverse colon is mobilized, the duodenum will come into view and must be gently swept downward. The omentum will either be taken with the specimen or, more commonly, dissected off the transverse colon.

The splenic flexure is most easily mobilized if the peritoneum of the descending colon is divided (Figs. 8-13 to 8-15) and the omentum is swept upward. The remaining attachments to the spleen can then be divided under direct vision without danger of traction on the spleen (see Figs. 8-8 and 8-9). Behind the splenic flexure, Gerota's fascia overlying the left kidney comes into view (see Fig. 8-9).

The descending colon is readily mobilized by incising the peritoneal reflection (see Figs. 8-13 to 8-15). Muscles of the posterior abdominal wall and the left ureter come into view (see Figs. 8-14 and 8-15).

Laparoscopic Approach to the Rectum

Laparoscopic mobilization of the rectum first requires incision along the peritoneal reflection and then circumferential dissection much like that done during open surgery. The left ureter, ductus deferens, internal iliac artery, and middle rectal artery may be seen (Figs. 8-16 to 8-21).

The right ureter is also at risk and must be identified. It is often visible under the peritoneum as it crosses over the iliac artery at its bifurcation (see Fig. 8-5). Some laparoscopic surgeons use fiberoptic lighted ureteral stents to facilitate identification of the ureters. The areolar tissue surrounding the ureters and creating the sheath tends to be adherent to the peritoneum, so the ureter must be gently mobilized downward off the peritoneum as a flap of peritoneum is developed.

The sympathetic and parasympathetic nerves that innervate the bladder and genital organs run along the internal iliac vessels and line the pelvic sidewall. Damage to these nerves is best avoided by confining the plane of dissection to the region close to the bowel wall.

BIBLIOGRAPHY

Anatomic References

1. Garcia-Ruiz A, Milsom JW, Ludwin KA, Marchesa P. Right colonic arterial anatomy: implications for laparoscopic surgery. *Dis Colon Rectum* 1996;39:906–911.
2. Ger R. Surgical anatomy of the pelvis. *Surg Clin North Am* 1988;68:1201–1216.
3. Keighley MRB, Williams NS. Anatomy and physiology. In: Keighley MRB, Williams NS, eds. *Surgery of the anus, rectum, and colon.* London: WB Saunders, 1993:1–17.
4. Moskowitz M, Zimmerman H, Felson B. The meandering mesenteric artery of the colon. *Am J Roentgenol* 1964;92:1088–1099.
5. VanDamme J-PJ. Behavioral anatomy of the abdominal arteries. *Surg Clin North Am* 1993;73:699–725.
6. Wind GG. The colon. In: Wind GG, ed. *Applied laparoscopic anatomy: abdomen and pelvis.* Baltimore: Williams & Wilkins, 1997:217–246.

Surgical Techniques

1. Bogen GL, Mancino AT, Scott-Conner CEH. Laparoscopy for staging and palliation of gastrointestinal malignancy. *Surg Clin North Am* 1996;76:557–569.
2. Darzi A, Super P, Guillou PJ, Monson JR. Laparoscopic sigmoid colectomy: total laparoscopic approach. *Dis Colon Rectum* 1994;37:268–271.
3. Hoffman GC, Baker JW, Fitchett CW, Vansant JH. Laparoscopic-assisted colectomy: initial experience. *Ann Surg* 1994;219:732–743.
4. Lange V, Meyer G, Schardey HM, Schildberg FW. Laparoscopic creation of a loop colostomy. *J Laparoendosc Surg* 1991;1:307–312.
5. Lointier PH, Lautard M, Massoni C, Ferrier C, DaPoigny M. Laparoscopically assisted subtotal colectomy. *J Laparoendosc Surg* 1993;3:439–453.
6. Monson JRT, Darzi A, Carey PD, Guillou PJ. Prospective evaluation of laparoscopic-assisted colectomy in an unselected group of patients. *Lancet* 1992;340:831–833.
7. Phillips EH, Franklin M, Carroll BJ, Fallas MJ, Ramos R, Rosenthal D. Laparoscopic colectomy. *Ann Surg* 1992;216:703–707.
8. Stalter KD. Utilization of Silastic vessel loop to maintain visualization of a ureter during laparoscopic sigmoid colectomy. *J Laparoendosc Surg* 1994;4:289–290.
9. Wexner SD, Johansen OB, Nogueras JJ, Jagelman DG. Laparoscopic total abdominal colectomy: a prospective trial. *Dis Colon Rectum* 1992;35:651–655.

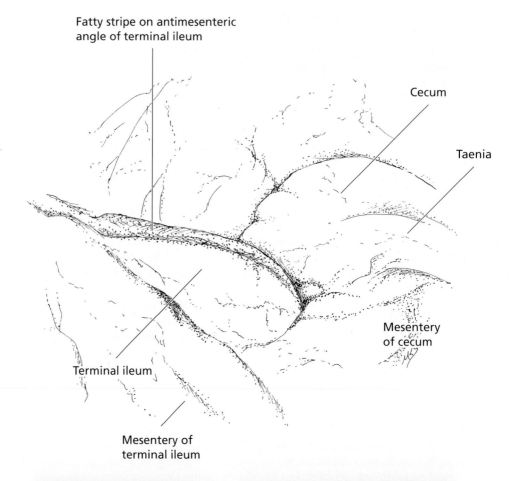

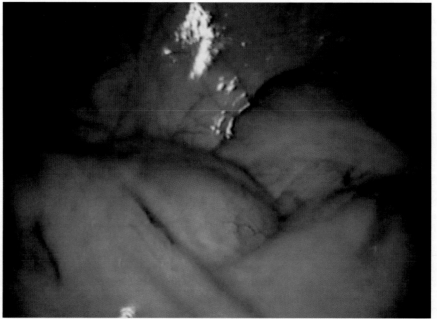

Fig. 8-1. Cecum and terminal ileum. The initial laparoscopic view of the right lower quadrant demonstrates the cecum and terminal ileum. Mesenteric fat obscures visualization of most of the circumference of the terminal ileum. Note the difference in color between the small and large intestine. One of the taeniae is visible.

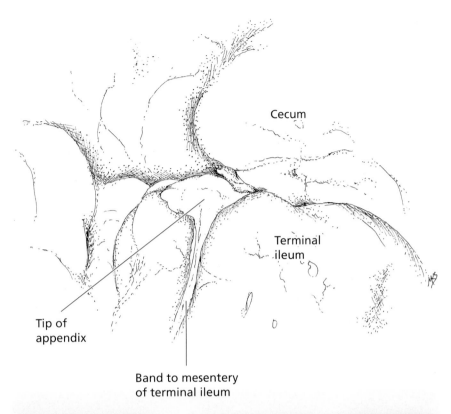

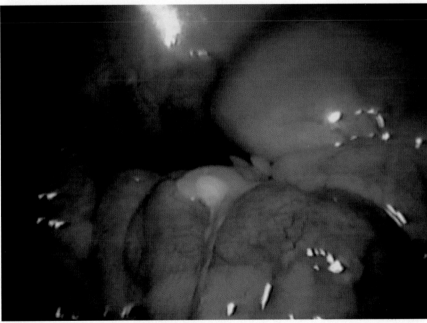

Fig. 8-2. Cecum and terminal ileum, tip of appendix. This view from another patient shows the tip of the appendix, tethered by a band that passes medially from the terminal ileum. The cecum and peritoneum of the abdominal wall occupy the background. The terminal ileum and associated mesentery are in the foreground.

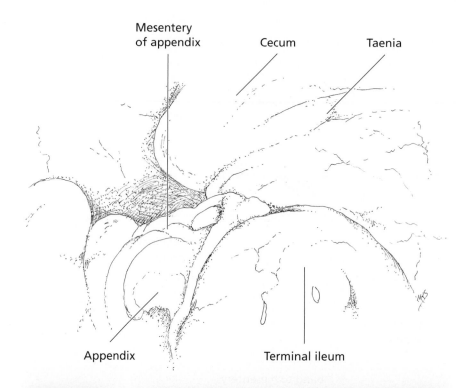

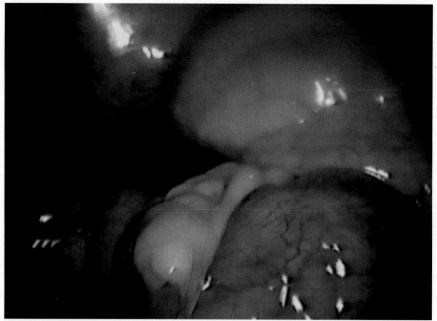

Fig. 8-3. Cecum and terminal ileum, appendix. Gentle traction on the band has elevated the appendix and cecum into better view. The cecum is seen to be asymmetrically enlarged, with prominence of the anterior sacculation. A taenia is visible. The terminal ileum and associated mesentery occupy the foreground.

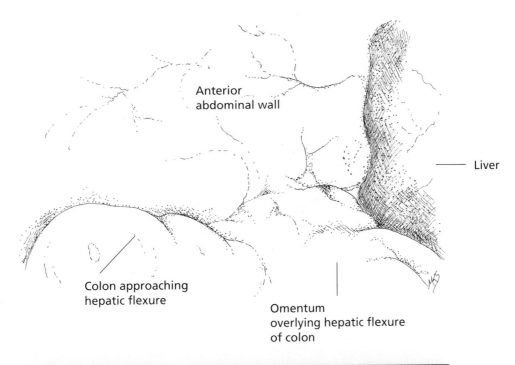

Anterior
abdominal wall

Liver

Colon approaching
hepatic flexure

Omentum
overlying hepatic flexure
of colon

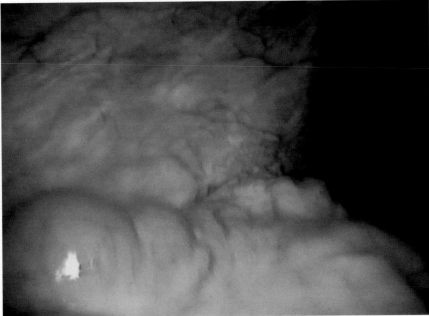

Fig. 8-4. Ascending colon at the hepatic flexure. Laparoscopic view of the ascending colon and hepatic flexure. The colon decreases in caliber as it makes transition from cecum to ascending colon. The hepatic flexure is obscured by overlying omentum. The liver is visible in the background.

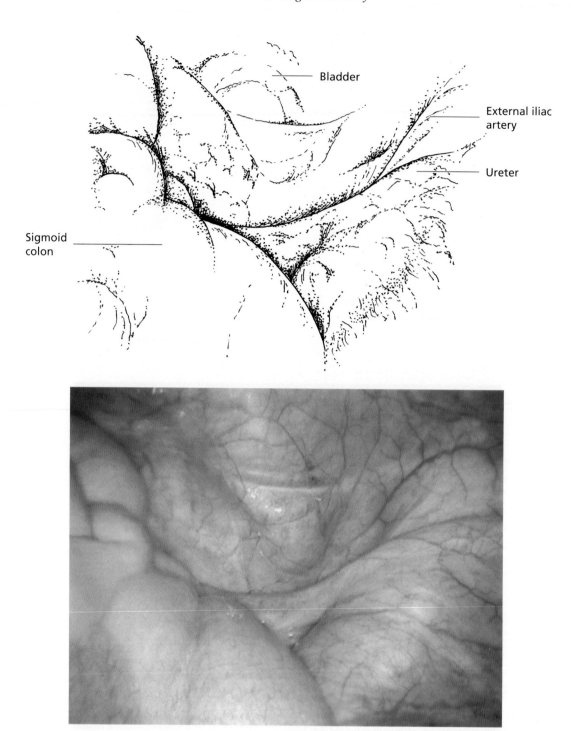

Fig. 8-5. Right ureter seen through the peritoneum. The right ureter is visualized through the intact peritoneum, crossing the iliac vessels on its way toward the bladder. The colon is seen in the foreground.

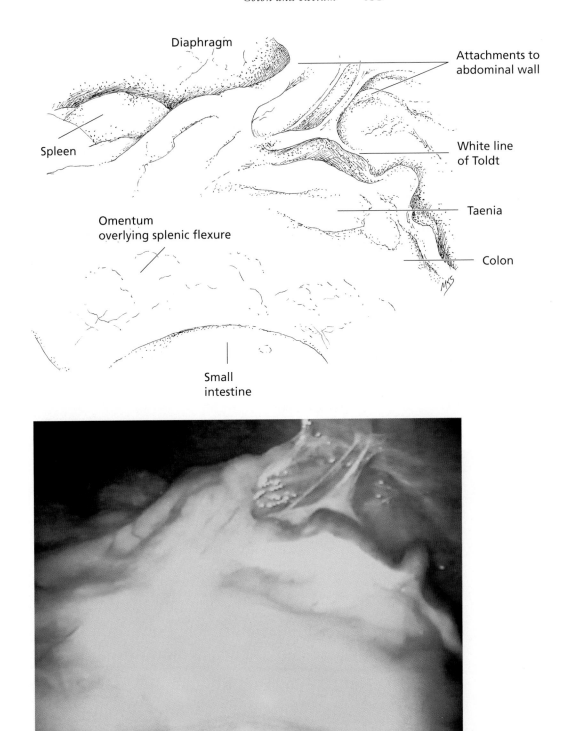

Fig. 8-6. Attachments of the splenic flexure to the anterior abdominal wall. The splenic flexure lies more cephalad and deeper in the abdomen than the hepatic flexure. This laparoscopic view was obtained with the patient turned so the left side faced upward, placing the splenic flexure and descending colon on traction, and illustrating the attachments to the lateral and anterior abdominal wall. The spleen and diaphragm are visible in the background.

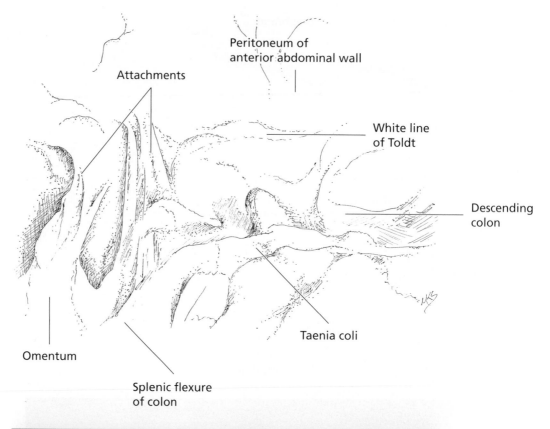

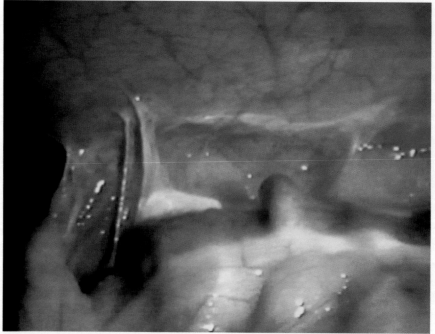

Fig. 8-7. Attachments of the splenic flexure and descending colon to the anterior abdominal wall. The white line of Toldt is visible, corresponding to the line of adherence of the colon. One of the taenia is seen.

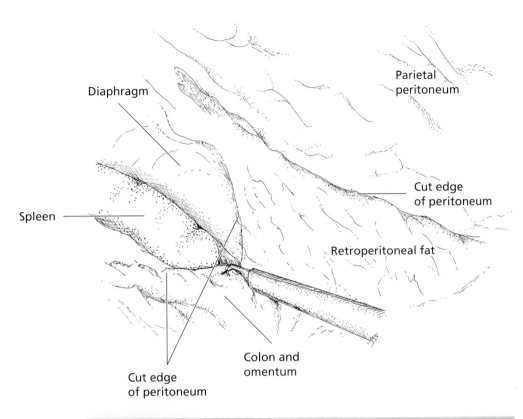

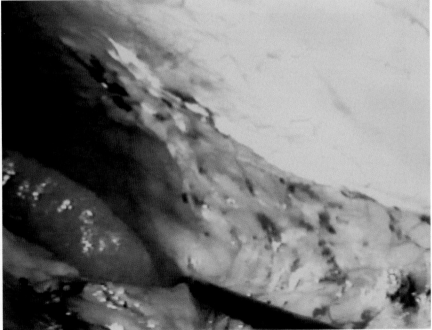

Fig. 8-8. Attachments of the splenic flexure to the spleen. The attachments of the splenic flexure to the anterior abdominal wall have been divided and the colon mobilized medially. The attachment of the splenic flexure to the spleen is being divided. The colon has been retracted medially and is out of view in the foreground. The diaphragm is visible in the background cephalad and lateral to the spleen.

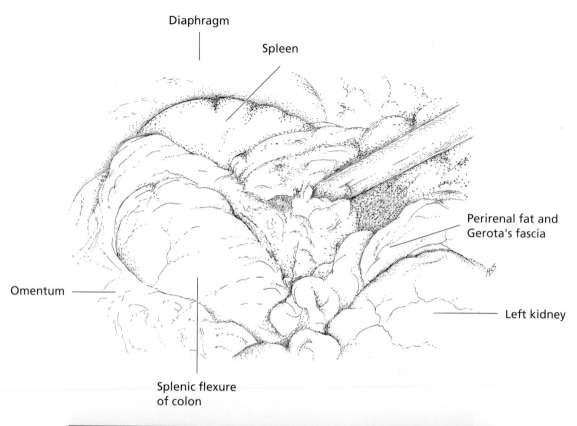

Diaphragm

Spleen

Perirenal fat and
Gerota's fascia

Omentum

Left kidney

Splenic flexure
of colon

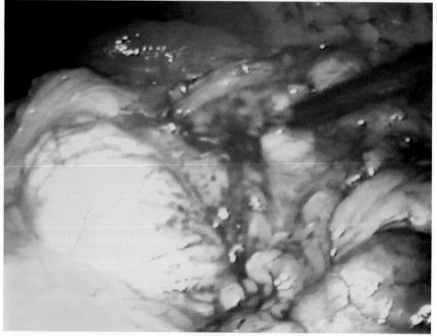

Fig. 8-9. Splenic flexure and descending colon being mobilized from Gerota's fascia. With further mobilization of the splenic flexure, Gerota's fascia and the left kidney come into view. The spleen, diaphragm, and anterior abdominal wall are visible in the background, and colon and omentum are in the foreground.

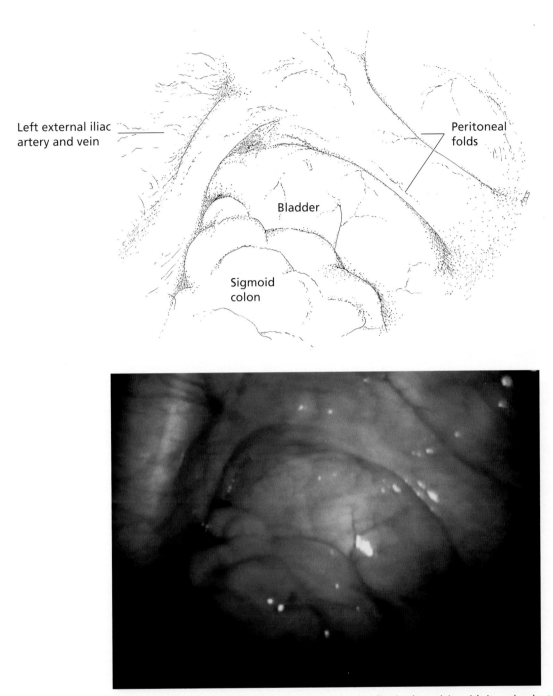

Left external iliac
artery and vein

Peritoneal
folds

Bladder

Sigmoid
colon

Fig. 8-10. Sigmoid colon in the male pelvis. The sigmoid colon lies in the pelvis, with its redundant portion touching the dome of the decompressed bladder. The lateral pelvic sidewall with iliac vessels is visible.

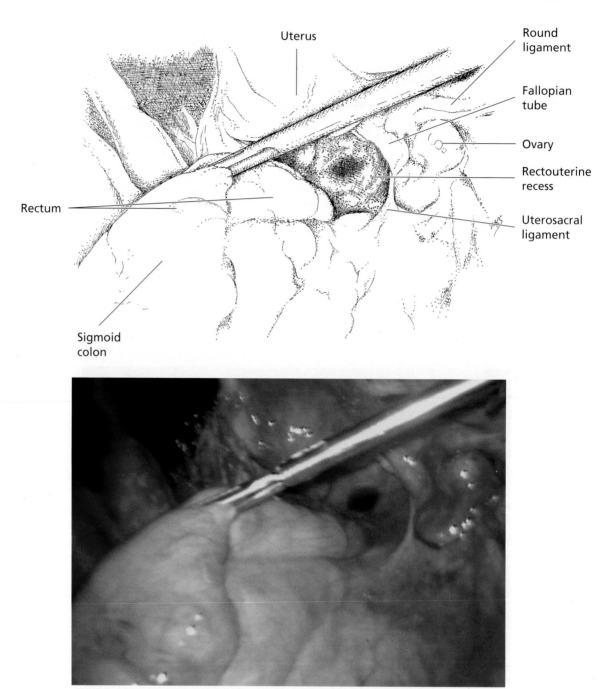

Fig. 8-11. Rectum descending into the female pelvis, rectouterine recess. The rectum begins where the tae-niae converge in the distal sigmoid colon. It is being elevated from the pelvis by gentle traction with an atrau-matic grasper. The rectouterine recess lies between the uterus and rectum. The uterus, ovary, round ligament, uterosacral ligament, and fallopian tube may be seen.

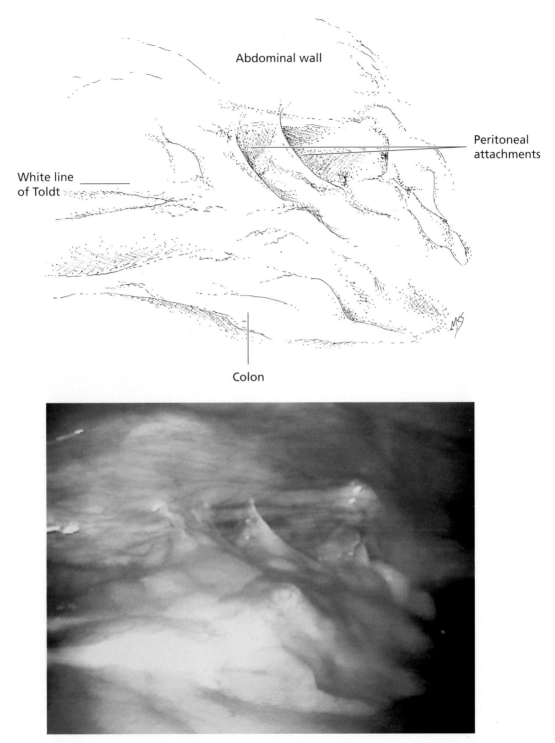

Fig. 8-12. Attachments of the descending and sigmoid colon. The attachments of the descending and sigmoid colon and the white line of Toldt are seen.

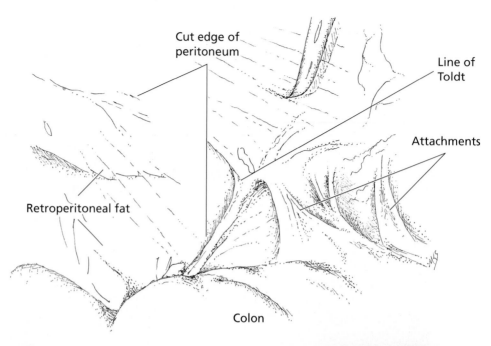

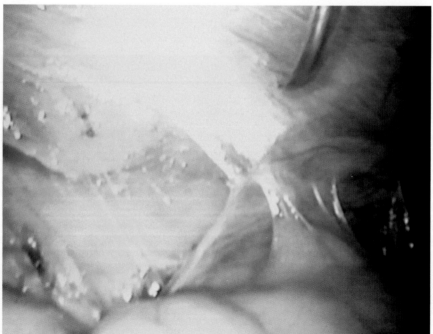

Fig. 8-13. Attachments of the descending colon. The white line of Toldt is being incised and the colon reflected medially. Attachments of the descending colon and sigmoid are visible to the right of the picture, where the incision has yet to be made.

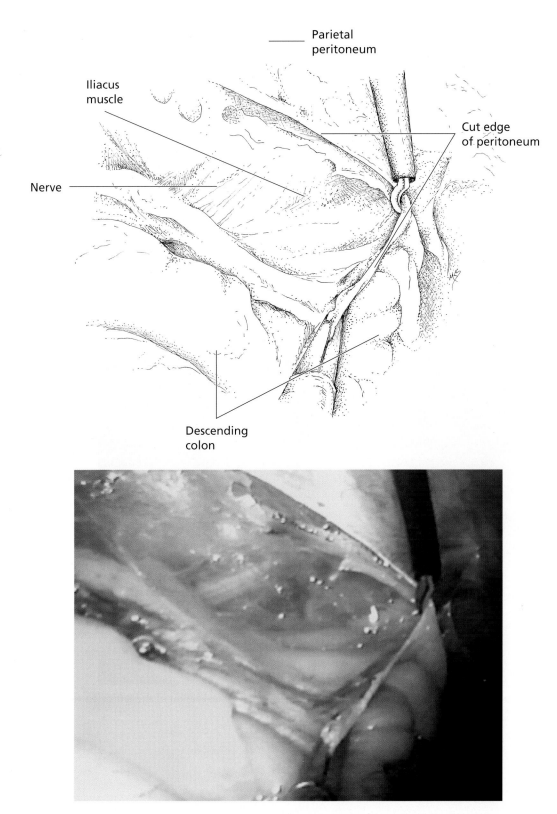

Parietal peritoneum

Iliacus muscle

Nerve

Cut edge of peritoneum

Descending colon

Fig. 8-14. Mobilization of the sigmoid colon to reveal underlying muscle and fascia. The incision of the white line of Toldt has been extended, and the colon is mobilized off the underlying iliacus muscle and fascia.

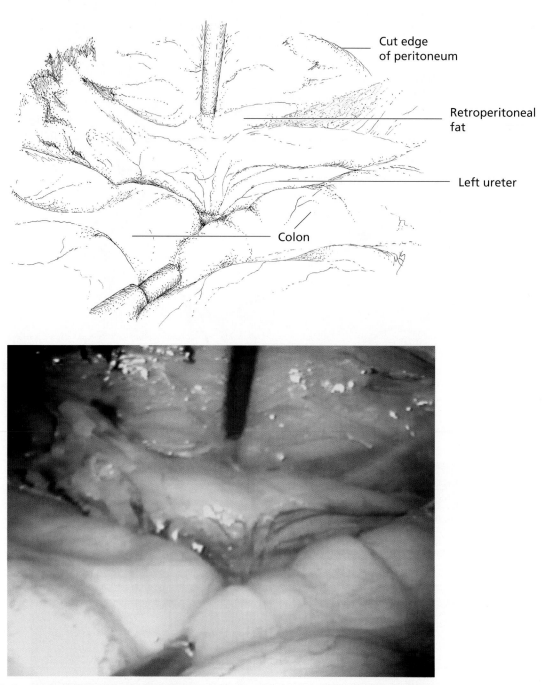

Fig. 8-15. Exposure of retroperitoneum under the left colon. Further mobilization of the left colon reveals retroperitoneal structures including left ureter.

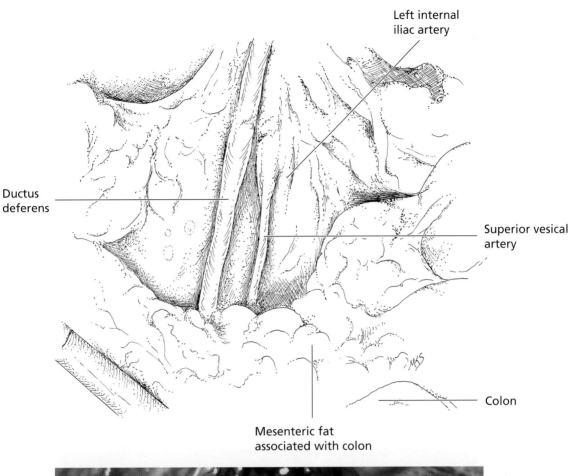

Left internal
iliac artery

Ductus
deferens

Superior vesical
artery

Colon

Mesenteric fat
associated with colon

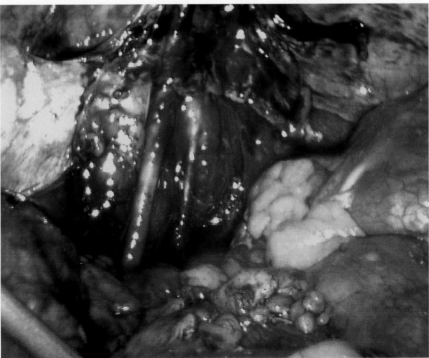

Fig. 8-16. Exposure of the left internal iliac artery and ductus deferens. The rectosigmoid has been mobilized to expose the left internal iliac artery and left ductus deferens along the pelvic sidewall. The colon is seen in the foreground. A small branch of the left internal iliac may be the superior vesical artery.

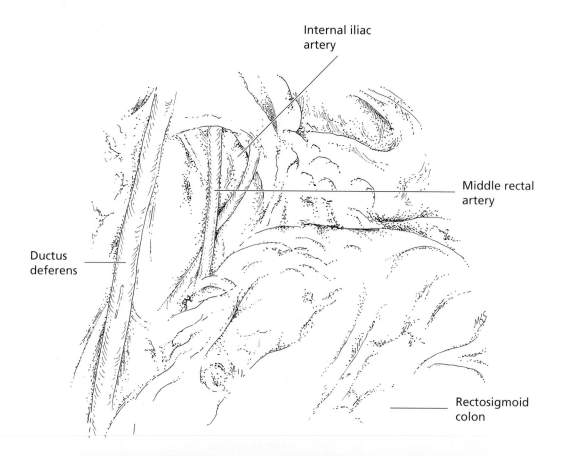

Internal iliac
artery

Middle rectal
artery

Ductus
deferens

Rectosigmoid
colon

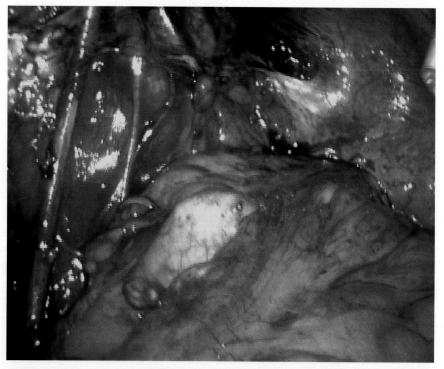

Fig. 8-17. Ductus deferens, internal iliac artery, middle rectal artery. The middle rectal artery is seen passing from the left internal iliac artery to the rectum. The rectosigmoid has been mobilized medially away from the pelvic sidewall.

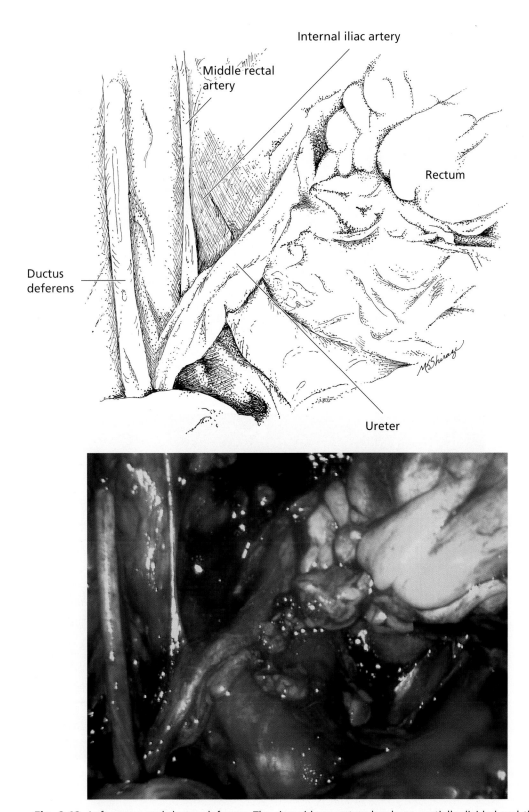

Fig. 8-18. Left ureter and ductus deferens. The sigmoid mesentery has been partially divided and the rectosigmoid retracted medially. The ureter is seen coursing toward the bladder. The ductus deferens is seen to the left of the frame.

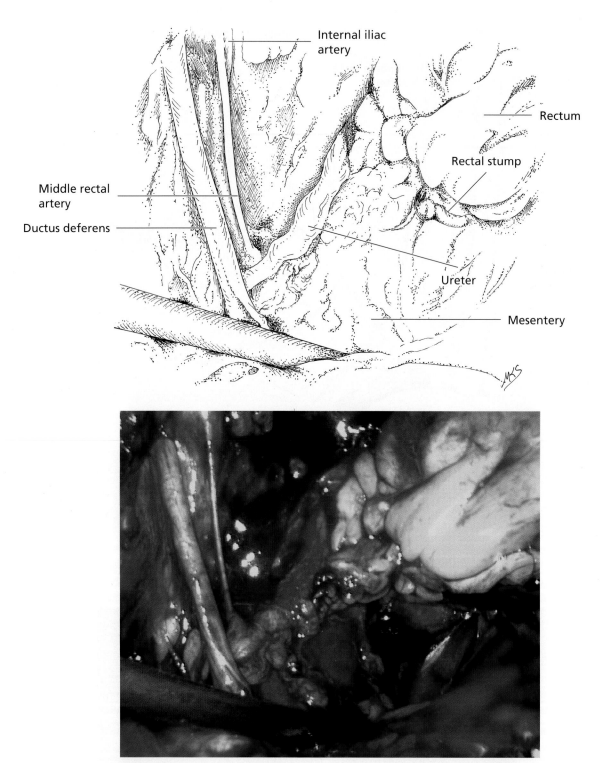

Fig. 8-19. Left ureter, ductus deferens, middle rectal artery, internal iliac artery. With the mesentery of the rectosigmoid divided and the rectosigmoid retracted medially away from the pelvic sidewall, the left ureter and ductus deferens are seen. The left internal iliac artery and middle rectal artery are noted.

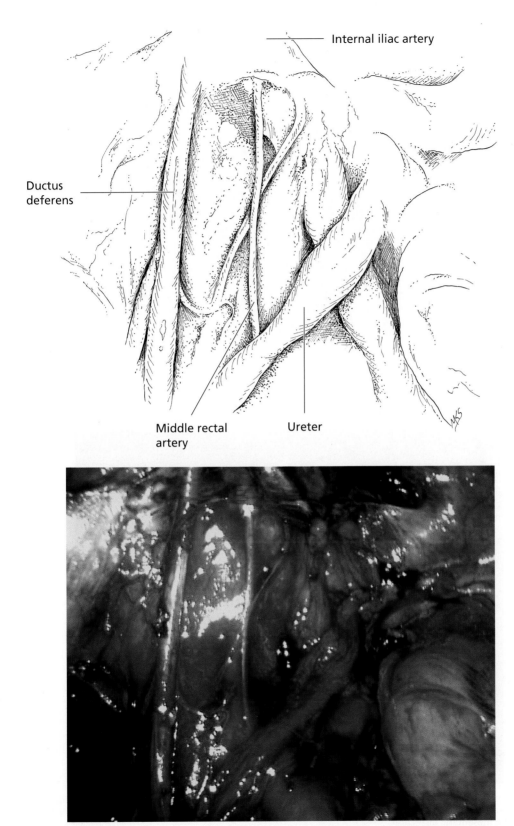

Fig. 8-20. Left ureter, ductus deferens, middle rectal artery. With further mobilization of the rectosigmoid, the ureter is more clearly seen.

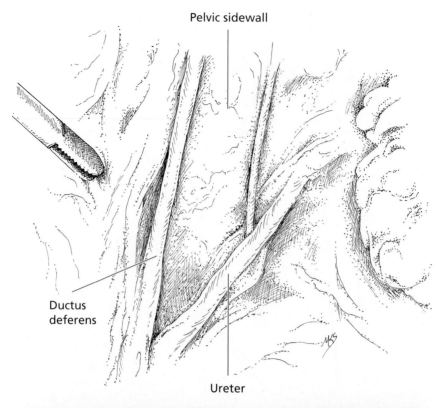

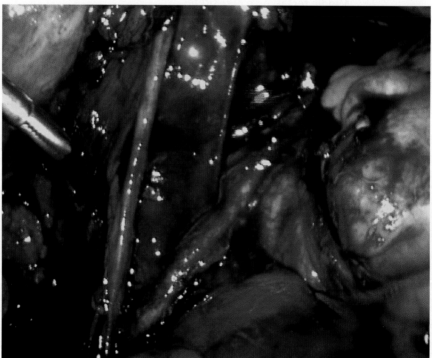

Fig. 8-21. Left ureter, ductus deferens. The rectosigmoid dissection has progressed with further mobilization of the bowel. The ureter is seen. Fatty areolar tissue containing nodes has been dissected off the pelvic sidewall with the mesenteric dissection.

9

PELVIS

SEAN P. HEDICAN

INITIAL LAPAROSCOPIC VIEW AND PRINCIPLES OF EXPOSURE

Laparoscopic visualization is typically obtained with an umbilically placed laparoscope. The patient is placed in steep Trendelenburg position, and loops of bowel are gently swept out of the pelvis. Gynecologic laparoscopists frequently place the patient in stirrups to facilitate access to the perineum. Pressure on the cervix can then be used to elevate the uterus and adnexae out of the pelvis. It is prudent to ensure that the patient's bladder is empty before pelvic laparoscopy. This serves to increase the working space and to minimize the chance of injury. Roll gauze can be wrapped around the scrotum to minimize pneumoscrotum in male patients.

ANATOMY AND SPECIFIC SURGICAL PROCEDURES

Because of the obvious differences in male and female pelvic anatomy, each is discussed separately. The simpler male pelvic anatomy is described first and forms a conceptual framework for the subsequent description of female pelvic anatomy.

Male Pelvis

Topographic Relations

The initial laparoscopic view of the male pelvis gives the impression of a spacious cavity, even though the male pelvis is relatively narrow (Fig. 9-1). The major topographic features are peritoneal folds or ligaments that subdivide the visual space and are thus extremely useful landmarks. These are discussed in detail in Chapter 1 and are briefly reviewed here from the standpoint of pelvic anatomy.

The location of the bladder can be inferred by the paired medial umbilical ligaments (see Figs. 1-8 to 1-11). These delineate the supravesical fossa. The bladder, typically collapsed by an indwelling bladder catheter or by preoperative straight catheterization, lies at the base of this fossa. The urachal remnant or median umbilical fold arises from the dome of the bladder and may also be visible (see Fig. 10-2).

The paired lateral umbilical folds correspond to the location of the inferior epigastric vessels (see Fig. 10-3). The space between the medial and lateral umbilical folds is the paravesical fossa. Although the lateral umbilical folds point to the medial edge of the internal inguinal ring, a more useful visual landmark is the convergence of the ductus deferens and gonadal vessels (Figs. 9-2 and 9-3). The detailed anatomy of the inguinal region and internal ring is discussed in Chapter 10. The lateral umbilical fossae overlie the internal rings and are lateral to the umbilical ligaments. Thus, indirect hernias exit the abdomen through the lateral umbilical fossae, and direct inguinal hernias exit through the paravesical fossa.

Posteriorly, the paired sacrogenital folds originate from the bladder and run laterally to the sacrum. The rectum (see Chapter 8) occupies the posterior portion of the male pelvis.

None of these folds or "ligaments" provide structural support to the pelvic organs. The actual supporting ligaments of the bladder include the lateral ligament (derived from pelvic fascia) and the puboprostatic and posterior ligaments. None of these structures are visible to the laparoscopist. The pelvic organs rest on the levator ani sling, which forms a musculofascial floor to the pelvic space.

Shiny peritoneum covers the surface of the pelvic viscera and sidewalls. The peritoneum dips down between bladder and rectum to form the rectovesical pouch. In thinner patients, the underlying superior aspects of the seminal vesicles may be visible as paired swellings beneath the peritoneum near the base of the bladder. The anterior layer of Denonvillier's fascia is not visible, but it may be conceptualized as an extension from the most extreme depth of the rectovesical pouch. This layer forms from residual extraperitoneal connective tissue that fuses in the space between the bladder and the rectum.

Ductus Deferens, Seminal Vesicles, and Bladder

The ductus deferens originates in the scrotum as a continuation of the duct of the epididymis, then ascends in the spermatic cord to enter the laparoscopic field of view at the internal ring. The presence of the ductus deferens at the internal ring is not sufficient evidence of descent of the testes out of the abdomen during laparoscopy for undescended testicle. The surgeon must visualize the gonadal vessels exiting the internal ring. The presence of blind-ending gonadal vessels is pathognomic for absence of the testis.

The internal ring is the visual apex of a triangle from which the ductus deferens and gonadal vessels diverge (see Figs. 9-2, 9-6, and 10-3 to 10-6). The ductus curves around the inferior epigastric vessels to pass medially (see Figs. 9-2 and 9-3; Figs. 9-4 and 9-5); the gonadal vessels pass laterally. From the laparoscopic perspective, the ductus crosses obliquely over the external iliac vessels to dive deep into the pelvis (see Figs. 8-16 to 8-21).

The ureter crosses under the ductus as both approach the bladder (see Figs. 8-18 to 8-21 and 9-4 and 9-5; Fig. 9-6). At the base of the bladder, in the extraperitoneal space and therefore invisible to the laparoscopist, the ureters enter the bladder, and the ductus deferens enters the seminal vesicles.

Arteries, Veins, and Lymphatic Drainage

The iliac arteries form a frame around the lateral rim of the pelvis. Both the common and external iliac arteries are visible by their position and prominent arterial pulsations (see Figs. 1-12 and 8-10). Large veins accompany the arteries but are less visible, particularly when collapsed because of the Trendelenburg position and elevated intraabdominal pressure. The veins are found deep and slightly lateral to the corresponding arteries.

The aorta bifurcates into common iliac arteries (see Fig. 8-5), which then bifurcate at approximately the level of the sacroiliac joint into internal and external iliac arteries. The external iliac arteries look like direct extensions of the common iliac arteries (see Figs. 1-10 and 1-12) and pass through, giving off few branches, to exit the pelvis at the femoral canal (see Figs. 10-8 to 10-10).

The internal iliac arteries provide most of the blood supply to the pelvis. From the anterior trunk of the internal iliac artery are derived the superior and inferior vesical arteries, the middle rectal artery, the uterine and vaginal arteries in the female, and the obturator artery. The obliterated umbilical artery or medial umbilical ligament arises at the continuation of the anterior trunk.

Lymphatic trunks accompany the named vessels, with groups of nodes named for the nearest contiguous major vessel. Because pelvic lymph node sampling and dissection are increasingly being performed laparoscopically, the anatomy of the pelvic nodes is discussed in some detail. In addition to anatomic knowledge of lymphatic pathways and major vessels, the laparoscopist must also know whether a diagnostic or therapeutic dissection is planned and for what malignancy. Often nodes are sampled to assess whether a patient is a candidate for definitive radiotherapy or extirpative surgery with curative intent. The laparoscopic surgeon must know which node group to sample to make the correct decision.

The lower extremities and perineum drain to superficial and deep inguinal nodes, well outside the laparoscopic field of view. The deep inguinal nodes and lymphatics pass through the femoral canal (see Fig. 10-12) into the pelvis to join the external iliac nodes, which then converge with internal iliac nodes to comprise the common iliac nodes. As the common iliac nodes converge and ascend medially, they join the paraaortic nodes. The external iliac nodes are subdivided into the following: an external group, which is found in the groove lateral to the external iliac artery, between that artery and the psoas major muscle; a middle group, which lies on the pelvic surface of the external iliac artery; and an internal group, which lies against the pelvic wall beneath the external iliac vein.

The obturator nodes are part of the internal iliac group (Figs. 9-7 to 9-14). They are laparoscopically important because involvement of these nodes may preclude radical resection for several neoplasms. These nodes are contiguous with the internal group of the external iliac nodes. The other nodes of the internal iliac group are found around the various branches of the internal iliac vessels (Fig. 9-15).

The key to laparoscopic identification of specific node groups is the identification of visual landmarks, and peritoneal templates that correspond to the desired excision groups have been described (see Bibliography). Packets of node-bearing tissue are dissected from underlying structures, which must be identified and protected. Injury to major veins, temporarily collapsed by the pressure of the pneumoperitoneum, may result in torrential hemorrhage when the intraabdominal pressure is lowered.

Two nerves are also at potential risk during these dissections. The genitofemoral nerve (see Figs. 11-12 to 11-14) runs on the psoas major muscle between the ureter (medially) and gonadal vessels (laterally). The obturator nerve leaves the medial border of psoas major muscle to pass beneath the iliac vessels near their bifurcation (see Figs. 9-9 to 9-13). This nerve is at risk during obturator node dissection. The ureter is also at risk, particularly as node dissection progresses proximally.

Pelvic Lymph Node Sampling or Dissection

Laparoscopic sampling or formal dissection can be used in any region of the iliac or paraaortic node chains. Lymph nodes are rarely identifiable unless enlarged, so the surgeon excises a packet of fat, lymphatics, and lymph nodes based on anatomic landmarks. Templates for the peritoneal incision and extent of dissection have been described for all the major node groups. References at the end of this chapter give additional information for specific malignancies. Obturator node dissection is described here.

The patient is positioned supine, and the laparoscopist stands to the contralateral side. It may be necessary to incise the peritoneal reflection and to mobilize the cecum (on the right) (see Figs. 7-14 and 7-15) or the sigmoid colon (on the left) to expose the retroperitoneum (see Figs. 8-12 to 8-15). The landmarks are as follows: the internal ring, visually identified by the convergence of ductus and gonadal vessels previously mentioned; the external iliac artery, visible by its pulsations; and the medial umbilical ligament. The pubic ramus is palpable to a probe or blunt grasper as an unyielding structure under the peritoneum and provides an additional laparoscopic landmark. The obturator node chain begins just lateral to the pubic ramus, overlying the bone. The limits of the dissection are the medial border of the external iliac vein and pelvic sidewall (laterally), the obturator nerve (posteriorly), the circumflex iliac vein (distally), and the point where the obturator nerve passes behind the external iliac vein (proximally). An incision is made in the peritoneum at the internal ring and carried proximal over the pulsation of the iliac artery (see Figs. 9-5 and 9-6). The ductus is divided below the internal ring to enhance exposure to the apex of the node packet (see Fig. 9-7). The obturator nerve, artery, and vein lie inferior to the pubic ramus along the posterior aspect of the obturator nodes and must be protected (see Figs. 9-8 to 9-10). An aberrant obturator vein (or artery, less common) running from the lower border of the external iliac vein straight down toward the obturator fossa should be assumed to be present, buried within the node packet, until proven otherwise (see Figs. 10-9, 10-19, and 10-20). Nodal tissue is detached and peeled away from the external iliac vein, artery, and obturator nerve. The internal iliac vein lies immediately deep to the dissection field. It is essentially invisible to the laparoscopist, but it can cause significant hemorrhage if it is torn. Dissection is terminated just posterior to the bifurcation of the common iliac vein (see Fig. 9-11).

More extended iliac dissections for bladder and urethral cancers are performed by beginning on both sides of the external iliac artery and working distally to proximally. The ureters must be identified and protected as they cross over the common iliac artery and vein just proximal to their bifurcation (see Figs. 8-5 and 8-18 to 8-21).

Female Pelvis

Topographic Relations

Although the female pelvis is wider than the male, the uterus and adnexal structures fill much of the space, creating a laparoscopic impression of crowding (see Fig. 2-15). Elevation of the uterus and adnexae by manipulation of the cervix from below or by traction on the round ligaments is crucial for enhanced exposure (see Fig. 8-11; Figs. 9-16 to 9-22). The uterus and adnexae visually divide the pelvic space. An anterior pelvic recess lies between the uterus and bladder. This relatively shallow fossa is termed the vesicouterine pouch or anterior cul-de-sac. A much deeper peritoneal recess lies posterior to the uterus, between it and the rectum. This is the rectouterine pouch (of Douglas) or posterior cul-de-sac (see Figs. 9-16 and 9-17). This is not only significant as a site of metastatic deposits, but also as a site sometimes used for specimen removal by posterior colpotomy.

In addition to the umbilical ligaments, several ligaments are associated with the uterus and adnexae. Most obvious are the round ligaments, which extend from the uterus just inferior to the junction with the fallopian tube in a curvilinear fashion to each internal ring (see Figs. 9-16 through 9-22). At the internal ring, the round ligaments exit through the inguinal canal in a manner analogous to the ductus deferens. Thus, the attachment of the round ligament to the pelvic sidewall is a useful visual landmark to the location of the internal ring in the female patient. The round ligaments must be distinguished from the fallopian tubes, which are generally pinker and lie below the round ligaments (see Figs. 9-17, 9-18, and 9-22).

Peritoneum covers the round ligaments and passes down to the pelvic floor on each side of the uterus, encasing the broad ligaments. These peritoneal layers come in closest apposition along the lateral walls of the uterus. Progressing inferiorly, the peritoneal layers diverge, becoming continuous with peritoneum of the vesicouterine and rectouterine pouches. Structures of importance in the broad ligaments are the uterine arteries and ureters. These peritoneal ligaments are crucial visual landmarks and must be divided during many gynecologic procedures, but they provide little actual support. Structural support for the pelvic organs comes from the pelvic and urogenital diaphragms and the uterosacral ligaments. Additional ligaments are described with the adnexal structures.

Uterus, Ovaries, and Fallopian Tubes

The normal nonpregnant uterus is approximately 8 cm in length and angled forward so the fundus lies over the posterior surface of the bladder. It is covered with peritoneum, except where the bladder touches the lower uterine segment at the anterior cul-de-sac and laterally at the broad ligaments.

The adnexal structures (ovaries, fallopian tubes) and broad ligaments lie lateral to the uterus. In order, from anterior to posterior, the round ligaments, fallopian tubes, and ovaries are seen. The ovaries are generally obvious laparoscopically because of their whiteness and knobby texture and because they hang down into the laparoscopic field. A normal ovary is white, almond-shaped, and approximately 3 cm in greatest dimension. The ovaries attach to the pelvic sidewall by the infundibulopelvic ligaments (which convey the gonadal vessels). The ovarian ligaments run from the ovaries to the lateral border of the uterus (see Figs. 9-20 and 9-22).

The fallopian tubes arise from the superior portion of the uterus just above the attachment points of the round ligament. Laparoscopically, the round ligaments tend to overhang the fallopian tubes and can be easily mistaken for them. The fallopian tubes curve out laterally to encircle the ovaries partially with their fimbriated ends.

Arteries, Veins, and Lymphatic Drainage

In addition to the vessels previously discussed with regard to the male pelvis (see earlier), the uterine and ovarian arteries are of great significance to the gynecologic laparoscopist. The uterine arteries arise from the internal iliacs in a variable fashion, and they pass medially on the levator ani, crossing over the ureter and ultimately dividing into ascending and descending branches. These trunks run in a tortuous but approximately parallel course to the uterus and vagina within the broad ligament. These vessels must be identified and secured in the course of laparoscopic-assisted vaginal hysterectomy. The ascending branch of the uterine artery terminates by anastomosing with the ovarian artery in the hilus of the ovary.

The ovarian (gonadal) arteries arise from the aorta to descend lateral to the ureter and genitofemoral nerve. The artery and accompanying veins cross over the external and internal iliac vessels to enter the pelvis. The left ovarian vein drains into the left renal vein, the right into the inferior vena cava.

Lymph node drainage of the upper vagina is to the common iliac nodes. The uterine cervix drains to all three iliac node groups, the uterine corpus drains to external iliac and paraaortic nodes, and the ovaries drain to either iliac or paraaortic nodes. The obturator nodes receive lymphatics from the cervix and uterus. Nodes in the sacral concavity also receive branches from the cervix and uterus.

The ureters enter the pelvis in close proximity to the female pelvic organs and are at risk for injury during laparoscopic surgery of this region. Intimate knowledge of pelvic anatomy and careful identification of the ureters are crucial. As the ureters course medially over the bifurcation of the iliac vessels, they pass obliquely under the ovarian vessels and then run in close proximity to the uterine artery. The right ureter actually forms the posterior limit of the right ovarian fossa.

Gynecologic Laparoscopy

Laparoscopy has been part of the gynecologic armamentarium for a long time, and a large body of literature is available describing these procedures. Laparoscopic surgery of adnexal structures is straightforward. In order, from anterior to posterior, the following tubular structures are encountered crossing the brim of the true pelvis: the round ligament of the uterus, the infundibulopelvic ligament (which contains the gonadal vessels), and the ureter. The ovary and fallopian tubes lie between the round ligaments and the infundibulopelvic ligaments. The main perils in laparoscopic adnexal surgery are mistaking the round ligament for the fallopian tube (which should not occur if the laparoscopic surgeon simply traces each structure proximal and distal and is aware of the possibility) and injury to the ureter during dissection of the infundibulopelvic ligaments. Deviation of the uterus to the contralateral side spreads out the structures of this region, creating the pelvic sidewall triangle (see Figs. 9-17 and 9-18) and facilitating identification. The base of this triangle is the round ligament; the medial side is the infundibulopelvic ligament, and the lateral side is the external iliac artery. The apex of the triangle is the point at which the infundibulopelvic ligament crosses the external iliac artery. The ureter enters the pelvis medial to this triangle and may be visible under the peritoneum overlying the external iliac artery (see Fig. 9-16).

Laparoscopic hysterectomy requires careful dissection in the retroperitoneum. An incision is made in the peritoneum overlying the pelvic sidewall triangle, between the fallopian tubes (medially) and the iliac vessels laterally. The ureter is identified and mobilized medially, away from the uterine vessels, which are mobilized laterally. Details of this dissection are given in Kadar (see Bibliography).

Pelvic node dissection may be included as part of a radical hysterectomy or as a separate sampling or dissection procedure. Nodes as far distal as Cloquet's node (in the femoral triangle) may be included (see Fig. 10-12), and dissection may be carried proximally to include the paraaortic nodes. Standing between the patient's legs facilitates the proximal part of the dissection.

BIBLIOGRAPHY

Anatomic References

1. Ger R. Surgical anatomy of the pelvis. *Surg Clin North Am* 1988;68:1201–1216.
2. Hinman F. *Atlas of urosurgical anatomy.* Philadelphia: WB Saunders, 1993:517–524.
3. Kadar N. Surgical anatomy and dissection techniques for laparoscopic surgery. *Curr Opin Obstet Gynecol* 1996;8:266–277.
4. Scott-Conner CEH, Dawson DL. *Operative anatomy.* Philadelphia: JB Lippincott, 1993:489–495.
5. Wind GG. *Applied laparoscopic anatomy: abdomen and pelvis.* Baltimore: Williams & Wilkins, 1997:249–299.

Surgical References

1. Canis M, Mage G, Chapron C, Wattiez A, Pouly JL, Bruhat MA. Laparoscopic hysterectomy: a preliminary study. *Surg Endosc* 1993;7:42–45.
2. Das S. Laparoscopic staging pelvic lymphadenectomy: extraperitoneal approach. *Semin Surg Oncol* 1996;12:134–138.
3. Gill IS. Laparoscopic pelvic lymphadenectomy: transperitoneal approach. *Semin Surg Oncol* 1996;12:126–133.
4. Grainger DA, Soderstom RM, Schiff SF, et al. Ureteral injuries at laparoscopy: insights into diagnosis, management, and prevention. *Obstet Gynecol* 1990;75:839–844.
5. Griffith DP, Schuessler WW, Nickell KG, Meaney JT. Laparoscopic pelvic lymphadenectomy for prostatic adenocarcinoma. *Urol Clin North Am* 1992;2:407–415.
6. Hass CA, Resnick MI. Laparoscopic pelvic and para-aortic/retroperitoneal lymph node dissection. *Semin Laparosc Surg* 1996;3:63–74.
7. Hsieh Y-Y, Lin W-C, Chang C-C, Yeh L-S, Hsu T-Y, Tsai H-D. Laparoscopic radical hysterectomy with low paraaortic, subaortic, and pelvic lymphadenectomy: results of short-term follow-up. *J Reprod Med* 1998;43:528–534.
8. Maher PJ, Wood EC, Hill DJ, Lotatgis NA. Laparoscopically-assisted hysterectomy. *Med J Aust* 1992;156:316–318.
9. Melvin WS, Blumgardner GI, Davies EA, Elkhammas EA, Henry ML, Ferguson RM. The laparoscopic management of post-transplant lymphocele: a critical review. *Surg Endosc* 1997;11:245–248.
10. Parker WH. Management of adnexal masses by operative laparoscopy: selection criteria. *J Reprod Med* 1992;37:603–606.
11. Possover M, Krause N, Plaul K, Kuhne-Heid R, Schneider A. Laparoscopic para-aortic and pelvic lymphadenectomy: experience with 150 patients and review of the literature. *Gynecol Oncol* 1998;71:19–28.
12. Reich H, McGlynn F, Sekel L, Taylor P. Laparoscopic management of ovarian dermoid cysts. *J Reprod Med* 1992;37:640–644.
13. Saye WA, Cohen MB, Winfield HN. Inverted V peritoneotomy significantly improves nodal yield in laparoscopic pelvic lymphadenectomy. *J Urol* 1993;149:772–775.
14. Shingleton WB. Laparoscopic pelvic lymphadenectomy. *Surg Clin North Am* 1996;76:585–593.
15. Spiritos NM, Schlaerth JB, Kimball RE, Leiphart VM, Ballon SC. Laparoscopic radical hysterectomy (type III) with aortic and pelvic lymphadenectomy. *Am J Obstet Gynecol* 1996;174:1763–1768.
16. Summit RL, Stovall TG, Libscomb GH, Ling FW. Randomized comparison of laparoscopy-assisted vaginal hysterectomy with standard vaginal hysterectomy. *Obstet Gynecol* 1992;80:895–901.

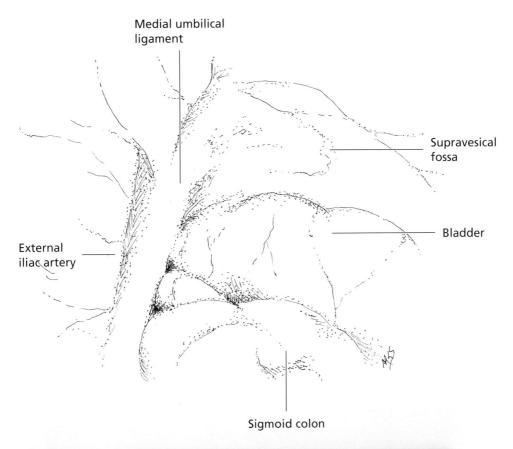

Medial umbilical
ligament

Supravesical
fossa

Bladder

External
iliac artery

Sigmoid colon

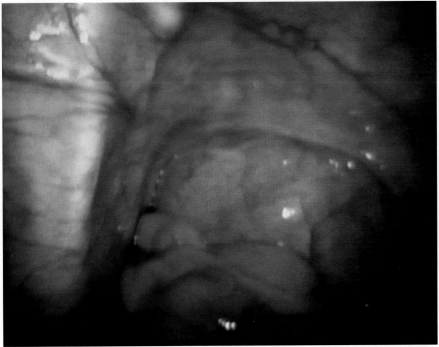

Fig. 9-1. View of the male pelvis. To the left, the external iliac artery is visible under the parietal peritoneum. The medial umbilical ligament arches upward, defining the left side of the supravesical fossa. The bladder is seen at the base of the supravesical fossa. The sigmoid colon occupies the foreground.

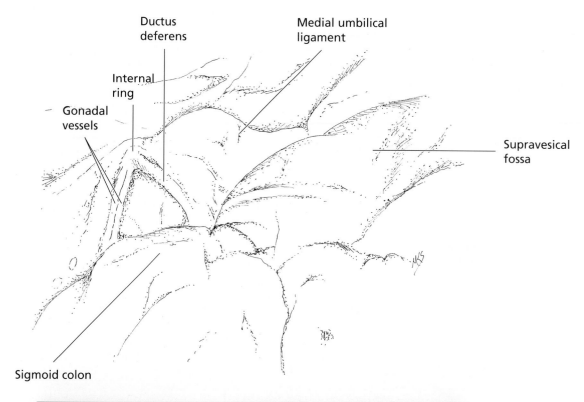

Ductus deferens

Medial umbilical ligament

Internal ring

Gonadal vessels

Supravesical fossa

Sigmoid colon

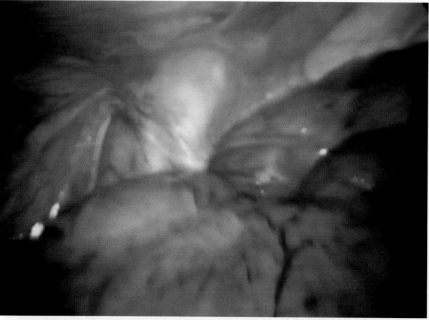

Fig. 9-2. Left internal ring, ductus deferens, gonadal vessels, and medial umbilical ligament. The gonadal vessels and ductus deferens are seen to converge at the internal ring, which is at the apex of a triangle. The sigmoid colon is in the foreground. The medial umbilical ligament defines the supravesical fossa, seen to the extreme right.

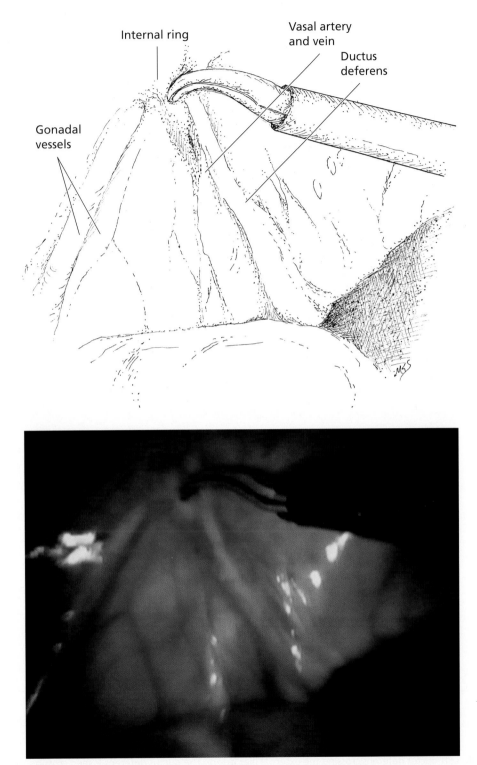

Fig. 9-3. Left internal ring. The ductus deferens and gonadal vessels form the apex of a triangle that points to the internal ring. The sigmoid colon is seen in the foreground, and the supravesical fossa is seen to the right. The vasal artery and vein may be seen accompanying the ductus deferens.

Ductus deferens

Transverse
peritoneal fold

External iliac
artery

Supravesical fossa

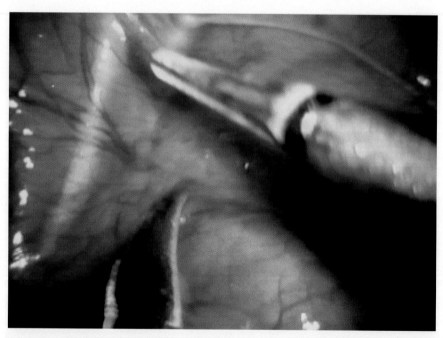

Fig. 9-4. Left ductus deferens crossing the external iliac artery. The ductus deferens is seen crossing the external iliac artery. Peritoneum of the supravesical fossa has been drawn into a transverse fold (of no anatomic significance) to the right. These folds frequently appear during laparoscopy and should not be confused with fixed anatomic structures such as the medial umbilical ligament.

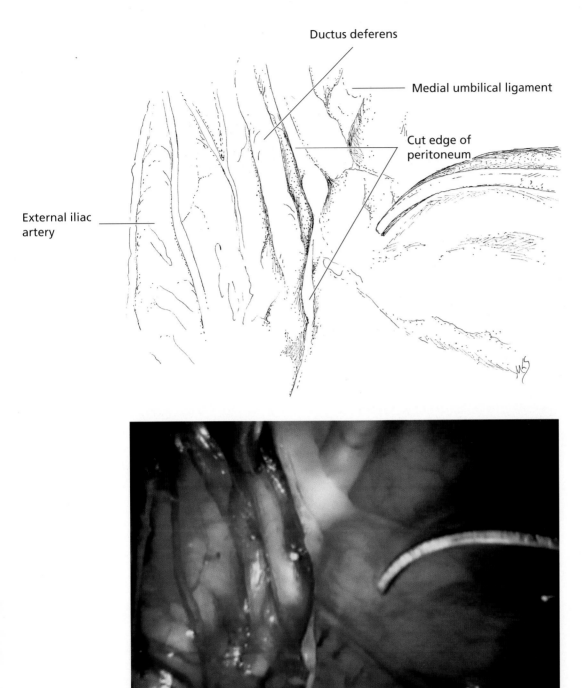

Ductus deferens

Medial umbilical ligament

Cut edge of peritoneum

External iliac artery

Fig. 9-5. Left ductus deferens and external iliac artery. The peritoneum has been incised for obturator node dissection, exposing the ductus deferens. This incision is made along the peritoneal surface of the external iliac artery, and a flap of peritoneum is developed medially, allowing the medial umbilical ligament to be reflected medially to expose the contents of the obturator foramen.

Cut edge of peritoneum

Medial umbilical ligament

Ductus deferens

Gonadal vessels

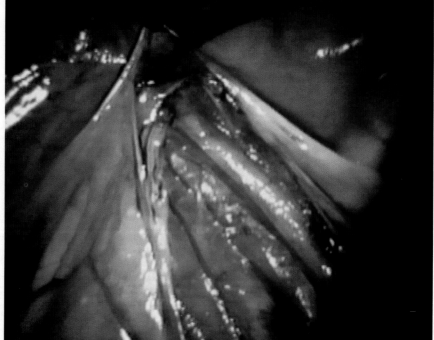

Fig. 9-6. Left internal ring with the peritoneum removed. Cephadal traction on the peritoneal incision reveals the convergence of the gonadal vessels and ductus deferens on the internal ring. The medial umbilical ligament is seen to the right.

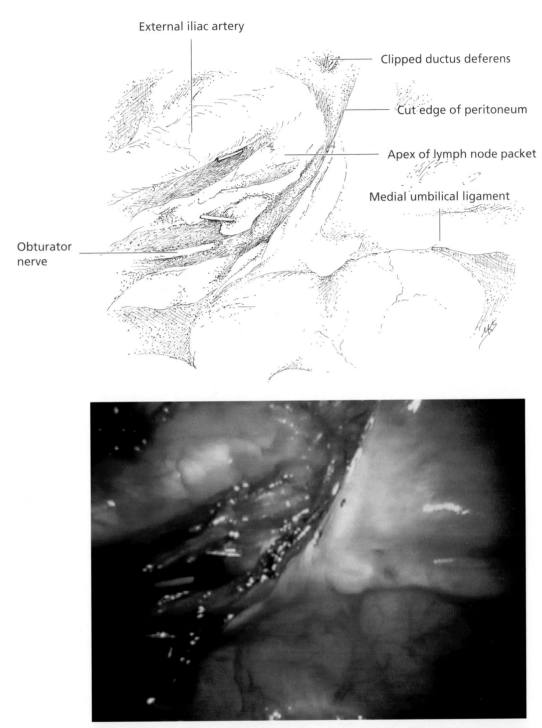

External iliac artery

Clipped ductus deferens

Cut edge of peritoneum

Apex of lymph node packet

Medial umbilical ligament

Obturator nerve

Fig. 9-7. Apex of the obturator node packet (left side). The ductus deferens has been divided and a segment excised to improve exposure. The distal end of the ductus is visible near the apex of the dissection. The external iliac artery forms one boundary of the dissection. The apex of the node packet is identified near the ductus. The obturator nerve can be glimpsed beneath the node packet. The medial umbilical ligament is noted to the right, forming another boundary of the dissection.

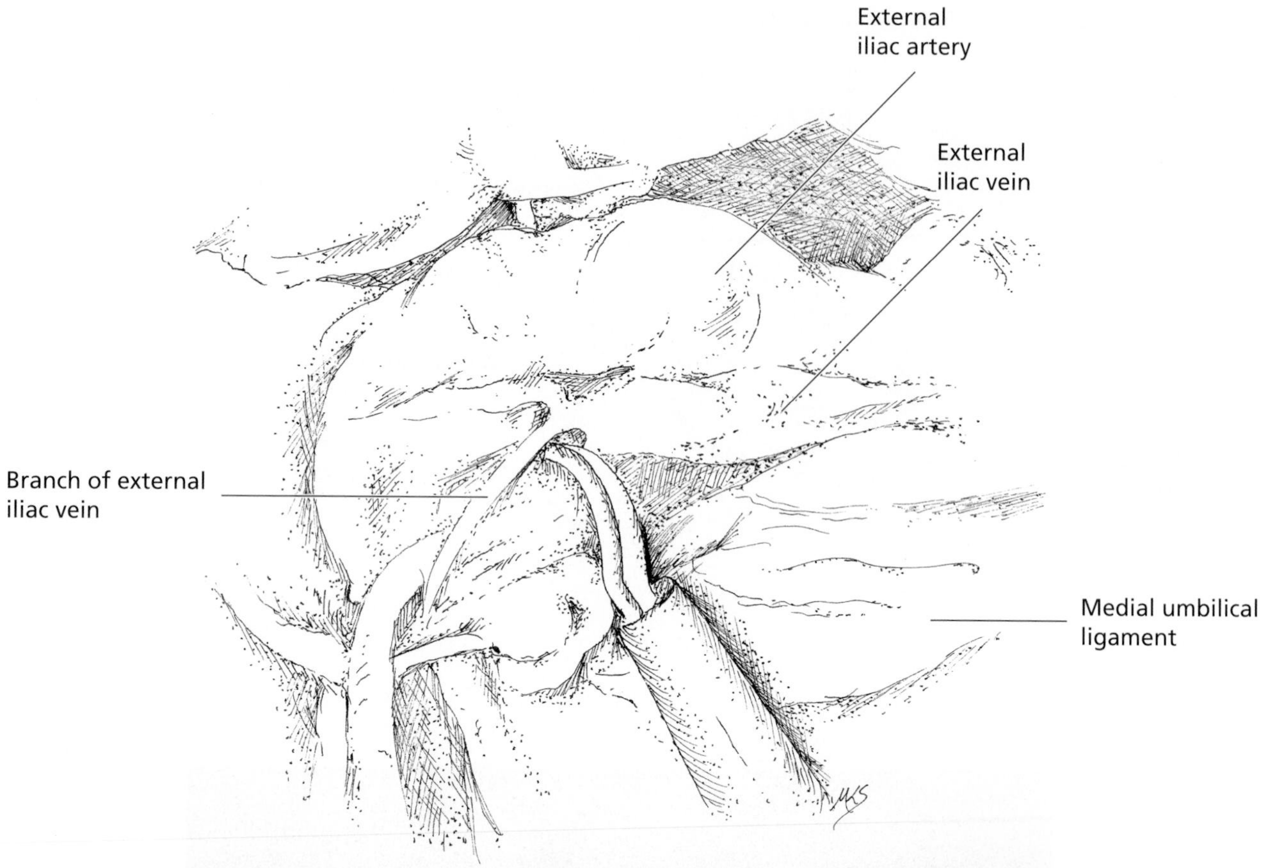

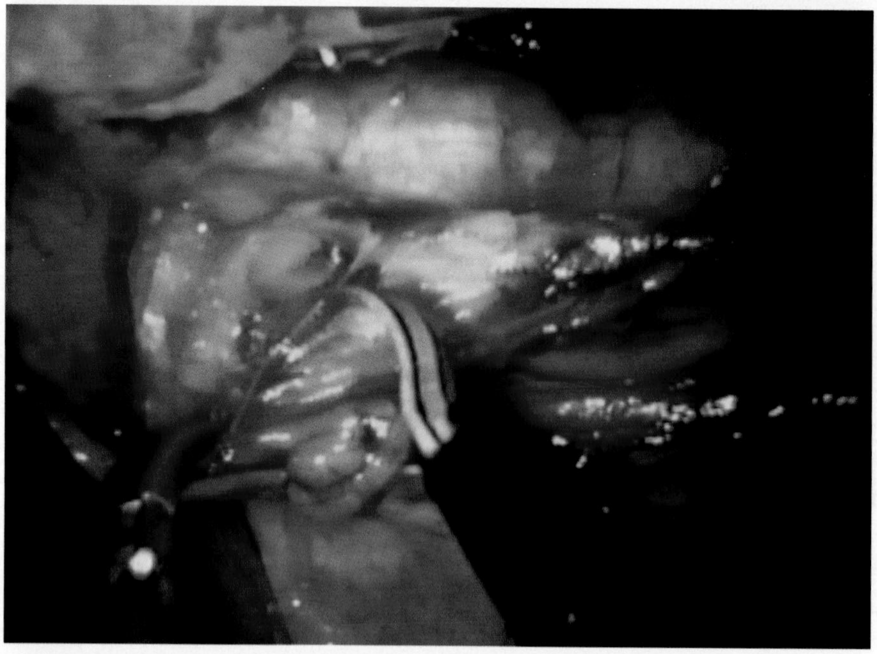

Fig. 9-8. Node packet being separated from the external iliac vein (left side). The external iliac vein is glimpsed deep to the external iliac artery. A small branch of the external iliac vein to the node packet is being defined and must be secured. Dissection will progress proximal, peeling the node packet out from beneath the external iliac artery and vein.

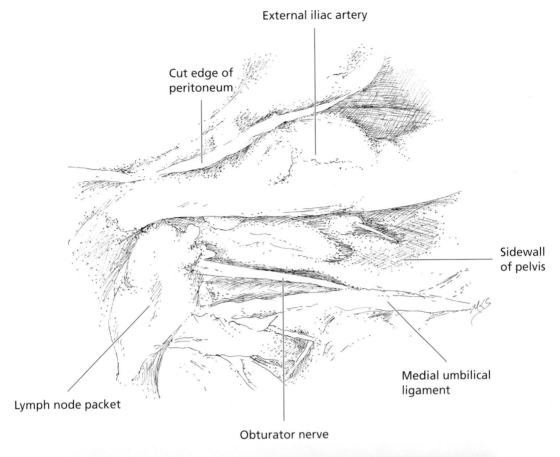

External iliac artery

Cut edge of
peritoneum

Sidewall
of pelvis

Medial umbilical
ligament

Lymph node packet

Obturator nerve

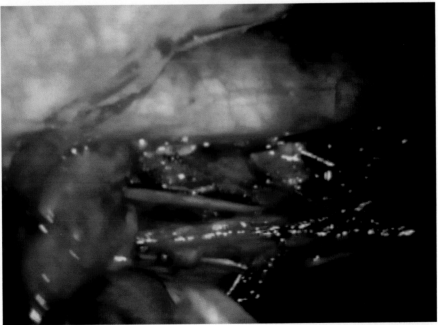

Fig. 9-9. Obturator nerve exposed (left side). The lymph node packet is being retracted downward to continue the dissection proximal. The external iliac artery is clearly seen; the external iliac vein is deep to the artery and is not visible. The floor of the dissection is the pelvic sidewall. The medial umbilical ligament is seen.

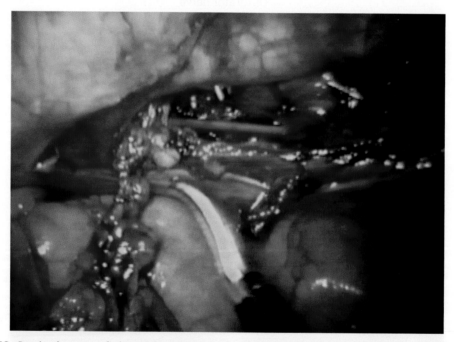

Fig. 9-10. Proximal extent of obturator node dissection (left side). The external iliac artery and obturator nerve are well seen. The medial umbilical ligament is obscured by the cut edge of the peritoneum, which overlies this important landmark.

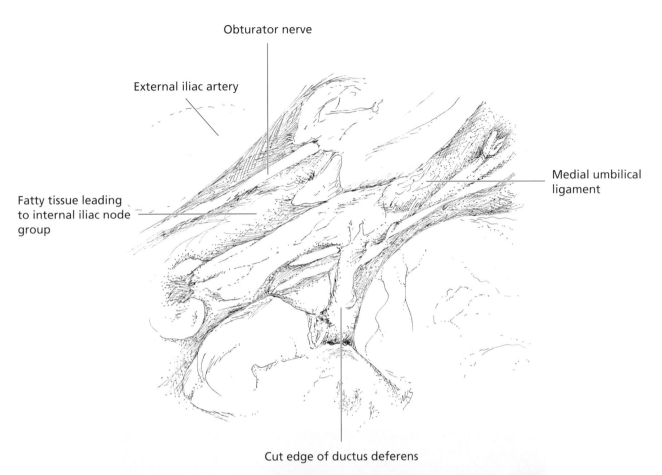

Obturator nerve

External iliac artery

Medial umbilical ligament

Fatty tissue leading to internal iliac node group

Cut edge of ductus deferens

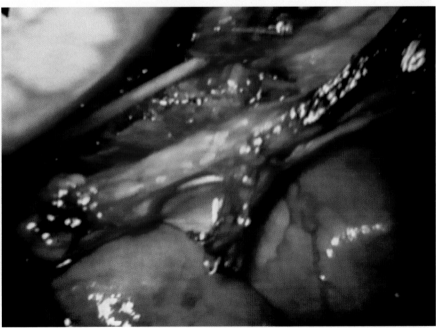

Fig. 9-11. Left obturator nerve, internal iliac node group (view with 30-degree laparoscope). At completion of the obturator node dissection, the fatty tissue connecting the obturator nodes with the deeper internal iliac node group may be seen. The divided end of the ductus deferens lies in the foreground, crossing the medial umbilical ligament.

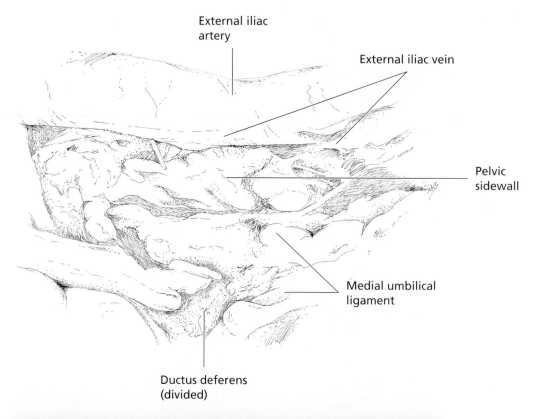

External iliac
artery

External iliac vein

Pelvic
sidewall

Medial umbilical
ligament

Ductus deferens
(divided)

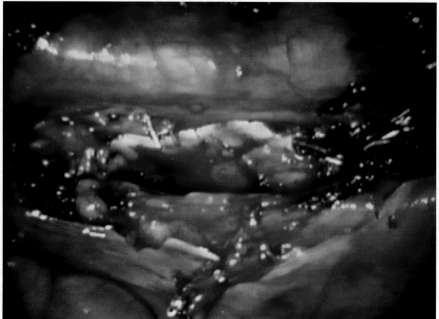

Fig. 9-12. Left obturator nerve, external iliac artery and vein. The external iliac vein may be glimpsed deep to the external iliac artery. The divided end of the ductus deferens and the medial umbilical ligament are seen.

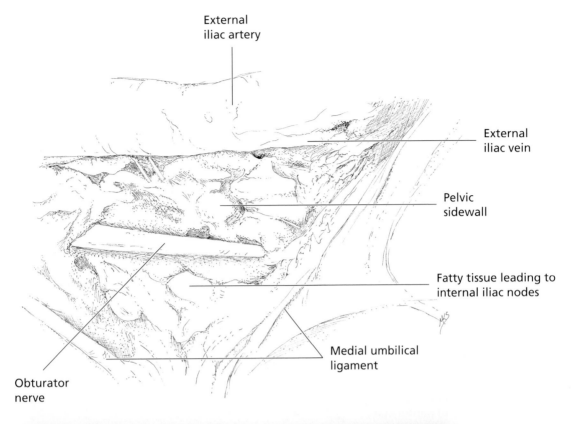

External
iliac artery

External
iliac vein

Pelvic
sidewall

Fatty tissue leading to
internal iliac nodes

Medial umbilical
ligament

Obturator
nerve

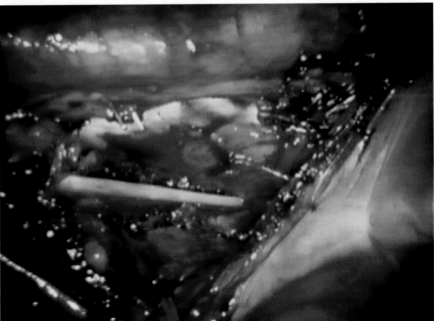

Fig. 9-13. Left obturator nerve, external iliac artery and vein. Traction on the medial umbilical ligament reveals the obturator nerve (after obturator node dissection), pelvic sidewall, and fatty tissue leading to the internal iliac node group.

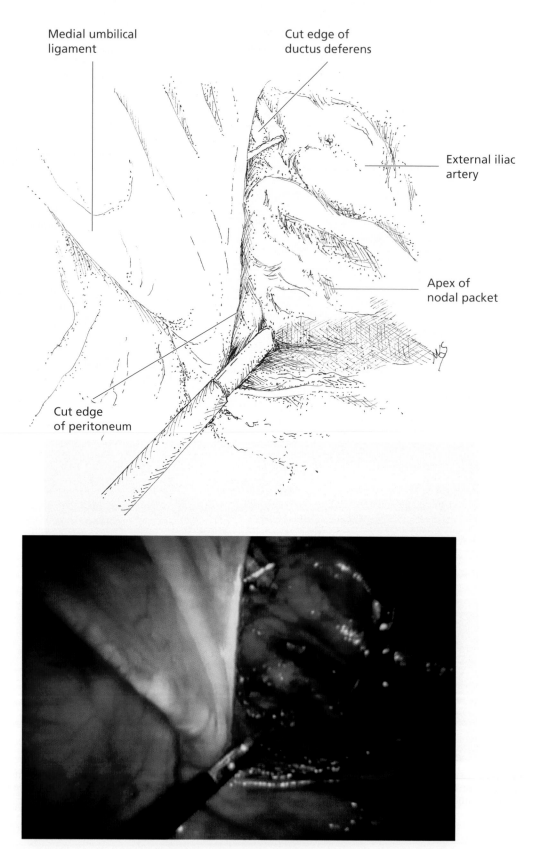

Fig. 9-14. Obturator node dissection (right side). The ductus deferens has been divided and is visible at the apex of the obturator node packet. The external iliac artery and medial umbilical ligaments are seen.

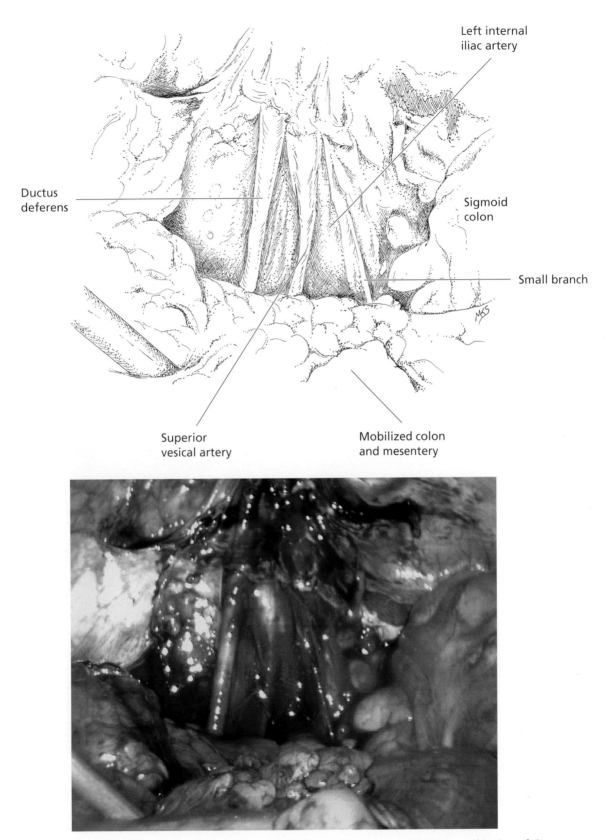

Fig. 9-15. Ductus deferens, internal iliac artery, and middle rectal or superior vesical artery. This view of the left pelvic sidewall was obtained after mobilization of the rectosigmoid colon, which is seen in the foreground. The ductus deferens and internal iliac artery are exposed against the pelvic sidewall. Two small branches of the internal iliac artery (the superior vesical artery and another branch) are seen.

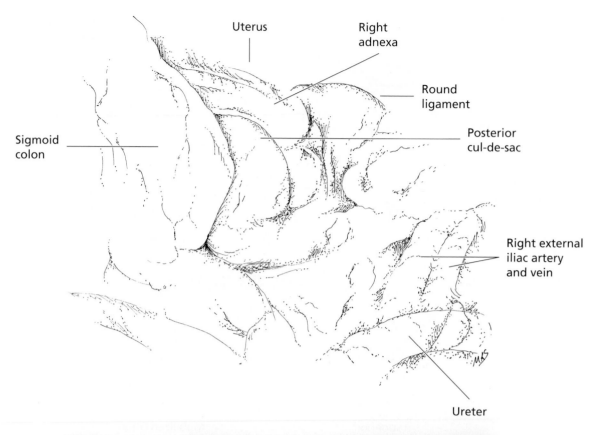

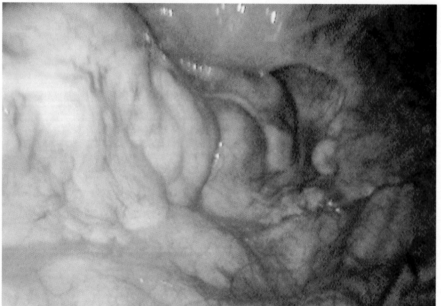

Fig. 9-16. Initial view of the female pelvis. The uterus and sigmoid colon fill the pelvis. The posterior cul-de-sac is seen between uterus and rectosigmoid. The round ligament is glimpsed arching off to the right. The right external iliac artery and vein form part of the frame of the pelvis on the right. The ureter crosses the iliac vessels in the foreground to dive into the pelvis.

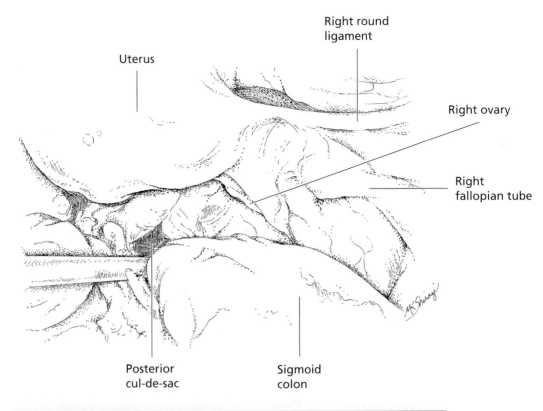

Uterus

Right round
ligament

Right ovary

Right
fallopian tube

Posterior
cul-de-sac

Sigmoid
colon

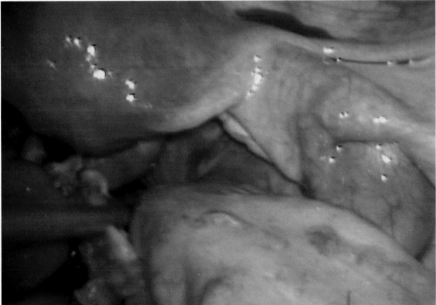

Fig. 9-17. Female pelvis; uterus and right adnexa. A probe is depressing the sigmoid colon, widening the posterior cul-de-sac and facilitating visualization of the uterus. The right round ligament curves off toward the right internal ring (not seen). The right adnexal structures are coming into view. These include the right fallopian tube, which is seen beneath the round ligament, and the ovary. The pelvic sidewall triangle is starting to be defined.

Bladder

Medial umbilical
ligament

Round
ligament

Sigmoid
colon

Uterus   Ovary   Fallopian   Pelvic sidewall
                               tube   triangle

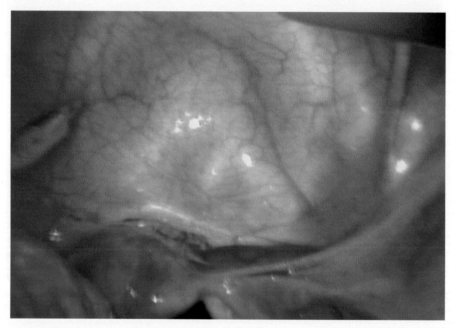

Fig. 9-18. Round ligament approaching the internal ring, pelvic sidewall triangle. The medial umbilical ligaments and bladder are noted. The lateral umbilical ligaments (out of the field of view) mark the entrance of the inferior epigastric vessels. The round ligament is seen arching off to the right to exit through the internal ring. The uterus, fallopian tubes, and adnexal structures are seen. The pelvic sidewall triangle is well delineated.

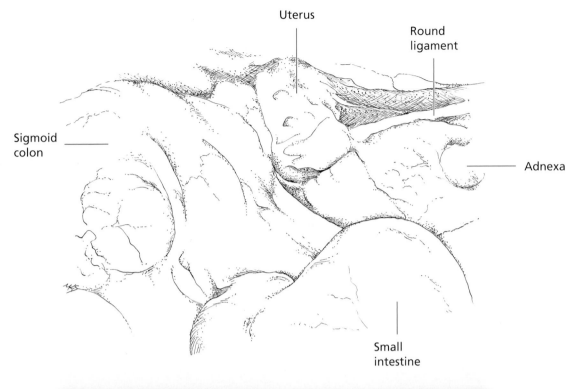

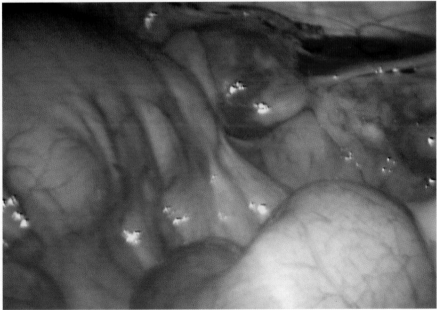

Fig. 9-19. Round ligament and adnexal structures. The sigmoid colon and small intestine occupy the foreground. The uterus, round ligament, and adnexa are noted. Better exposure of these structures requires retraction of the uterus to the contralateral side, pressure on the cervix from below (to elevate uterus and adnexa), or gentle traction on the adnexal structures.

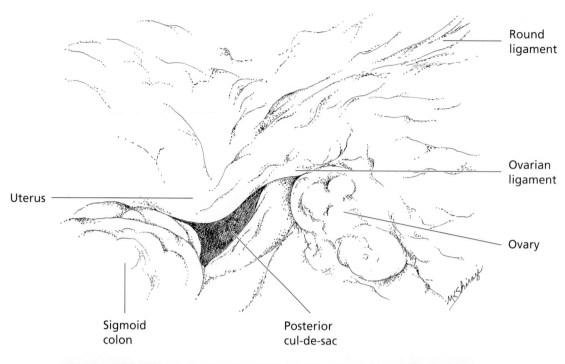

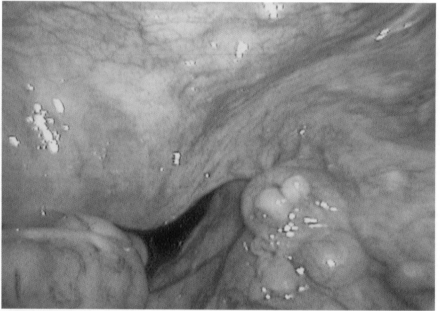

Fig. 9-20. Round ligament, uterus, ovarian ligament, and ovary. In this view of the female pelvic organs *in situ*, the ovarian ligament tethering the ovary to the uterus is noted. The round ligament is in the background. The sigmoid colon and posterior cul-de-sac are seen in the foreground.

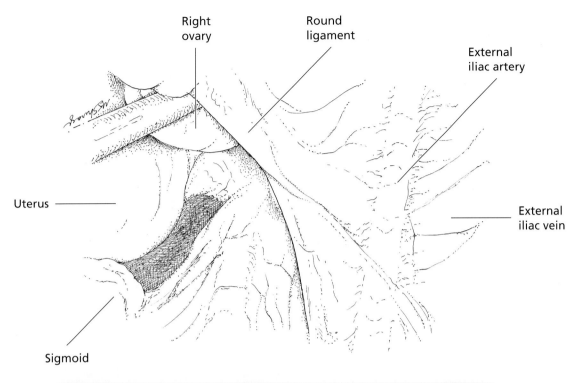

Right ovary

Round ligament

External iliac artery

External iliac vein

Uterus

Sigmoid

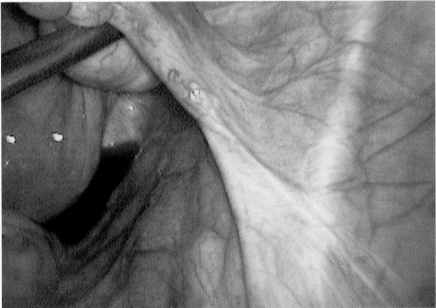

Fig. 9-21. Round ligament, pelvic sidewall, and external iliac artery and vein. This view of the pelvic sidewall in a female patient demonstrates the round ligament crossing the external iliac artery and vein. The right ovary is elevated by a probe. The uterus, posterior cul-de-sac, and sigmoid colon are noted.

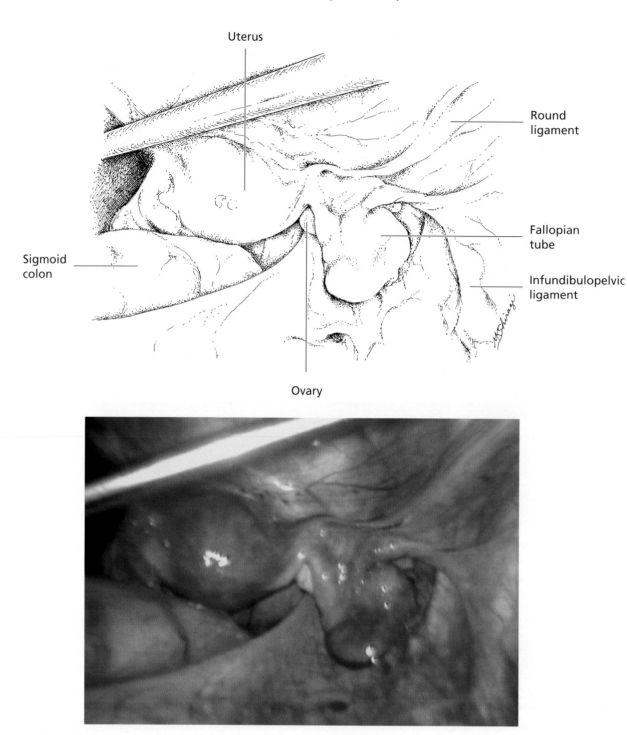

Fig. 9-22. Round ligament, uterus, adnexal structures, and infundibulopelvic ligament. The uterus is gently elevated by a probe passed beneath the left round ligament. The pelvic sidewall triangle on the right is exposed. Round ligament curves off to the right. The infundibulopelvic ligament containing the gonadal vessels is seen to pass from the pelvic sidewall to the ovary. The ovary and fallopian tube are noted. The sigmoid colon and posterior cul-de-sac are glimpsed.

10

INGUINAL REGION

GENE L. COLBORN AND WENDY GRAM BRICK

INITIAL LAPAROSCOPIC VIEW AND PRINCIPLES OF EXPOSURE

The inguinal region may be approached transperitoneally or extraperitoneally. The transperitoneal view is described first, followed by the extraperitoneal view.

Transperitoneal View

The internal surface of the anterior abdominal wall, visible through the laparoscope, is lined with glistening parietal peritoneum. In the lower abdomen, five peritoneal folds may be seen converging on the underside of the umbilicus. Rarely seen or appreciated during open surgery, these prominent "umbilical folds" or ligaments are useful laparoscopic landmarks. In the midline, the median umbilical fold extends from the apex of the bladder to the underside of the umbilicus and contains the obliterated urachus. The paired medial umbilical folds correspond to the position of the embryologic umbilical arteries, obliterated to fibrous remnants except where the superior vesical arteries are found in the pelvic portion. These folds sometimes hang down and obscure the laparoscopic view of the lateral abdominal wall unless they are retracted toward the abdominal wall. The location of these folds is variable (as discussed in Chapter 1), but they are reliable landmarks for the lateral extent of the bladder (see Figs. 1-8 to 1-11, 1-13, and 1-14; Figs. 10-1 to 10-4). An umbilically placed laparoscope must be passed beneath these for adequate inspection of the lateral anterior abdominal wall.

More laterally, the less prominent paired lateral umbilical folds contain the inferior epigastric artery and veins (see Figs. 1-8 and 10-1 to 10-4). These mark the lateral extent of Hesselbach's triangle and hence are useful landmarks (Fig. 10-5).

Associated with these folds bilaterally are three shallow spaces or fossae. The most medial of these are the paired supravesical fossae (see Figs. 1-8 to 1-11, 10-1, and 10-2). The bladder forms the base, decompressed by an indwelling catheter whose balloon may be visible through the bladder wall. Hernias in these fossae are rare, owing to the rectus abdominis muscle and associated aponeurotic sheaths. Between the medial and lateral umbilical folds, the medial umbilical fossa is the site of direct inguinal hernias. Preperitoneal fat may camouflage a large direct hernia defect. In this instance, the angle between the medial and lateral umbilical ligaments decreases, and these two folds become more nearly parallel. After a peritoneal incision is made, blunt dissection between the medial and lateral umbilical folds exposes the region required for visualization of most direct hernia defects.

The lateral umbilical fossa, site of indirect hernias, lies lateral to the lateral umbilical folds (Figs. 1-13, 1-14, 10-3, and 10-4). This fossa overlies the deep (internal) inguinal ring and indicates the site where the processus vaginalis extends into the anterior abdominal wall. A small dimple may be visible at the junction of the internal spermatic vessels and ductus deferens, marking the location of this landmark. A hernia appears as an evagination of the peritoneum away from the laparoscope. Additionally, a large indirect hernia pushes the inferior epigastric vessels medially.

The femoral fossa is below and slightly medial to the lateral inguinal fossa, separated from it by the medial end of the iliopubic tract internally and the inguinal ligament externally. The femoral fossa overlies the femoral ring. Generally, a femoral hernia is evident as an evagination of peritoneum through the femoral canal. Occasionally, preperitoneal fat obscures the hernia, which is then evident only when the lower peritoneal flap is dissected.

Extraperitoneal Approach

The correct plane is usually identified by a combination of direct visualization and blunt dissection, followed by balloon dissection. Small direct hernias may actually reduce during dissection, but because the general surgical approach involves placing a large patch of prosthetic material, it is not crucial to visualize the exact defect. Extraperitoneal dissection may be extremely difficult and/or hazardous if prior extraperitoneal urologic surgery on the bladder or prostate has been performed.

Landmarks that are used during extraperitoneal dissection include the bony and musculoaponeurotic layers of the abdominal wall, the bladder, Cooper's ligament and the iliopubic tract, the inferior epigastric artery and vein, the gonadal vessels, and the ductus deferens (see Fig. 10-5; Figs. 10-6 and 10-7).

ANATOMY AND SPECIFIC SURGICAL PROCEDURES

The laparoscopic anatomy of the inguinal canal may be considerably simplified and divided into the anatomy of the fascial defects and their repair and the anatomy of nerves and vascular structures to be avoided and protected (see Fig. 10-7; Figs. 10-8 to 10-10).

Hernias begin as protrusions of peritoneum through fascial defects (Figs. 10-11 to 10-15). The laparoscopic view of the inguinal canal deals primarily with the peritoneal surfaces, the structures within the preperitoneal space, and the transversalis fascia and its thickenings (the so-called transversalis fascia analogs).

The transversalis fascia lines the interior of the muscular wall of the abdomen (see Figs. 10-4 to 10-6). This fascial layer and aponeurotic tissue of the transversus abdominis provide the "posterior wall" of the inguinal canal. Direct inguinal hernias result from attenuation and weakening of these combined tissues (see Figs. 10-13 and 10-14) and emerge through Hesselbach's triangle, medial to the inferior epigastric vessels (Fig. 10-16).

The preperitoneal (properitoneal or extraperitoneal) space lies between the transversalis fascia and the peritoneum. It contains fatty areolar tissue, the umbilical artery remnant, and inferior epigastric vessels. In most cases, a condensation of extraperitoneal connective tissue can be observed just internal to the transversalis fascia (see Figs. 10-5 and 10-6). This layer invests the inferior epigastric vessels and is continuous with the thick, adipose-rich vesicoumbilical fascia that passes with the urachus superiorly toward the umbilicus, medial to the obliterated umbilical arteries (see Fig. 10-14). The space of Retzius lies between the vesicoumbilical fascia posteriorly and the posterior rectus sheath and pubic bones anteriorly, extending from the muscular pelvic floor upward to the level of the navel. This is the space generally first entered in extraperitoneal laparoscopy for inguinal hernia repair.

The fascial covering of the inferior epigastric vessels is sometimes regarded as a separate layer, termed the posterior or deep transversalis fascia. Laterally, this fascial layer often overlies and fuses with the iliopubic tract, increasing its density and its reflectiveness with laparoscopic illumination.

After entering the internal inguinal ring, the ductus deferens separates from other structures of the spermatic cord, curves around the lateral side of the inferior epigastric artery, and descends into the true pelvis. Within the pelvis, the ductus deferens runs posteriorly on the medial side of the obliterated umbilical artery (medial umbilical folds), crosses the ureter, and runs medially toward the posterior surface of the bladder and seminal vesicles (see Figs. 1-10 and 10-3 to 10-7). For the laparoscopic surgeon, the confluence of the ductus deferens and the testicular vessels forms a visible landmark corresponding to the internal inguinal ring when no indirect hernia exists (see Figs. 10-3 and 10-4). When an indirect hernia is present, it is usually seen as an evagination of peritoneum between these structures (see Fig. 10-13). The visible presence of gonadal vessels entering the internal ring is presumed evidence of testicular descent into the inguinal canal and is a useful landmark when laparoscopy is performed for undescended testes.

The iliopubic tract is a variably bright-appearing band that often provides an extremely important laparoscopic landmark (see Fig. 10-14). The tract consists primarily of aponeurotic transversus abdominis fibers and the associated transversalis fascia. As noted earlier, however, its thickness is often enhanced by the reinforcement of an adherent lamina of extraperitoneal connective tissue (or the internal lamina of transversalis fascia). Finally, a falciform extension of connective tissue derived from the psoas sheath regularly contributes to the complexity of the tract.

The iliopubic tract extends approximately from the anterior superior iliac spine to the pubic tubercle. A sense of distance can be gained from Figs. 10-7 and 10-10, where a centimeter ruler has been placed with its free edge corresponding to the anterior superior iliac spine. The iliopubic tract runs approximately parallel to the inguinal ligament, lies anterior to the femoral sheath, and is associated with the inferior edge of the inguinal ligament (which is not seen laparoscopically). Thickenings of fascia associated with the iliopubic tract curve around the medial surface of the femoral sheath and border the internal inguinal ring. The iliopubic tract terminates by fanning out to attach to the medial portion of Cooper's ligament and the pubic tubercle. This layer is not strong enough to be useful in laparoscopic hernia repair, but it is an extremely important landmark. The region below the iliopubic tract should be avoided, because numerous vessels and nerves may be encountered (see Figs. 10-10 and 10-16; Figs. 10-17 to 10-20). Variations in the pattern of insertion of the iliopubic tract on the superior pubic ramus result in differences in size of the femoral ring and may predispose to femoral hernia when the resulting ring is broad. The femoral canal may be visualized laparoscopically (see Fig. 10-12).

Cooper's ligament is easily seen laparoscopically as a shiny, fibrous ligamentous band covering the pectineal ridge or line of the superior pubic ramus (see Fig. 10-1). To probe palpation, it is perceived as a firm, unyielding structure. The ligament is composed of the tendinous origin of the pectineus muscle of the thigh and the insertion of aponeurotic fibers derived principally from the lacunar part (ligament of Gimbernat) of the inguinal ligament and the medial insertion of the iliopubic tract or transversus abdominis.

The inferior epigastric artery leaves the external iliac artery and curves medially and anteriorly, initially hugging the medial margin of the internal inguinal ring as it ascends in the extraperitoneal tissues (see Figs. 1-13 and 1-14). This useful laparoscopic landmark is seen in Figs. 10-4 and 10-5 and most of the remaining figures throughout this chapter. It pierces the transversalis fascia in the region of the arcuate line. Branches of the inferior epigastric artery include retropubic and suprapubic branches, the cremasteric artery, small twigs to the rectus muscle, and even smaller peritoneal branches.

The retropubic branch of the inferior epigastric artery normally passes lateral to the femoral ring as it runs toward the obturator foramen, where it may anastomose with the obturator artery, in addition to providing supply to tissues of the posterior aspect of the pubic bone and pelvic sidewall. In 20% to 40% of anatomically normal individuals, the retropubic branch replaces the obturator artery, providing an aberrant obturator artery (see Figs. 10-9, 10-10, and 10-12). In many cases, the vessel can be large and descends almost vertically, curving along the free margin of the lacunar ligament or even passing across the femoral ring before descending across the pectineal ligament. In this location, it may be displaced medially or laterally by a femoral hernia. A retropubic vessel or an aberrant obturator vessel can give origin to branches of significant size to the urinary bladder or its associated tissues.

Vascular variations are of extreme importance to the laparoscopic surgeon working in the inguinofemoral area. Careful identification of anatomy and gentle atraumatic dissection in the extraperitoneal plane ensure that inadvertent trauma to these vessels does not occur. Retropubic veins accompany the retropubic artery and course deep to the iliopubic tract. The term "circle of death" or corona mortis refers to the vascular ring formed by the anastomosis of an aberrant obturator artery with a normal obturator artery arising from a branch of the internal iliac artery (see Fig. 10-20). When such a vessel is cut or torn, both segments of the vessel can bleed profusely, because each arises from a major artery. Injury to an aberrant obturator vein may be more insidious during laparoscopic herniorrhaphy, because the vein may be collapsed by pressure of insufflation and may provide an unseen source of postoperative bleeding. The possible presence of an aberrant vessel should be remembered whenever the pectineal ligament must be exposed or used to secure a piece of mesh.

Although the laparoscopic approach to hernias in this region should provide excellent visualization of vascular anomalies and should thus preclude inadvertent injury, fatty tissue medial to the external iliac vessels can easily hide an aberrant obturator artery and vein crossing Cooper's (or pectineal) ligament (see Figs. 10-18 to 10-20), where these vessels may be injured by staples placed in the pectineal ligament. Additionally, an aberrant obturator vein draining directly into the external iliac vein is easily avulsed if tissues are handled roughly. Other small venous tributaries are found in this region, including retropubic veins.

Suprapubic branches of the inferior epigastric artery and vein course medially along the upper border of the superior pubic ramus, the pectineal ligament, and the pubic crest to supply the vesicoumbilical tissues. These vessels vary in size from less than half a millimeter to—in the case of suprapubic veins—more than half a centimeter in diameter. The suprapubic veins receive contributions from veins draining the rectus, the connective tissues of the rectus sheath, and the peritoneum.

The cremasteric or external spermatic artery accompanies the spermatic cord through the internal ring. It generally arises from the inferior epigastric artery at the lower, medial aspect of the internal inguinal ring, then crosses the preperitoneal space to join the spermatic cord in the inguinal canal. The cremasteric artery is accompanied by the genital branch of the genitofemoral nerve, which provides motor supply to the cremasteric muscle and sensory fibers to the urogenital region. In the female, the cremasteric artery often provides origin for the artery of the round ligament (Sampson's artery), in addition to the contribution from the uterine artery. Thus, the round ligament must be doubly clipped or ligated if it is divided.

The deep circumflex iliac artery and vein cross laterally over the femoral sheath, running between the iliopubic tract and iliopectineal arch, piercing the transversalis fascia to run in the space between the transversus abdominis and internal oblique muscles (see Fig. 10-17). A large ascending branch passes upward between these muscles near the anterior superior iliac spine to supply the lower anterolateral abdominal wall. Significant hematomas can occur if these vessels are traumatized by staples or suturing.

The gonadal vessels (testicular arteries—male; ovarian arteries—female) arise from the front of the aorta just below the renal arteries. These gonadal vessels pass obliquely downward in the retroperitoneum, crossing the genitofemoral nerve, ureter, and lower part of the external iliac artery (see Figs. 1-12 and 10-3 to 10-20). In the male, the testicular artery enters the spermatic cord at the internal inguinal ring. In the female, the ovarian artery enters the pelvic cavity at the pelvic brim after crossing the external iliac artery and vein, then runs medially in the suspensory ligament of the ovary to enter the broad ligament of the uterus. Thus, the ovarian artery is not in close proximity to the internal inguinal ring in the female.

Because laparoscopic inguinal hernia repair proceeds from the "inside out," even when done extraperitoneally, the common superficial nerves of the groin (such as the ilioinguinal and iliohypogastric nerves) are not seen. The genitofemoral nerve may or may not be visualized. It is shown clearly in the figures that accompany this chapter for illustrative purposes. This clear display was obtained by cadaver dissection, and the laparoscopic surgeon rarely glimpses the numerous nerves of the region. Thus, the surgeon must proceed based on "probable locations" of sensory nerves to avoid postoperative nerve entrapment syndromes. These nerves include the femoral nerve, the lateral cutaneous nerve of the thigh, the genitofemoral nerve and its genital and femoral branches, the obturator nerve, the ilioinguinal nerve, and the iliohypogastric nerve (see Figs. 10-7 to 10-10, 10-12, and 10-16 to 10-19). These nerves are considered in sequence.

The femoral nerve is the largest branch of the lumbar plexus. It descends within the fibers of the psoas major muscle, emerging from the lower lateral border of the muscle about 6 cm above the iliopubic tract to pass between the psoas and iliacus muscles deep to the iliac fascia (see Figs. 10-10, 10-16, and 10-19). The nerve passes behind the inguinal ligament to enter the thigh. Behind the inguinal ligament, the femoral nerve splits into anterior and posterior divisions. It is the most lateral of the three (nerve, artery, vein) structures to pass beneath the inguinal ligament into the thigh and is separated from the femoral artery (which lies medial to it) by some muscle slips of the psoas major muscle. Irrespective of its depth and position, the femoral nerve is at risk during laparoscopic herniorrhaphy. It can be injured by staples placed lateral to the external iliac vessels, close to the iliopectineal arch, resulting in pain and/or muscle weakness in the anterior thigh. The anterior cutaneous branch of the femoral nerve arises early, not uncommonly, and is at risk as it passes beneath or through the iliopubic tract in a more superficial position just lateral to the external iliac vessels (see Figs. 10-9, 10-12, and 10-16).

The lateral femoral cutaneous nerve (or lateral cutaneous nerve of the thigh) is one of the two most commonly injured nerves when inguinal herniorrhaphy is performed laparoscopically. It emerges from the lateral border of the psoas major muscle, crosses the iliacus, and runs obliquely toward the anterior superior iliac spine, sending branches to the parietal peritoneum. It enters the pelvis by passing behind and lateral to the cecum on the right and behind the lower portion of the descending colon on the left. At a variable distance (0 to 4.0 cm) medial to the anterior superior iliac spine, the nerve then passes either behind or through the inguinal ligament to enter the thigh in the vicinity of the sartorius muscle. Entrapment of this nerve causes considerable morbidity. The intrapelvic course is variable, but the nerve can generally be found within 1 cm of the anterior superior iliac spine, and staple placement in the vicinity of the anterior superior iliac spine should be avoided (see Figs. 10-10, 10-12, and 10-16). In 18% of instances in one series reported by Dibenedetto and associates (see Bibliography), the nerve was either in the vertical plane of the anterior superior iliac spine or in the plane of the iliopubic tract. In 11%, it was within 1 cm of the anterior superior iliac spine. In 14 of 78 (18%) cadaveric specimens dissected in our laboratory, the ilioinguinal nerve was partially or entirely combined with the lateral femoral cutaneous nerve until they separated in their passage through the abdominal wall.

The genitofemoral nerve passes obliquely forward and downward through the psoas major muscle to emerge near the medial border of this muscle. It descends on the surface of the psoas major muscle, crossing behind the ureter to divide (at a variable distance) above the inguinal ligament into the genital and femoral branches (see Fig. 10-8). The genital branch can often be seen lying on the surface of the distal segment of the external iliac artery until, near the origin of the inferior epigastric artery, the nerve enters the inguinal canal through the internal inguinal ring (see Figs. 10-6, 10-9, 10-10, and 10-17). It supplies the cremaster muscles and gives a few fibers to the skin of the scrotum in the male. In the female, it accompanies the round ligament to terminate in the skin of the mons veneris and labium majus.

In a common anatomic variant, the genital branch passes below the iliopubic tract in the vicinity of the internal inguinal ring to enter the inguinal canal from below. The nerve is clearly at risk in these cases, when staples are placed in this region, as noted by Annibali and colleagues (see Bibliography). The femoral branch of the genitofemoral nerve descends on the lateral aspect of the external iliac artery, crosses the deep circumflex iliac artery, and passes behind the inguinal ligament to enter the femoral sheath (see Fig. 10-16). This branch is superficial in an area where staples are usually applied to tack the inferomedial border of the mesh, according to Annibali and associates. The genital branch of the genitofemoral nerve is occasionally damaged when the sac of an indirect hernia is reduced. Annibali and associates also report that it is one of the two nerves most likely to be injured in laparoscopic inguinal hernia repair. Genitofemoral neuralgia results in burning or sharp pain in the inguinal region and radiation to the genitalia and medial upper thigh. In 6 of 78 specimens (7.7%) dissected in our laboratory, the genitofemoral and ilioinguinal nerves were combined.

The ilioinguinal nerve, smaller than the iliohypogastric nerve, actually lies in a plane superficial to the preperitoneal space. Most experienced surgeons are accustomed to visualizing this nerve just deep to the external oblique aponeurosis on the anterior surface of the cord. During open herniorrhaphy, this nerve is carefully sought, identified, mobilized, and protected. In laparoscopic herniorrhaphy, the nerve is rarely seen and rarely injured. In approximately 25% of cases, all or part of the ilioinguinal nerve crosses the iliac fossa just beneath the iliac fascia. In such instances, the nerve can be impaled by staples placed through the iliopubic tract. Vigorous bimanual techniques during staple placement (using pressure on the external abdominal wall to produce resistance and to ensure deep staple placement) may place the nerve at risk. The surgeon should avoid placing deep staples lateral to the internal inguinal ring. Fibers of the nerve distribute to the superomedial area of the thigh, the skin over the root of the penis and upper part of the scrotum in the male, and the mons pubis and adjacent labium majus in the female. There is considerable overlap in territory among the iliohypogastric, ilioinguinal, lateral femoral cutaneous, and genitofemoral nerves. Overzealous attempts to protect nerves by anatomic identification are neither advisable nor feasible.

The iliohypogastric nerve perforates the posterior part of the transversus abdominis muscle just above the iliac crest, running between that muscle and the internal oblique, where it divides into lateral and anterior cutaneous branches. This course, between two muscle layers, places the nerve in a plane superficial to the preperitoneal space. Similar to the ilioinguinal nerve, this nerve is never seen and is rarely injured during laparoscopic herniorrhaphy, unless vigorous bimanual counterpressure is used. The ilioinguinal and iliohypogastric nerves vary from individual to individual with respect to relative size and territory. The iliohypogastric nerve commonly supplies the skin of the abdomen above the pubis.

The obturator nerve passes behind the common iliac vessels at the pelvic brim, runs along the lateral side of the internal iliac vessels, then turns downward as it passes over the obturator internus, in front of the obturator vessels, to exit through the obturator foramen. It lies below the pectineal ligament medially.

Two triangles (of "doom" and of "pain") and a "trapezoid of doom" have been described as regions to avoid when staples are placed to secure mesh. Placing staples within these designated regions may imperil one or more nerves, as described earlier. The "triangle of doom" (see Fig. 10-18) is defined by the ductus deferens medially, the testicular vessels laterally, and the external iliac vessels inferiorly. This triangle contains the external iliac artery and vein, the deep circumflex iliac vein, the genital branch of the genitofemoral nerve, and the femoral nerve (not seen, covered by fascia). No staples should ever be placed within this triangle.

A second "triangle of pain" is demarcated by the testicular vessels, the iliopubic tract, and the inferior edge of the peritoneal incision (see Fig. 10-17). This triangle contains the lateral femoral cutaneous and anterior femoral cutaneous nerves, the femoral branch of the genitofemoral nerve, and (hidden by fascia) the femoral nerve. The triangle often contains unnamed small nerves, presumably motor to the lower anterior abdominal wall. It may also contain an aberrant ilioinguinal nerve. Some have expanded this "triangle" to a trapezoidal region demarcated by the ductus deferens medially, the anterior superior iliac spine laterally, and the entire area below the iliopubic tract. This "trapezoid of doom" encompasses both triangles.

A basic rule in laparoscopic herniorrhaphy has been stated simply thus, by Seid and Amos (see Bibliography): "Never place a staple below the iliopubic tract anywhere lateral to the ductus (all the way to the anterior superior iliac spine)." Nerves in this region are variable in location, difficult to see, and easily entrapped by staples placed in this area. Most nerves pass below the iliopubic tract, but occasionally nerve fibers pass directly through the iliopubic tract, making staple placement within the iliopubic tract itself potentially problematic as well. The lateral femoral cutaneous nerve, genitofemoral nerve, and an aberrant ilioinguinal nerve are particularly likely to send fibers within the iliopubic tract. The femoral nerve can be injured where it lies in a relatively superficial position just lateral to the gonadal vessels.

Laparoscopic Inguinal Herniorrhaphy

The inguinal region is easily visualized with an umbilically placed 30- to 45-degree angled laparoscope. The surgeon visualizes the lateral and medial umbilical ligaments. The internal inguinal ring can be identified as a dimple (in anatomically normal individuals) or as a hole if an indirect hernia is present. Next, the surgeon identifies the ductus deferens and testicular vessels. The inferior epigastric vessels course along the medial side of the internal ring and then run in the lateral umbilical folds.

An incision is made in the peritoneum transversely above the level of the internal ring extending from the midline to a point lateral to the internal ring. The plane immediately behind the peritoneum is dissected, thus teasing preperitoneal fat and associated structures back onto the abdominal wall. Once an adequate area of peritoneum has been mobilized, the pubic tubercle, Cooper's ligament, and the medial portion of the iliopubic tract are sought. The pubic tubercle is often obscured by preperitoneal fat and the medial umbilical ligaments. It can always be palpated with the tip of a blunt instrument or probe. The surgeon should identify this structure as early as possible in the dissection. Cooper's ligament is similarly easy to palpate and may be seen as a shiny, firm structure, once the overlying preperitoneal fat is stripped away. One should beware accidental injury to aberrant obturator vessels. Following Cooper's ligament inferolaterally from the pubic tubercle, the external iliac vessels are seen. The medial aspect of the iliopubic tract can be seen crossing the inferior border of the internal ring and separating the inguinal canal from the femoral canal. The juncture of the transversus abdominis arch, iliopubic tract, and Cooper's ligament at the pubic tubercle forms a starting point to confirm the location of the iliopubic tract.

The basic principles of laparoscopic hernia repair are remarkably similar to those of open herniorrhaphy. All peritoneal extrusions are reduced, usually during insufflation and dissection, and the fascial defect is closed. This fascial closure is achieved by laying a piece of mesh over all potential weak points. The surgeon should select points of mesh fixation superiorly, laterally, and medially. One should remember the "trapezoid of doom" and not place staples within this region. The mesh is covered with peritoneum at the conclusion of the procedure.

Ligation of Varicocele

Most (90%) of varicoceles occur on the left side. Laparoscopic ligation begins by inspecting the area of the internal inguinal ring and identifying the ductus deferens and testicular vessels that converge on the internal ring (see Figs. 10-3 and 10-4). The dilated testicular veins (generally two, accompanying a single artery) are identified. The peritoneum overlying the vessels is opened and the veins are teased away from the artery. The artery is usually posterior and medial to the veins and can be identified by visible pulsations. Occasionally, a laparoscopic Doppler probe is needed. The artery is preserved, and all other vascular tissue is clipped and divided. There may be smaller veins accompanying the two main venous trunks, and it is wise to ligate all tissues but the artery.

Exploration for Undescended Testis

Initial exploration begins with inspection of the internal ring to determine whether the ductus deferens and testicular vessels can be seen converging on and exiting the abdomen through the internal ring (see Figs. 10-3 and 10-4). If the ductus deferens enters the cord at the internal ring, then the testis is presumed to have entered the inguinal canal.

BIBLIOGRAPHY

Anatomic References

1. Ahlberg NE, Bartly O, Chidekel N. Right and left gonadal veins: an anatomical and statistical study. *Acta Radiol* 1966;4:593–601.
2. Brick WG, Colborn GL, Gadacz TR, Skandalakis JE. Crucial anatomic lessons for laparoscopic herniorrhaphy. *Am Surg* 1995;61:172–177.
3. Broin EO, Horner C, Mealy K, et al. Meralgia paraesthetica following laparoscopic inguinal hernia repair: an anatomical analysis. *Surg Endosc* 1995;9:76–78.
4. Colborn GL, Brick WG, Gadacz TR, Skandalakis JE. Inguinal anatomy for laparoscopic herniorrhaphy. I. The normal anatomy. *Surg Rounds* 1995;May:189–198.
5. Colborn GL, Brick WG, Gadacz TR, Skandalakis JE. Inguinal anatomy for laparoscopic herniorrhaphy. II. Altered inguinal anatomy and variations. *Surg Rounds* 1995;June:223–232.
6. Dibenedetto LM, Lei Q, Gilroy AM, Hermey DC, Marks SC Jr, Page DW. Variations in the inferior pelvic pathway of the lateral femoral cutaneous nerve: implications for laparoscopic hernia repair. *Clin Anat* 1996;9:232–236.
7. Eubanks S, Newman L 3rd, Goehring L, Lucas GW, Adams CP, Mason E. Meralgia paresthetica: a complication of laparoscopic herniorrhaphy. *Surg Laparosc Endosc* 1993;3:381–385.
8. Ger R. Laparoscopic repair of groin hernias: a clinicoanatomic review. I. *Surg Rounds* 1994;May:345–350.
9. Ger R. Laparoscopic repair of groin hernias: a clinicoanatomic review. II. *Surg Rounds* 1994;June:395–401.
10. Keating JP, Morgan A. Femoral nerve palsy following laparoscopic inguinal herniorrhaphy. *J Laparoendosc Surg* 1993;3:557–559.
11. Kraus MA. Nerve injury during laparoscopic inguinal hernia repair. *Surg Laparosc Endosc* 1993;3:342–345.
12. Lechter A, Lopez G, Martinez C, Camacho J. Anatomy of the gonadal veins: a reappraisal. *Surgery* 1991;109:735–739.
13. Rosser J. The anatomical basis for laparoscopic hernia repair revisited. *Surg Laparosc Endosc* 1994;4:36–44.
14. Sampath P, Yeo CJ, Campbell JN. Nerve injury associated with laparoscopic inguinal herniorrhaphy. *Surgery* 1995;118:829–833.
15. Seid AS, Amos E. Entrapment neuropathy in laparoscopic herniorrhaphy. *Surg Endosc* 1994;8:1050–1053.
16. Skandalakis JE, Colborn GL, Androulakis JA, Skandalakis LJ, Pemberton LB. Embryologic and anatomic basis of inguinal herniorrhaphy. *Surg Clin North Am* 1993;73:799–836.
17. Woods S, Polglase A. Ilioinguinal nerve entrapment from laparoscopic hernia repair. *Aust N Z J Surg* 1993;63:823–824.

Surgical References

1. Annibali RG, Fitzgibbons RJ Jr, Filipi CJ, Litke BS, Salerno GM. Laparoscopic inguinal hernia repair. In: Greene FL, Ponsky JL, eds. *Endoscopic surgery*. Philadelphia: WB Saunders, 1994:352–386.
2. Chapman WHH, Crombie CH, Cox SS, Orlando DAP, Pories WJ. Laparoscopic inguinal hernia repair. *Curr Surg* 1996;53:477–485.
3. Heiss KF, Shandling B. Laparoscopy for the impalpable testes: experience with 53 testes. *J Pediatr Surg* 1992;27:175–179.
4. Mehan DJ, Andrus CH, Parra RO. Laparoscopic internal spermatic vein ligation: report of a new technique. *Fertil Steril* 1992;58:1263–1266.
5. Ramshaw BJ, Tucker JG, Duncan TD, et al. Technical considerations of the different approaches to laparoscopic herniorrhaphy: an analysis of 500 cases. *Am Surg* 1996;62:69–72.
6. Read RC. Anatomy of abdominal herniation: the parietoperitoneal spaces. In: Nyhus LM, Baker RJ, Fischer JF, eds. *Mastery of surgery,* vol 2, 3rd ed. Boston: Little, Brown, 1997:1795–1806.
7. Stanley KE, Winfield HN, Donovan JF. Laparoscopic varicocele ligation. *Surg Rounds* 1994;Feb:109–116.
8. Voeller GR, Mangiante EC Jr, Wilson C. Totally preperitoneal laparoscopic inguinal herniorrhaphy using balloon dissection. *Surg Rounds* 1995;Mar:107–112.

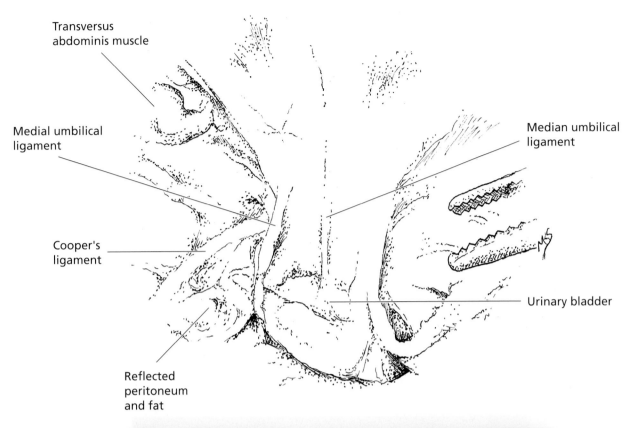

Transversus
abdominis muscle

Medial umbilical
ligament

Cooper's
ligament

Reflected
peritoneum
and fat

Median umbilical
ligament

Urinary bladder

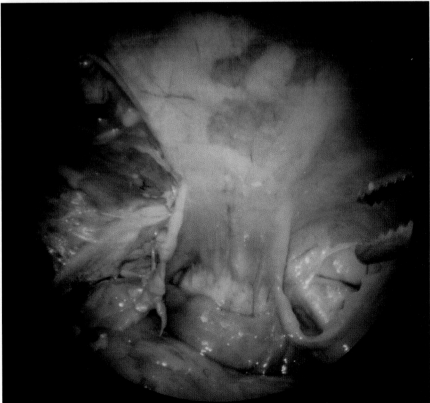

Fig. 10-1. Panoramic view of the inguinal region. Both inguinal regions are seen. The peritoneum has been divided and reflected from the left inguinal area to expose the transversus abdominis and Cooper's ligament. The median and medial umbilical ligaments and bladder are noted.

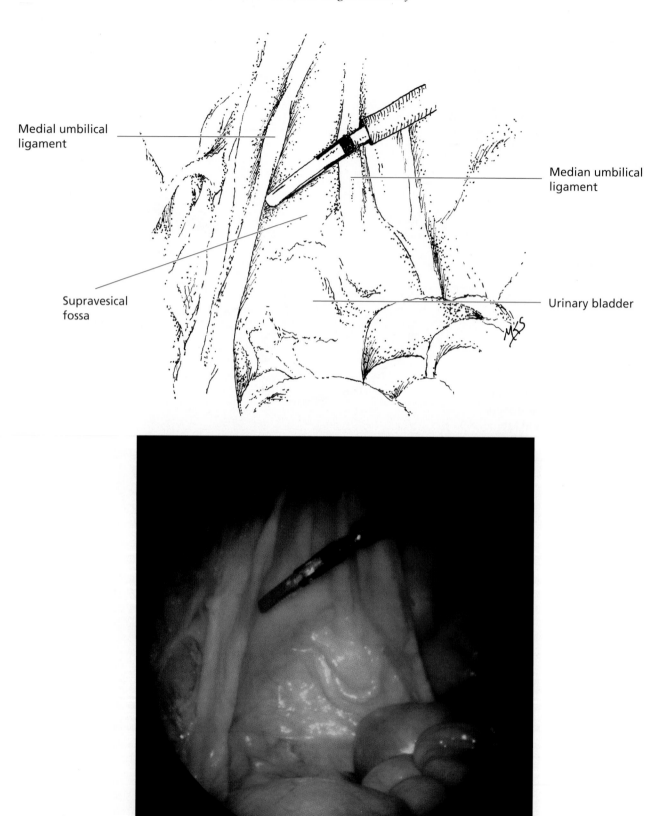

Fig. 10-2. Median and medial umbilical ligaments and supravesical fossa. The urinary bladder lies just medial to the medial umbilical ligaments.

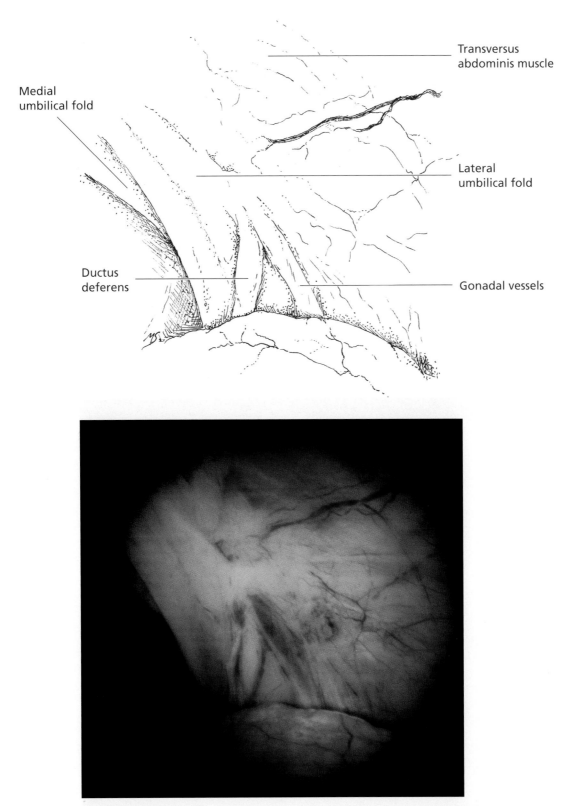

Transversus
abdominis muscle

Medial
umbilical fold

Lateral
umbilical fold

Ductus
deferens

Gonadal vessels

Fig. 10-3. Right inguinal region, peritoneum intact. The medial and lateral umbilical folds form useful land-marks. The junction of the ductus deferens and gonadal vessels marks the location of the deep inguinal ring.

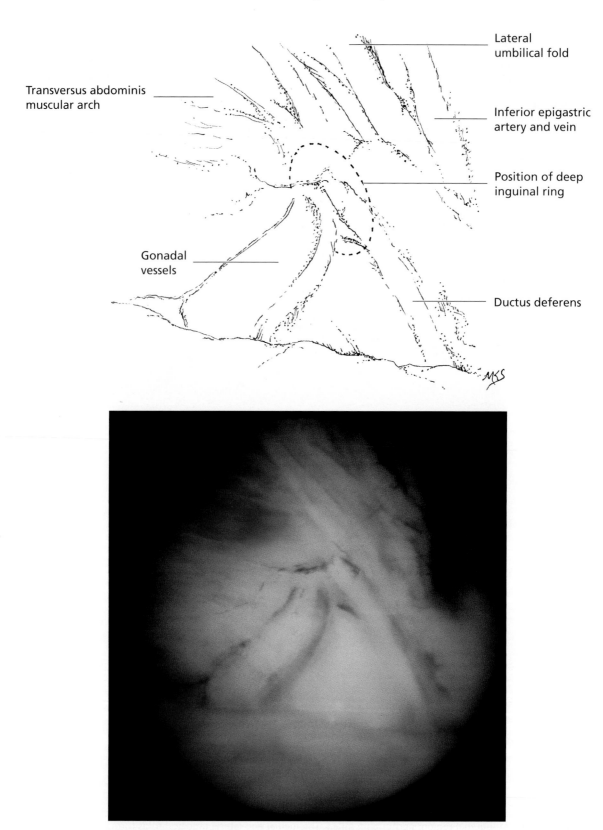

Fig. 10-4. Left inguinal region, peritoneum intact. The ductus deferens and gonadal vessels converge at the deep inguinal ring (*dotted line* indicates location of deep inguinal ring). The lateral umbilical fold is visible.

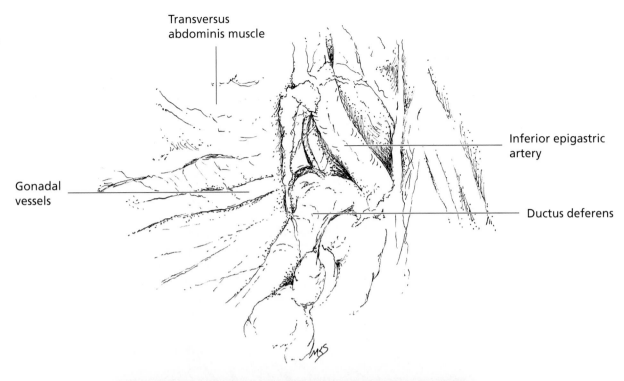

Transversus
abdominis muscle

Inferior epigastric
artery

Gonadal
vessels

Ductus deferens

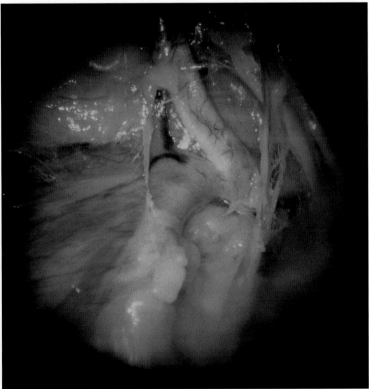

Fig. 10-5. Left deep inguinal ring. The peritoneum has been removed. The transversus abdominis muscle is visible through a thin layer of extraperitoneal connective tissue. At the deep inguinal ring, the ductus deferens and gonadal vessels converge. The inferior epigastric vessels are seen passing cephalad, delineating the lateral extent of Hesselbach's triangle (see Fig. 10-20).

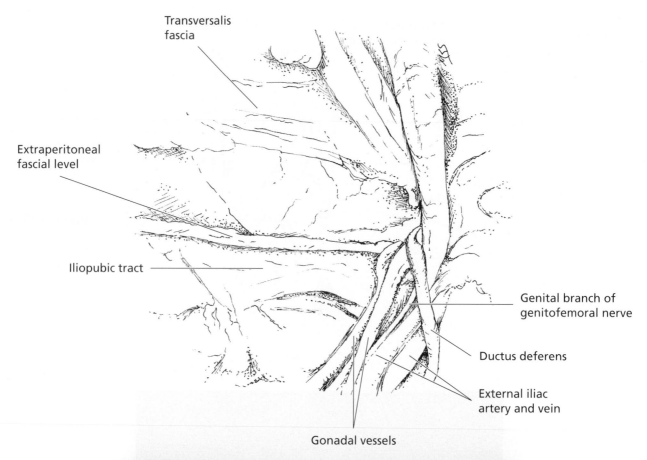

Transversalis
fascia

Extraperitoneal
fascial level

Iliopubic tract

Genital branch of
genitofemoral nerve

Ductus deferens

External iliac
artery and vein

Gonadal vessels

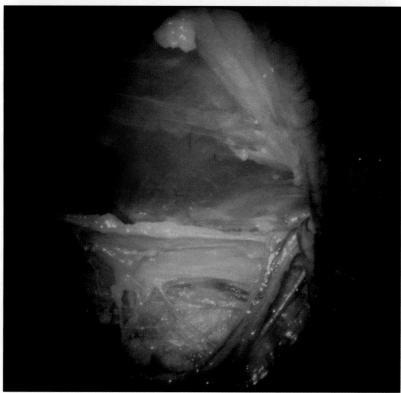

Fig. 10-6. Lateral inguinal fossa and structures converging on the left deep inguinal ring. In this view, with the peritoneum removed, the structures converging on the deep inguinal ring are clearly seen. The ductus deferens comes from medially, crosses over the external iliac artery and vein, and joins the gonadal vessels to form the spermatic cord at the deep ring. Extraperitoneal fascia, transversalis fascia, and the iliopubic tract are visible.

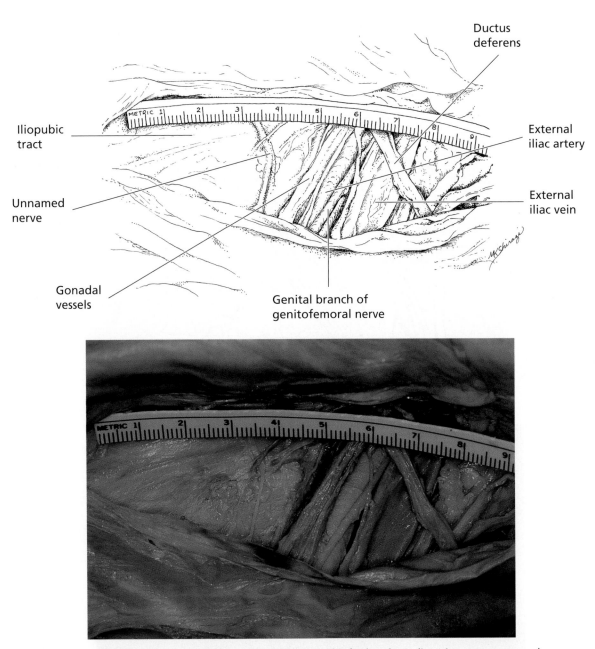

Fig. 10-7. Left inguinal fossa and the deep inguinal ring. In this fresh cadaver dissection, structures are shown as they would be encountered during laparoscopic exploration of the region. Cut edges of the peritoneum are visible at the superior and inferior borders of the field. The ruler demonstrates the distance in centimeters from the anterior superior iliac spine (not visible, deep to the free edge of the ruler). The iliopubic tract and iliac fascia are seen. The external iliac artery and vein and gonadal vessels are noted medially. The ductus deferens crosses these vascular structures. The genital branch of the genitofemoral nerve can be seen just lateral to the external iliac artery. An unnamed nerve is seen on the iliac fascia.

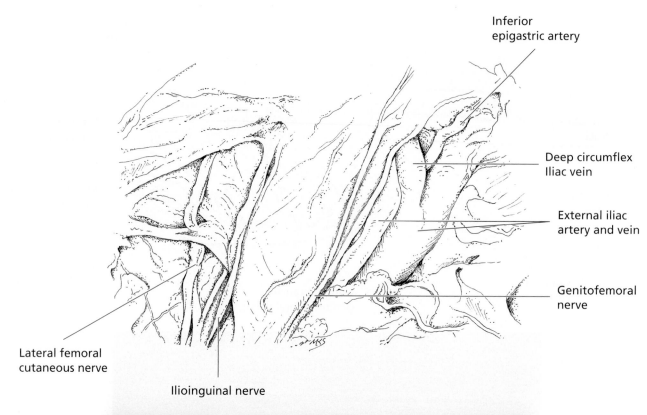

Inferior
epigastric artery

Deep circumflex
Iliac vein

External iliac
artery and vein

Genitofemoral
nerve

Lateral femoral
cutaneous nerve

Ilioinguinal nerve

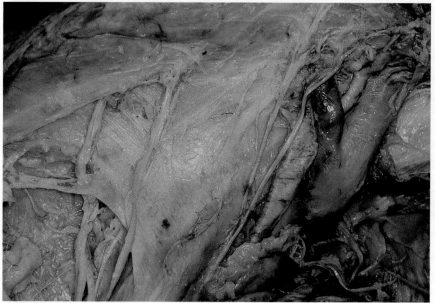

Fig. 10-8. Vessels and nerves of the triangle of doom and triangle of pain, left inguinal fossa. This cadaver dissection demonstrates, from the laparoscopic perspective, the complex anatomy and numerous important structures encountered below the iliopubic tract. These structures are at risk during laparoscopic hernia repair.

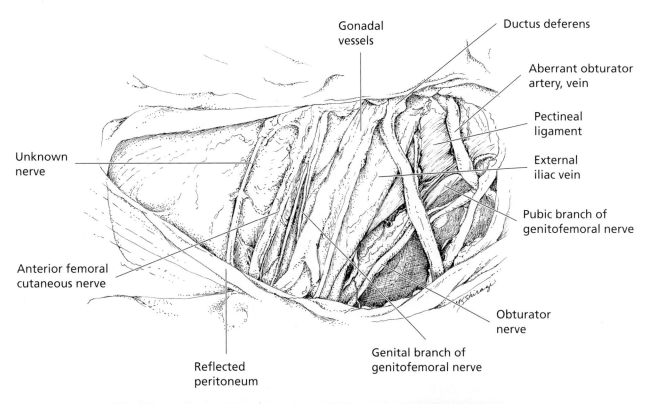

Gonadal vessels

Ductus deferens

Aberrant obturator artery, vein

Pectineal ligament

Unknown nerve

External iliac vein

Pubic branch of genitofemoral nerve

Anterior femoral cutaneous nerve

Obturator nerve

Genital branch of genitofemoral nerve

Reflected peritoneum

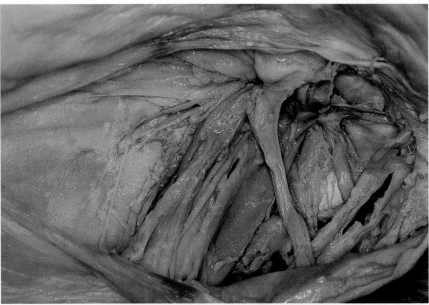

Fig. 10-9. Aberrant obturator vessels, left inguinal region. In this cadaver dissection, seen from the laparoscopic perspective, aberrant obturator vessels are seen passing across the pectineal ligament in the region of the inguinal floor. The obturator nerve, anterior femoral cutaneous nerve, pubic and genital branches of the genitofemoral nerve, and an unknown small nerve are well seen.

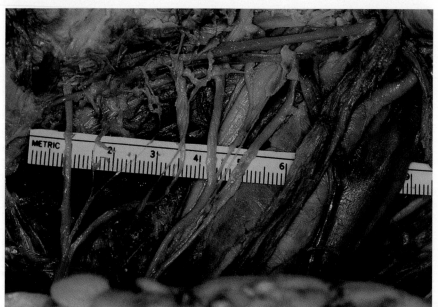

Inferior
epigastric artery

Genital branch of
genitofemoral nerve

Femoral
nerve

Deep circumflex
iliac artery

Aberrant
obturator artery

Ductus
deferens

Lateral femoral
cutaneous nerve

Obturator
nerve

Ilioinguinal and lateral
femoral cutaneous nerve

Gonadal vessels

External iliac
artery and vein

Fig. 10-10. Nerves of the triangle of pain, including variants, left iliac fossa. In this cadaver dissection, seen from the laparoscopic perspective, the ruler is again placed with its free edge at the anterior superior iliac spine. The iliopubic tract has been dissected. In this case, an aberrant obturator branch of the external iliac artery gives origin to the inferior epigastric artery. The femoral nerve, genital branch of the genitofemoral nerve, lateral femoral cutaneous nerve, and combined ilioinguinal and lateral femoral cutaneous nerve are noted.

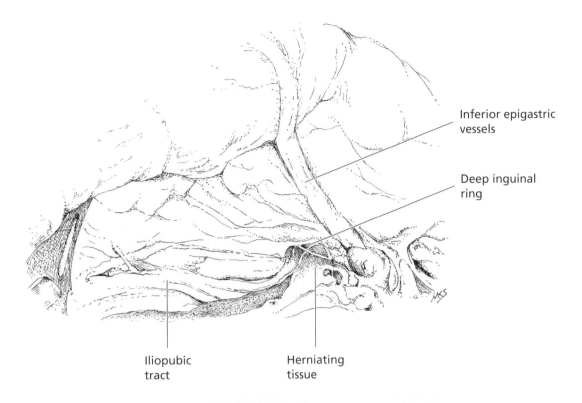

Inferior epigastric
vessels

Deep inguinal
ring

Iliopubic
tract

Herniating
tissue

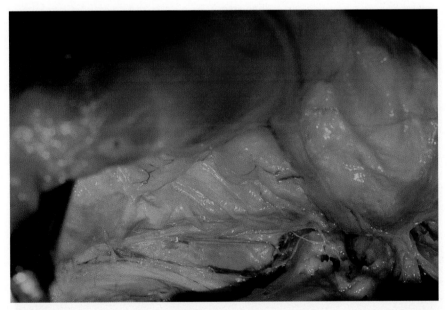

Fig. 10-11. Left indirect inguinal hernia, view of herniating tissues with the peritoneum and extraperitoneal connective tissue partially removed. The inferior epigastric vessels and the iliopubic tract are seen. This cadaver dissection was photographed from the laparoscopic perspective.

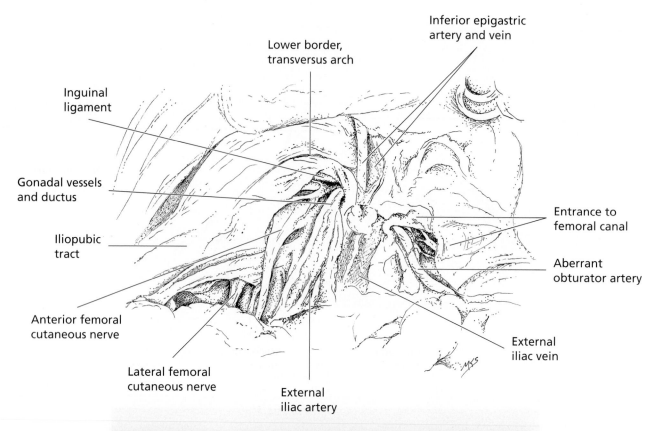

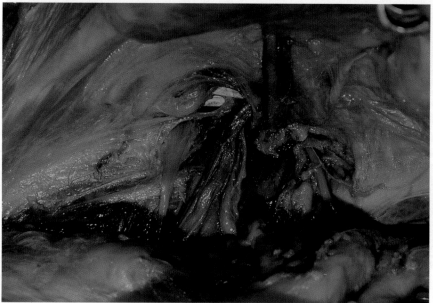

Fig. 10-12. Left-sided inguinal anatomy after retraction of an indirect inguinal hernia. The inguinal ligament can be seen through the dilated deep inguinal ring. The transversus abdominis aponeurosis and iliopubic tract provide the medial border of the femoral canal, which is here seen filled with lymphatic and adipose tissue. An aberrant obturator artery crosses the lateral border of the femoral canal.

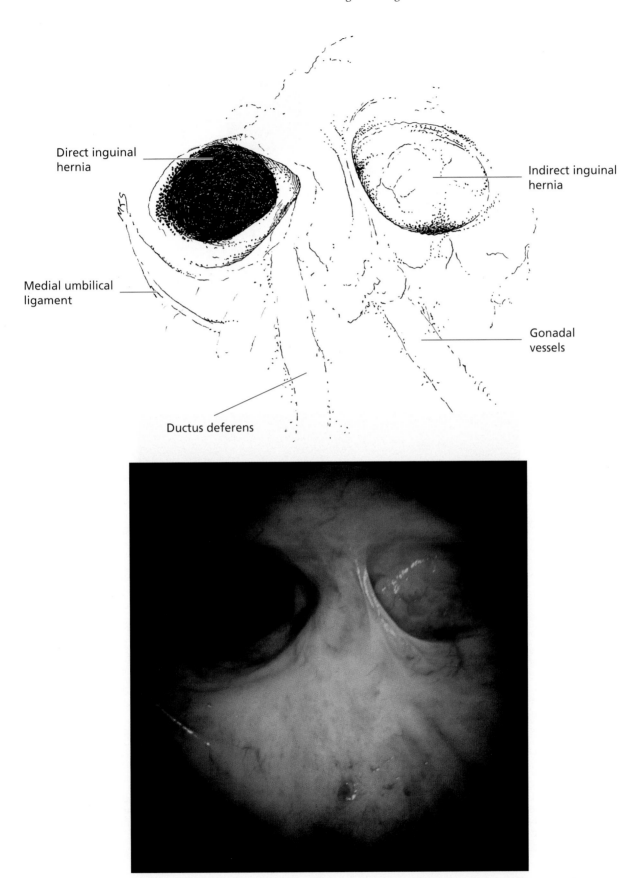

Fig. 10-13. Laparoscopic view of a right pantaloon hernia, peritoneum intact. Both an indirect hernia and a direct hernia are present, forming the two legs of the "pantaloon." The gonadal vessels and ductus deferens are seen to converge at the internal ring, which is dilated and distorted by the indirect hernia.

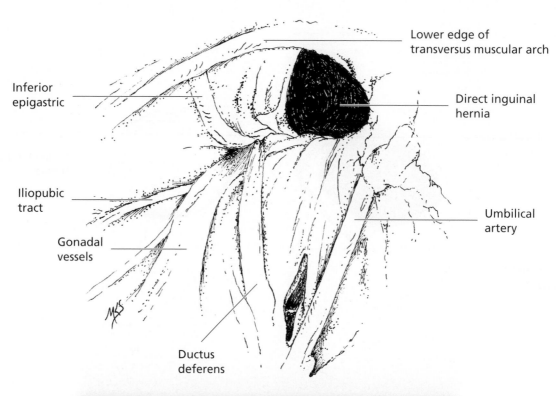

Lower edge of
transversus muscular arch

Inferior
epigastric

Direct inguinal
hernia

Iliopubic
tract

Umbilical
artery

Gonadal
vessels

Ductus
deferens

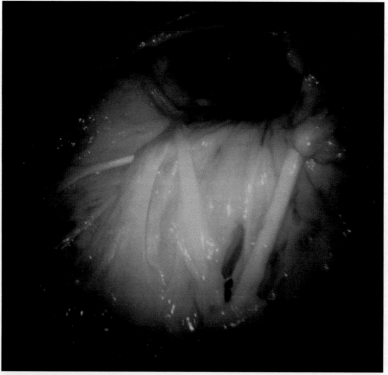

Fig. 10-14. Laparoscopic view of a left direct inguinal hernia. This large hernia is seen to protrude medial to the inferior epigastric vessels in the region of Hesselbach's triangle. The obliterated umbilical artery is seen passing medially. The ductus deferens and gonadal vessels converge on the region of the deep inguinal ring. The iliopubic tract and the muscular arch of the transversus abdominis are seen.

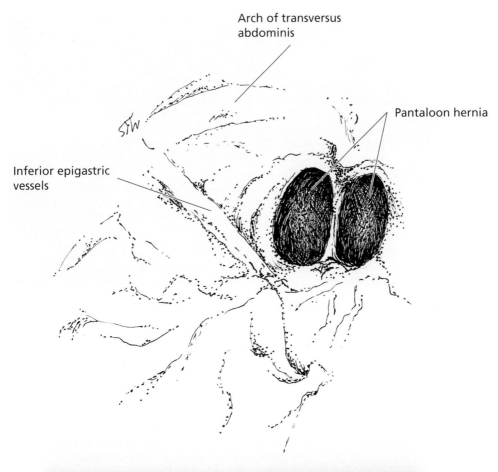

Arch of transversus
abdominis

Pantaloon hernia

Inferior epigastric
vessels

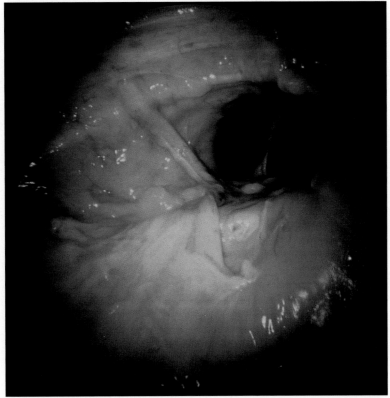

Fig. 10-15. Left direct pantaloon hernia. The arch of the transversus abdominis muscle is well delineated, and a pantaloon hernia is seen to emerge through Hesselbach's triangle. The inferior epigastric vessels are seen.

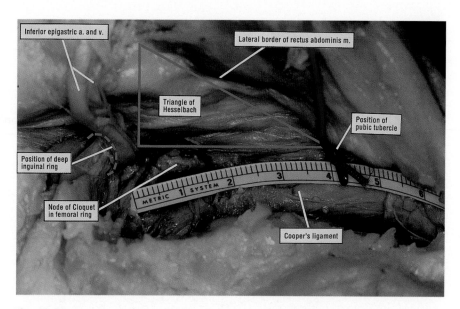

Fig. 10-16. Structures of Hesselbach's triangle, viewed from the laparoscopic perspective.

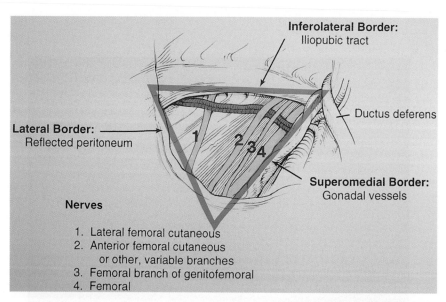

Fig. 10-17. Triangle of pain, modified from the initial description by Aniballi and colleagues (see Bibliography). Deep to the iliopubic tract, the positions of nerves cannot be seen or predicted with certainty. Hence the superior border of the triangle (iliopubic tract) is the most important landmark. (From Colborn GL, Brick WG, Gadacz TR, Skandalakis JE. Inguinal anatomy for laparoscopic herniorrhaphy. II. Altered inguinal anatomy and variations. *Surg Rounds* 1995;June:223–232, with permission.)

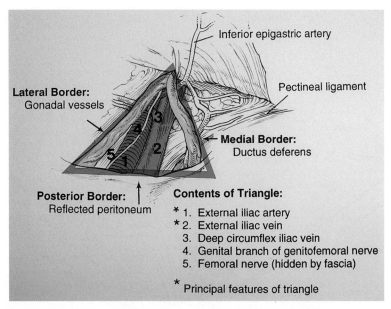

Fig. 10-18. Triangle of doom. The triangle of doom contains three major vessels and two nerves. The significant laparoscopic landmarks include the ductus deferens, which forms the medial border, and the gonadal vessels, which form the lateral border. The triangle of doom and triangle of pain together form a trapezoid. The important boundaries then become the ductus deferens medially and the iliopubic tract superiorly (From Colborn GL, Brick WG, Gadacz TR, Skandalakis JE. Inguinal anatomy for laparoscopic herniorrhaphy. I. The normal anatomy. *Surg Rounds* 1995;May:189–198, with permission.)

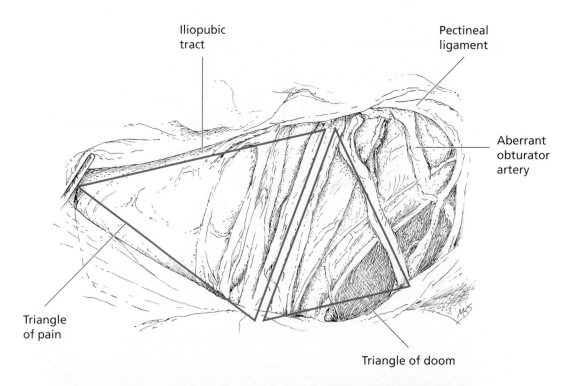

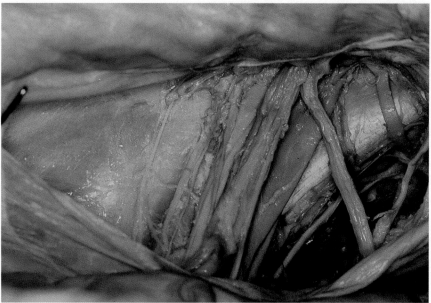

Fig. 10-19. Triangles of doom and pain seen from the laparoscopic perspective. This dissection demonstrates that, taken together, the triangles of doom and pain actually comprise a trapezoid. An aberrant obturator artery and vein are noted below the pectineal ligament and just medial to the triangle of doom. Thus, for all practical purposes, the dangerous region comprises the whole area that lies deep to the iliopubic tract or pectineal ligament. For simplicity, the numerous nerves and vessels of the two triangles are not individually labeled (see Figs. 10-9, 10-17 and 10-18).

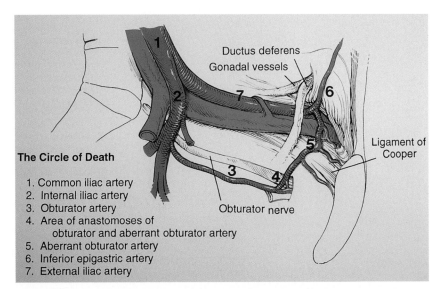

The Circle of Death

1. Common iliac artery
2. Internal iliac artery
3. Obturator artery
4. Area of anastomoses of
    obturator and aberrant obturator artery
5. Aberrant obturator artery
6. Inferior epigastric artery
7. External iliac artery

Ductus deferens
Gonadal vessels
Ligament of Cooper
Obturator nerve

Fig. 10-20. The "circle of death." Among the numerous components of the triangle of doom are significant vascular structures. Note how an aberrant obturator artery forms part of the so-called "circle of death." Because this is essentially an anastomotic arch, both sides of the vessel bleed vigorously if it is inadvertently transected. Injury may be unrecognized at the time of surgery. (From Colborn GL, Brick WG, Gadacz TR, Skandalakis JE. Inguinal anatomy for laparoscopic herniorrhaphy. II. Altered inguinal anatomy and variations. *Surg Rounds* 1995;June:223–232, with permission.)

11

KIDNEYS AND ADRENAL GLANDS

SEAN P. HEDICAN

INITIAL LAPAROSCOPIC VIEW AND PRINCIPLES OF EXPOSURE

The kidneys and adrenal glands are located deep in the retroperitoneum and are visible only after mobilization of the structures that lie anterior to them. Both intraperitoneal and extraperitoneal laparoscopic approaches have been described. The intraperitoneal route remains the most popular for two reasons: first, it goes through familiar territory and the anatomy is relatively straightforward; second, a much larger working space can be generated and maintained. This is the approach described here. Bibliographic references at the end of the chapter give information on the extraperitoneal route.

Access and exposure are enhanced by placing the patient in a semiflank or full lateral position. Elevating the kidney rest and hyperextending the patient by "breaking" the table increases the distance between the lower costal margin and the anterior superior iliac spine and facilitates trocar placement. An angled laparoscope is extremely helpful for adequate visualization. Because the veins are encountered first, venous anatomy is described before arterial anatomy in this chapter, a reversal of the conventional sequence of description.

ANATOMY AND SPECIFIC SURGICAL PROCEDURES

Fascial Spaces of the Retroperitoneum

Familiarity with fascial planes of the posterior abdomen is essential. The parietal peritoneum that lines the anterior abdominal wall reflects over the intraabdominal viscera and defines a space between the peritoneum and the anterior renal (Gerota's) fascia. This anterior pararenal space contains the pancreas on the left and part of the mesocolon. It is the space the laparoscopic surgeon must enter during initial exposure of the kidneys and adrenals through the transabdominal route. Access to the anterior pararenal space is obtained by mobilizing the colon medially after incising along the line of Toldt (see Figs. 8-6 to 8-9). If this initial dissection is taken too deep by incising the underlying fascia, the laparoscopic surgeon will elevate the kidney and adrenal prematurely by entering the posterior pararenal space. One should avoid this by visually confirming the smooth convexity of Gerota's fascia (Fig. 11-1) and by probe palpation of the kidney.

The anterior and posterior renal fasciae envelop the kidney to create the perirenal space. This space contains fat, kidney, and adrenal glands. Superiorly, the anterior and posterior renal fasciae fuse with each other and with the inferior aspect of the diaphragm. Anteriorly, the fascial layers are continuous across the midline and contain the great vessels. Inferiorly, the fascia remains open and contains the ureter, gonadal vessels, and periureteric fat.

Left Kidney and Adrenal Gland

Topographic Relations

The spleen, pancreas, left colon, and stomach overlie the left kidney and adrenal. Laparoscopic exposure is usually obtained by mobilizing the splenic flexure of the colon medially and dividing the splenocolic ligament (see Fig. 11-1; Fig. 11-2). Additional exposure is obtained by division of the phrenocolic, splenorenal, and renocolic ligaments, which are generally not perceived as discrete structures. The spleen and tail of pancreas may be fully mobilized if necessary, but generally these structures can simply be displaced upward. This maneuver exposes Gerota's fascia surrounding the kidney and adrenal. Seen through the laparoscope, this fascia should appear as a smooth, convex, well-encapsulated mass of fat. Gentle pressure with the tip of a probe or blunt grasper produces ballottement of the kidney and causes it to move within Gerota's fascia. This helps to confirm that dissection has been performed in the correct plane. It is important to note that the superior pole of the kidney and adrenal lie deeper than the lower pole of the kidney (Fig. 11-3).

Although it is theoretically possible to expose the left adrenal by creating a window in the lesser sac, the exposure is inadequate for laparoscopic surgery, and it is difficult to access the adrenal gland deep to the pancreas. The normal left adrenal is crescent shaped and nestles along the upper pole of the kidney. The color (deeper orange) and firm texture as well as the visible sharp edge make it easy for the laparoscopist to distinguish normal adrenal gland from fat (see Fig. 11-3; Fig. 11-4). When enlarged, the adrenal pushes the left kidney downward and loses its sharp edge, becoming more rounded. The color of an adrenal adenoma reflects the cell type of origin but is generally different from surrounding yellow fat. Laparoscopic ultrasound is a useful adjunct in locating the adrenal gland, especially in obese patients with small tumors (e.g., aldosteronomas).

Veins, Arteries, and Collecting System

The renal veins lie anterior to the arteries and are the first vascular structures encountered by the laparoscopist during hilar dissection. Because the inferior vena cava lies to the right of the aorta, the left renal vein (see Fig. 11-4; Figs. 11-5 to 11-9) is of necessity longer than the right and crosses anterior to the aorta to drain into the inferior vena cava. In rare cases, a double left renal vein forms a "renal collar" encircling the aorta with both an anterior and a posterior renal vein.

The left gonadal vein drains into the inferior aspect of the left renal vein and thus may be a useful laparoscopic landmark in the obese patient (see Fig. 11-6). Lumbar veins occasionally drain into the renal vein in the region of the vertebral bodies. These are particularly treacherous for the laparoscopic surgeon because they are deep to the vein and may bleed significantly if torn.

The left adrenal vein runs along the long axis of the leaf-shaped left adrenal (see Fig. 11-5). The left adrenal vein averages 2 to 3 cm in length, and there is usually ample length to clip or ligate. Ample venous collaterals allow ligation of this vein (for example, during laparoscopic donor nephrectomy) without causing venous infarction of the adrenal gland. In rare cases, the left adrenal vein receives drainage from a left inferior phrenic vein, which usually enters from the posterior aspect of the vein.

The renal arteries arise from the lateral aspect of the aorta (see Figs. 11-7 to 11-9). Anomalies are encountered in 25% to 33% of anatomically normal individuals and generally represent persistence of one of the five fetal segmental arteries. Double renal arteries, unilateral or bilateral, are the most common variant. These accessory renal arteries usually arise directly from the aorta, but they may come from any vessel in the vicinity (the renal artery, gonadal artery, or superior mesenteric artery). Accessory vessels to the lower pole are twice as common as those to the upper pole. An accessory vessel to the lower pole of the kidney crosses in front of the ureter and may cause hydronephrosis (Fig. 11-10). The left renal artery is shorter than the right. It lies deep to the vein, which is usually larger than the artery. The laparoscopic surgeon finds the left renal artery by mobilizing the left renal vein and elevating it gently. Although the artery lies slightly cephalad to the vein, laparoscopic perspective may cause it to be visualized below the vein (see Figs. 11-7 and 11-9). Double renal arteries are common, as previously mentioned, and should be suspected if an unusually small artery is easily visualized above or below the vein. This feature may not have been detected on preoperative studies. A potential pitfall, if the laparoscopist is disoriented, is mistaking the splenic artery for the renal artery. As with any surgery, careful identification and confirmation of all structures are mandatory. In the renal hilum, the renal artery divides into four or five branches, most of which lie between the renal vein and the pelvis of kidney.

The adrenal glands are supplied by multiple (more than 50) tiny arterial twigs derived from the inferior phrenic artery, renal artery, and aorta. These vessels are generally secured with electrocautery or ultrasonically activated scissors, rather than by individual identification. Potential pitfalls during laparoscopic adrenalectomy include damage to or ligation of a superior renal polar vessel, with resulting renovascular hypertension.

The pelvis of the kidney is the deepest of the three hilar structures (vein, artery, collecting system). It is much easier for the laparoscopic surgeon to identify the ureters in their midportion (Figs. 11-11 to 11-14) and to trace cephalad. The left gonadal vein is another useful landmark that can be traced back to the renal vein to help define the hilum. Although the appearance of the ureter with its surrounding plexus of vessels is characteristic to the experienced laparoscopist, the ureter is the only tubular structure in the retroperitoneum that vermiculates. The left ureter is longer than the right, owing to the more cephalad location of the left kidney. The left ureter passes over the medial portion of the psoas major muscle and genitofemoral nerve (see Fig. 11-13) and passes under the gonadal vessels to enter the pelvis near the bifurcation of the common iliac vessels (see Figs. 8-5 and 8-18 to 8-21). It tends to adhere to the peritoneum, particularly in the region of the sigmoid mesocolon, and it must be gently pushed down off the peritoneum as it is dissected free.

The blood supply of the ureter comes from regional vessels to form a rich plexus. Despite this characteristic, overzealous mobilization can devascularize the ureter (particularly if the periureteral tissues are stripped away). The rare duplicated ureter is detected on preoperative imaging studies. The distal portion of the ureter is supplied by vesical arteries with contributions from other internal iliac-derived regional vessels. The midportion has a more tenuous blood supply derived from the aorta.

Laparoscopic Nephrectomy

The technique of nephrectomy varies with the purpose for which the procedure is performed. Laparoscopic donor nephrectomy is usually performed on the left side. The line of Toldt is incised, and the left colon is mobilized medially. The ureter is identified and mobilized in its midportion. Dissection in Gerota's fascia reveals the kidney. The left renal vein and artery are identified, and adequate lengths of both are dissected. Typically, the origin of the left renal artery at the aorta is exposed. Gonadal and adrenal veins are clipped and divided. The ureter is dissected down to the iliac vessels, taking care to include the periureteral tissue with surrounding vessels. Finally, the dissection is completed by elevating the kidney from Gerota's fascia. Dissection of the upper pole is technically the most difficult because this is farthest from the umbilically placed laparoscope. The lateral attachments are maintained to prevent torsion on the vessels. These are divided last, after vascular structures have been secured.

Although laparoscopic radical nephrectomy has been described, it is still controversial, as are many laparoscopic resections for malignancy. Bibliographic references at the end of the chapter give further details on this and other laparoscopic renal procedures.

Left Adrenalectomy

Exposure is obtained as described earlier, with the additional necessity to mobilize spleen and pancreas gently cephalad or medially. Gerota's fascia is identified and incised.

Following the plane between the superior pole of the kidney and Gerota's fascia, the fat surrounding the left adrenal may be dissected from the kidney. Laparoscopic ultrasound may be useful if the adenoma is small or the patient is obese. Large adenomas are easier to recognize as relatively discrete rounded masses, generally differing in color from the surrounding fat.

The left adrenal vein is clipped and divided early, if possible (Figs. 11-15 to 11-18). The tissue surrounding the adrenal contains multiple tiny arterial branches and is best secured with electrocoagulation or ultrasonic scissors (Figs. 11-19 and 11-20). The surgeon should avoid grasping the adrenal or adenoma directly, because it is likely to tear. One should use the long axis of a grasper of suction cannula to displace the gland or tumor gently away from the region being dissected (see Fig. 11-18).

Right Kidney and Adrenal Gland

Topographic Relations

The right kidney and adrenal lie slightly lower than the left. They are covered by liver, colon, and duodenum. The laparoscopic surgeon must mobilize the hepatic flexure and right colon to expose the right kidney. Generally, it is only necessary to divide the right triangular ligament to expose the right adrenal gland. This allows the liver to be elevated, thus creating a working space in the subhepatic region, without risk of tearing the capsule of the liver. It is rarely necessary to mobilize the duodenum or right colon, but the laparoscopic surgeon must be prepared to do this if necessary.

The right adrenal is shaped like a triangle with its base curved concavely over the medial portion of the upper pole of the right kidney. Medially, the second side of the triangle nestles against the inferior vena cava and is curved to conform to its contour. The lateral border is the oblique third leg of the triangle; this conforms to the contour of the lower edge of the liver. Posteriorly, the right adrenal rests on the diaphragm.

Veins, Arteries, and Collecting System

The right renal vein is shorter and the right renal artery is longer than the left. Anomalies of both may occur. Duplication of the right renal vein is occasionally seen, and lumbar veins may drain into the renal vein. The right adrenal vein is short (0.5 to 1 cm), fat, and drains directly into the inferior vena cava. It is sometimes joined by an accessory hepatic vein, entering from the cephalad aspect. Multiple right adrenal veins occasionally occur. These may drain directly into the inferior vena cava or into the right renal vein.

The right renal artery passes behind the inferior vena cava as it runs from the aorta to the right kidney. The first branch point usually occurs just as the right renal artery emerges from behind the inferior vena cava, but it may occur behind the vena cava. For all practical purposes, the laparoscopic surgeon can assume the presence of two renal arteries to secure, rather than one, on the right side. The right ureter is slightly shorter than the left.

Laparoscopic Right Adrenalectomy

Mobilization is as previously described. The major hazard in laparoscopic right adrenalectomy is injury to the short, fat, fragile right adrenal vein. Dissection in the anterior adventitial plane of the inferior vena cava, rather than along the adrenal gland, reveals the entrance of the right adrenal vein onto the inferior vena cava (Fig. 11-21). Gentle lateral displacement of the adrenal gland generally yields sufficient length for control. An endoscopic linear stapler with a vascular cartridge is an excellent alternative to clip ligation if the vein is large. Once the adrenal vein is secured, the remainder of the adrenalectomy proceeds more or less as previously described.

BIBLIOGRAPHY
Anatomic References

1. Hinman F. *Atlas of urosurgical anatomy.* Philadelphia: WB Saunders, 1993:984–997.
2. Johnstone FFC. The surgical anatomy of the adrenal glands with particular reference to the suprarenal vein. *Surg Clin North Am* 1963;44:1315–1321.
3. Lei QF, Marks SC, Touliopoulos P, Raptopoulos V. Fascial planes and compartments of the posterior abdomen: the perirenal and pararenal pathways. *Clin Anat* 1990;3:1–15.
4. Merklin RJ, Michels NA. The variant renal and suprarenal blood supply with data on the inferior phrenic ureteral, and gonadal arteries: a statistical analysis based upon 185 dissections and a review of the literature. *J Int Coll Surg* 1958;29:41–76.
5. Wind GG. *Applied laparoscopic anatomy: abdomen and pelvis.* Baltimore: Williams & Wilkins, 1997:301–365.

Surgical References

1. Brunt LM, Doherty Gem, Norton JA, Soper NJ, Quasebarth MA, Moley JF. Laparoscopic adrenalectomy compared to open adrenalectomy for benign adrenal neoplasms. *J Am Coll Surg* 1996;183:1–10.
2. Chen RN, Moore RC, Kavoussi LR. Laparoscopic pyeloplasty: indications, technique and long-term outcome. *Urol Clin North Am* 1998;25:323–330.
3. Duh Q-Y, Siperstein AE, Clark OH, et al. Laparoscopic adrenalectomy: comparison of the lateral and posterior approaches. *Arch Surg* 1996;131:870–876.
4. Flowers JL, Jacobs S, Cho E, et al. Comparison of open and laparoscopic live donor nephrectomy. *Ann Surg* 1997;226:483–490.
5. Gagner M. Laparoscopic adrenalectomy. *Surg Clin North Am* 1996;76:523–537.
6. Gagner M, Lacroix A, Bolte E, Pomp A. Laparoscopic adrenalectomy: the importance of a flank approach in lateral decubitus position. *Surg Endosc* 1994;8:135–138.
7. Gill IS. Retroperitoneal laparoscopic nephrectomy. *Urol Clin North Am* 1998;25:343–360.
8. Kerbl K, Clayman RV, McDougall EM, et al. Transperitoneal nephrectomy for benign disease of the kidney: a comparison between laparoscopic and open surgical technique. *Urology* 1994;43:607–613.
9. Nakada SY, McDougall EM, Clayman RV. Laparoscopic extirpation of renal cell cancer: feasibility, questions, and concerns. *Semin Surg Oncol* 1996;12:100–112.
10. Petelin JB. Laparoscopic adrenalectomy. *Semin Laparosc Surg* 1996;3:84–94.
11. Smith PA, Ratner LE, Lynch FC, Corl FM, Fishman EK. Role of CT angiography in the preoperative evaluation for laparoscopic nephrectomy. *Radiographics* 1998;18:589–601.

Spleen

Gerota's
fascia

Splenic flexure
of colon

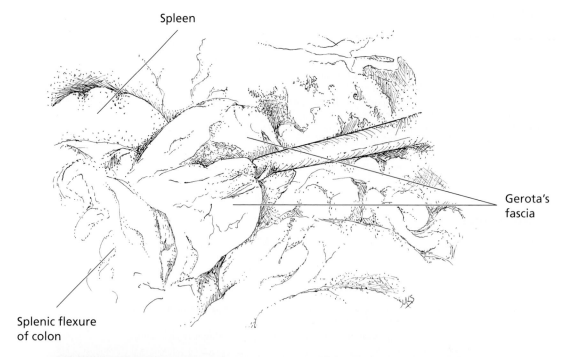

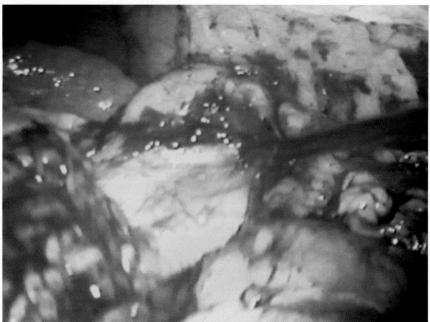

Fig. 11-1. Gerota's fascia (left side). The splenic flexure and descending colon have been mobilized medially and are visible to the left of the figure. The spleen is noted in the background.

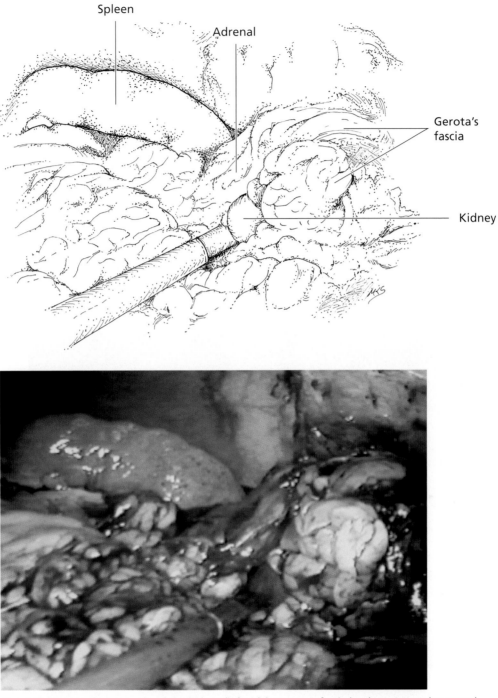

Fig. 11-2. Gerota's fascia and upper pole of the kidney (left side). Gerota's fascia has been opened to reveal the upper pole of the left kidney. The edge of the adrenal gland is seen, showing the characteristic color and texture that allow visual differentiation from surrounding fat.

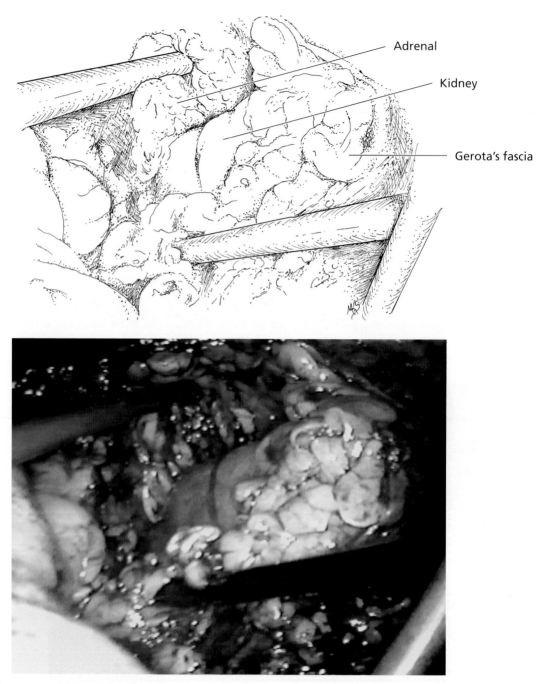

Fig. 11-3. Incision in Gerota's fascia to reveal the left kidney. The adrenal gland may be glimpsed.

Adrenal

Kidney

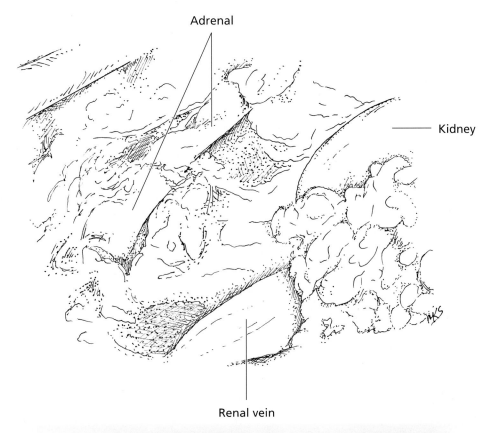

Renal vein

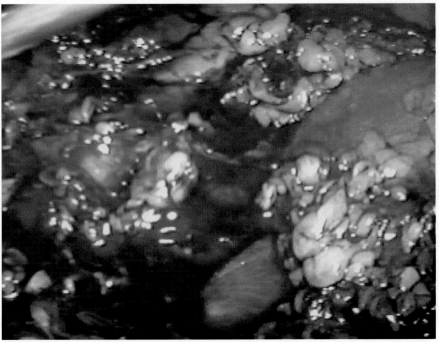

Fig. 11-4. Left renal vein and superior pole of the left kidney and left adrenal gland. Dissection medial to the kidney has exposed a portion of the renal vein, the most superficial structure in the renal hilum. The left adrenal gland is seen.

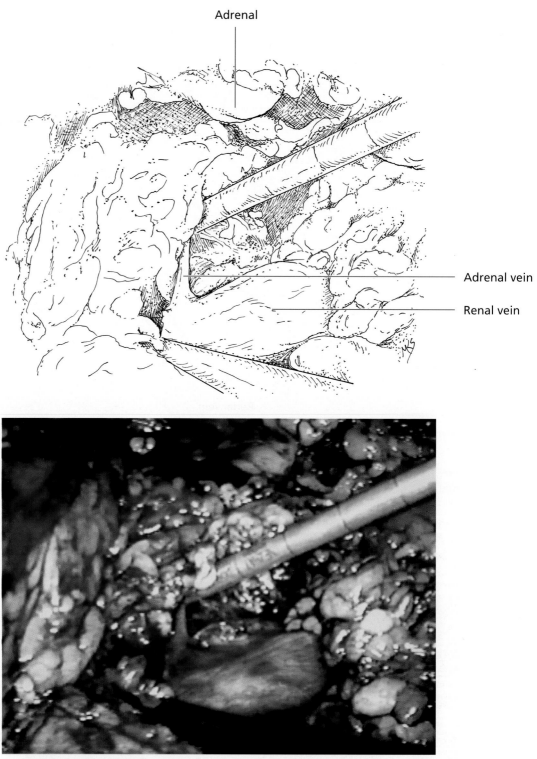

Adrenal

Adrenal vein

Renal vein

Fig. 11-5. Left renal vein and left adrenal vein. The left adrenal vein has been identified at its entrance into the left renal vein and is being elevated by an instrument.

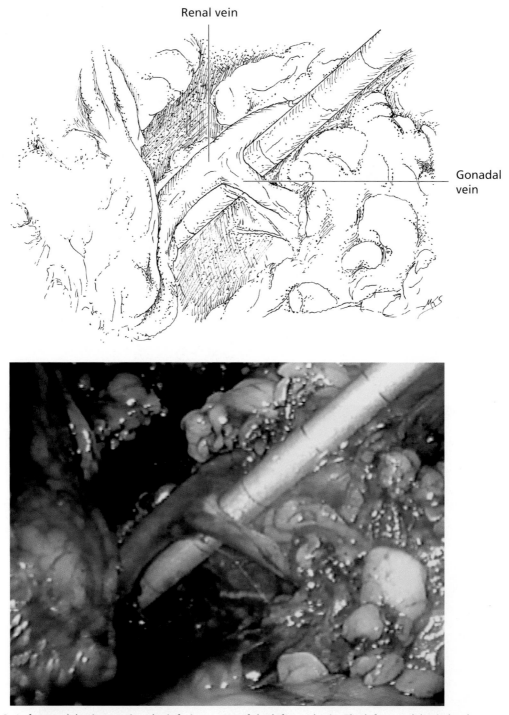

Fig. 11-6. Left gonadal vein entering the inferior aspect of the left renal vein. The left gonadal vein has been elevated by an instrument and traced to its termination on the left renal vein.

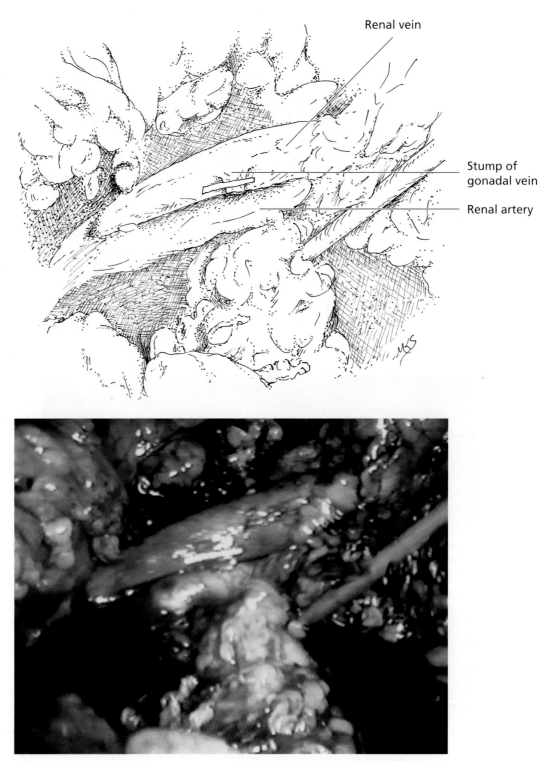

Renal vein

Stump of
gonadal vein

Renal artery

Fig. 11-7. Left renal artery seen deep to the left renal vein. The left gonadal vein has been clipped and divided.

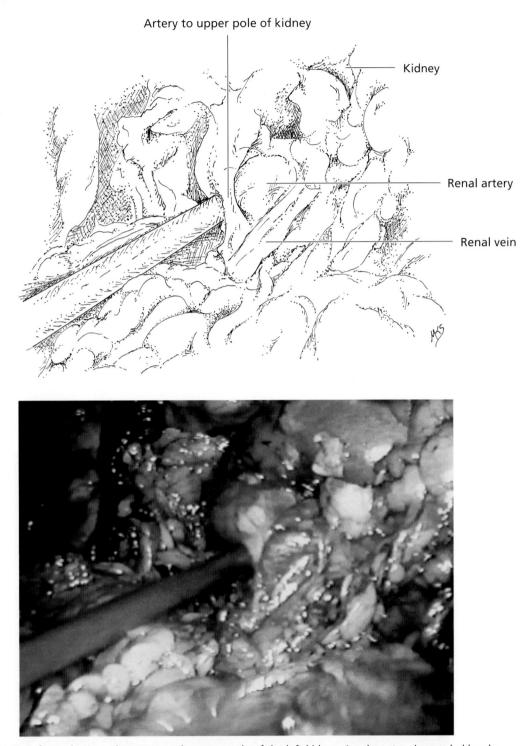

Artery to upper pole of kidney

Kidney

Renal artery

Renal vein

Fig. 11-8. Left renal vein, polar artery to the upper pole of the left kidney. A polar artery is revealed by elevating the upper pole of the left kidney. Left renal vein is seen in the foreground.

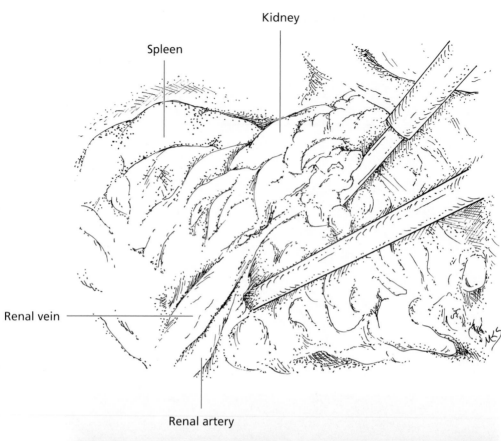

Spleen

Kidney

Renal vein

Renal artery

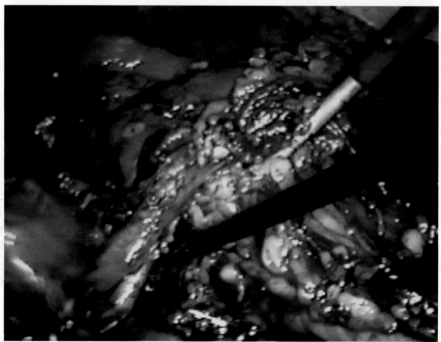

Fig. 11-9. Left renal vein and renal artery. The left kidney is being retracted to display the left renal vein and renal artery entering the hilum of the kidney. The colon is seen in the foreground, and the spleen is glimpsed in the background.

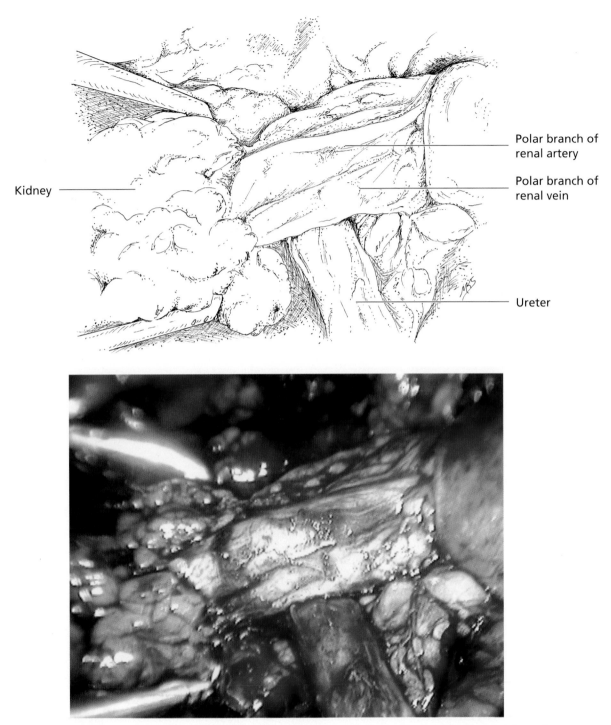

Kidney

Polar branch of renal artery

Polar branch of renal vein

Ureter

Fig. 11-10. Left ureter crossed by aberrant branches of the left renal artery and vein. These segmental vessels caused hydronephrosis. The kidney is seen in the background.

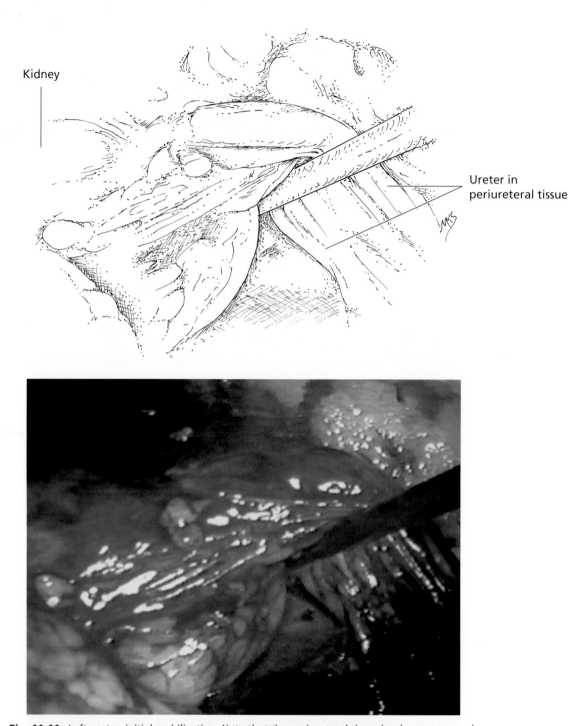

Fig. 11-11. Left ureter, initial mobilization. Note that the periureteral tissue has been preserved.

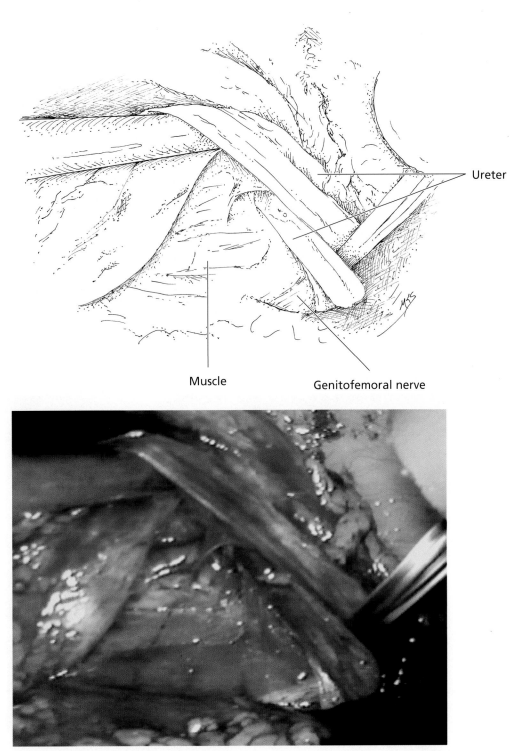

Fig. 11-12. Left ureter. Further dissection elevated the left ureter with periureteral tissue from the underlying muscle. The genitofemoral nerve may be glimpsed.

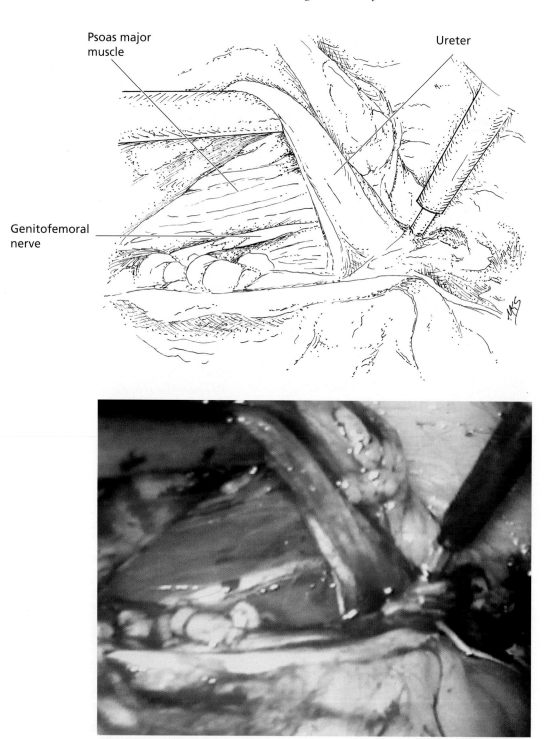

Fig. 11-13. Left ureter. The psoas major muscle and genitofemoral nerve are visualized.

Ureter

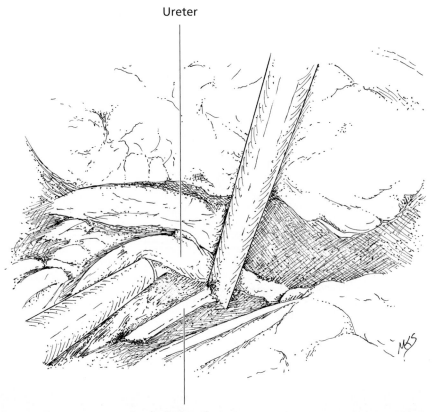

Genitofemoral nerve

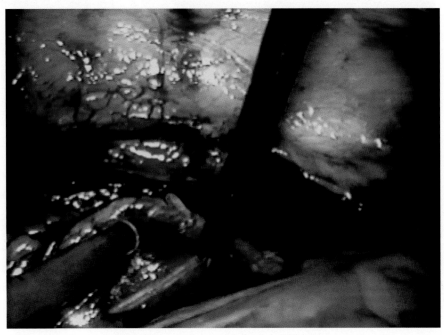

Fig. 11-14. Left ureter, distal mobilization.

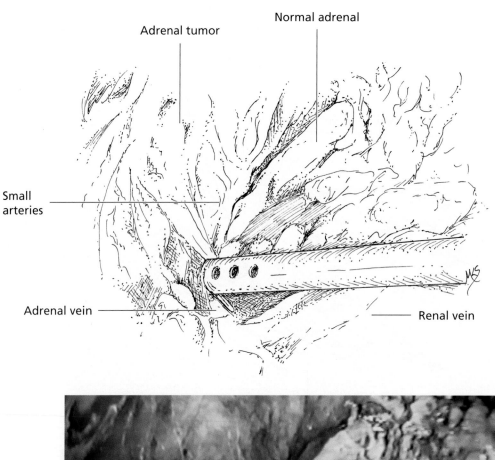

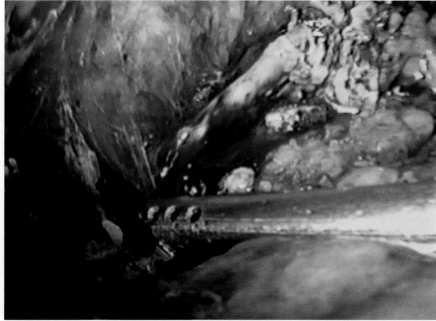

Fig. 11-15. Left adrenal vein and small arterial branches to the left adrenal gland. The left adrenal vein is shown as it enters the left adrenal gland.

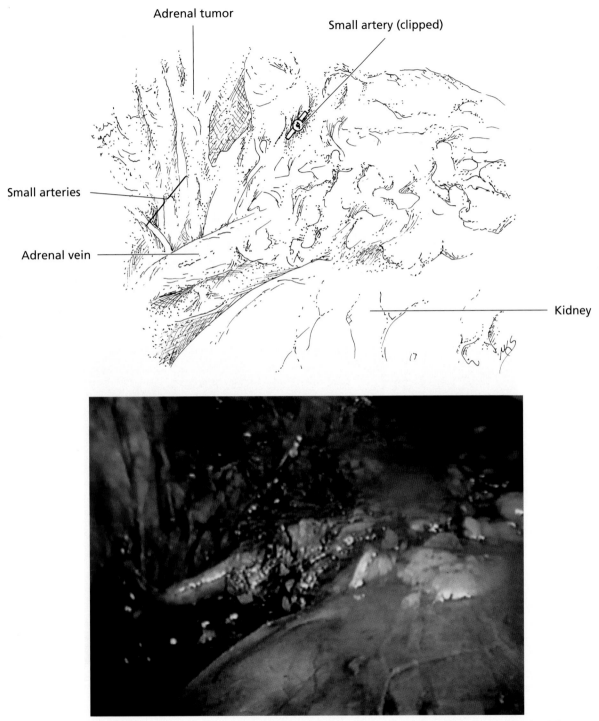

Fig. 11-16. Left adrenal vein. An adrenal tumor lies to the left; more normal adrenal gland is seen to the right.

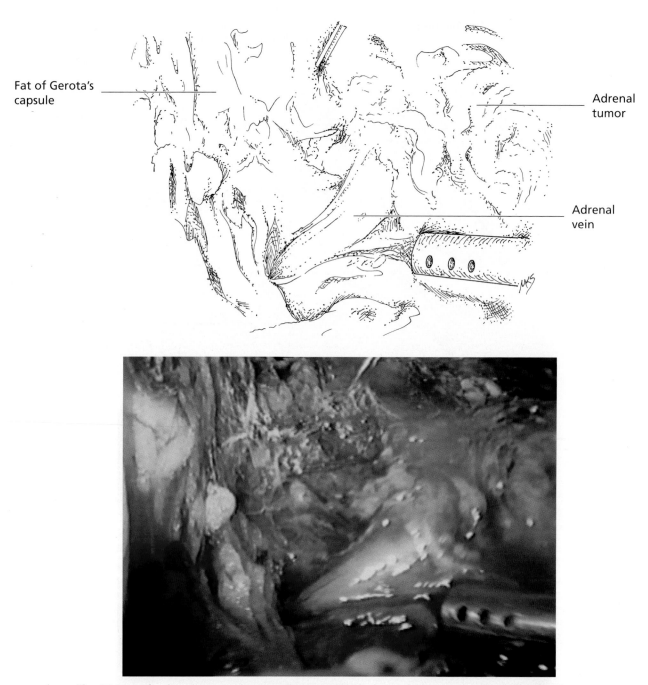

Fat of Gerota's
capsule

Adrenal
tumor

Adrenal
vein

Fig. 11-17. Left adrenal vein. In this example, an extremely short adrenal vein has been identified between the adrenal tumor and the renal vein (not seen).

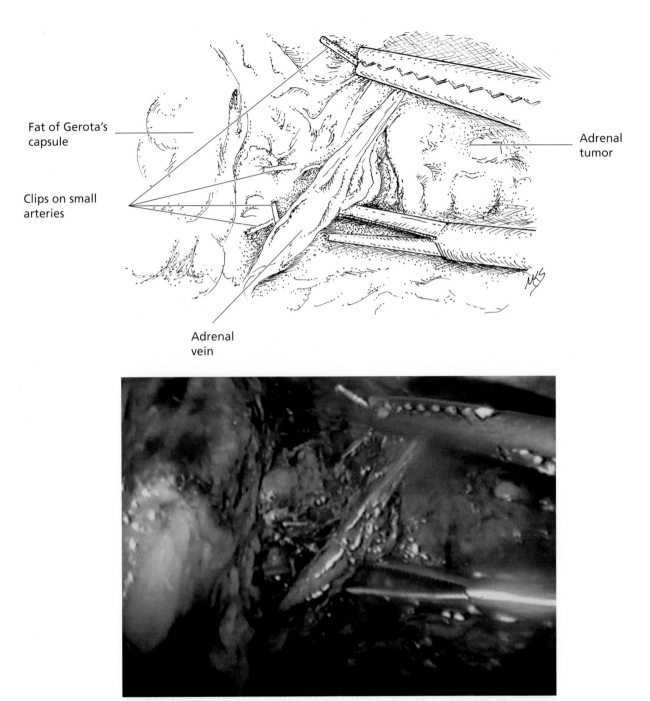

Fat of Gerota's capsule

Adrenal tumor

Clips on small arteries

Adrenal vein

Fig. 11-18. Left adrenal vein. Several small arterial branches have been clipped and divided.

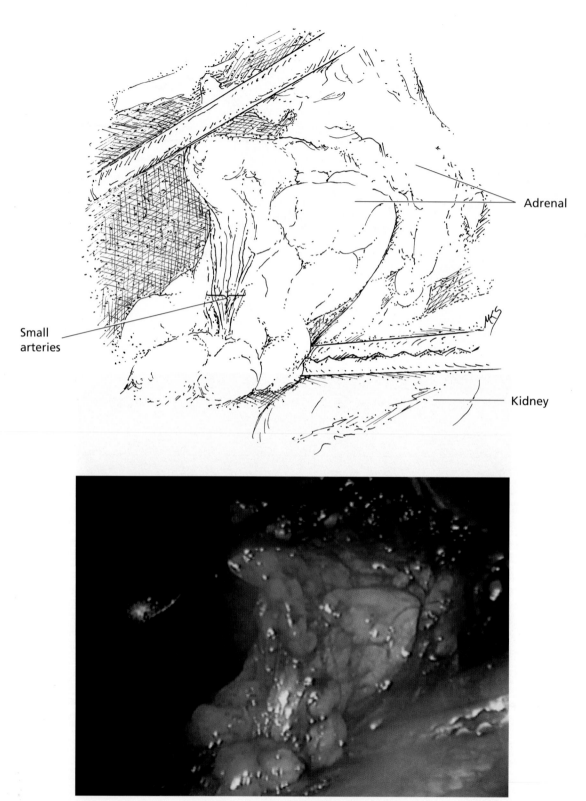

Fig. 11-19. Multiple small arterial twigs to the left adrenal gland. The left adrenal gland is being elevated surrounded by fat. Numerous tiny arterial branches must be secured with electrocautery or ultrasonic dissecting shears.

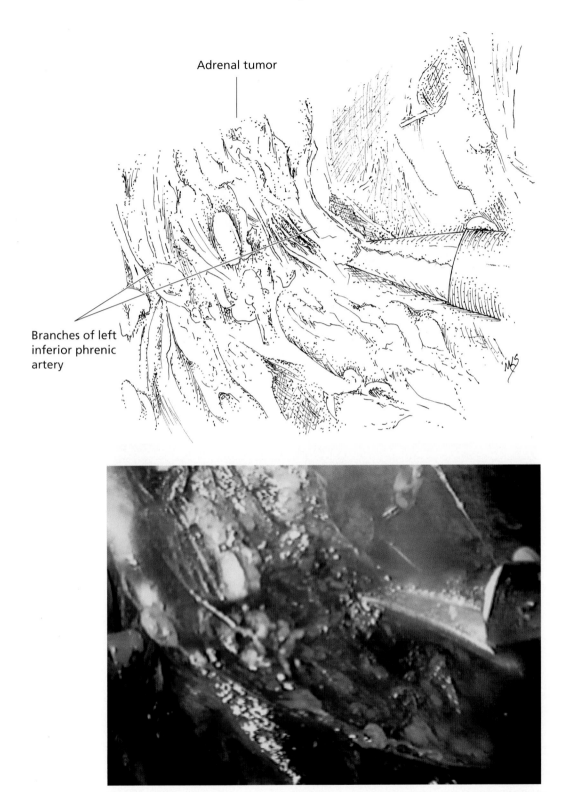

Fig. 11-20. Small vascular branches from the left inferior phrenic artery to the left adrenal gland. These multiple tiny vessels must be secured with electrocautery or ultrasonic shears.

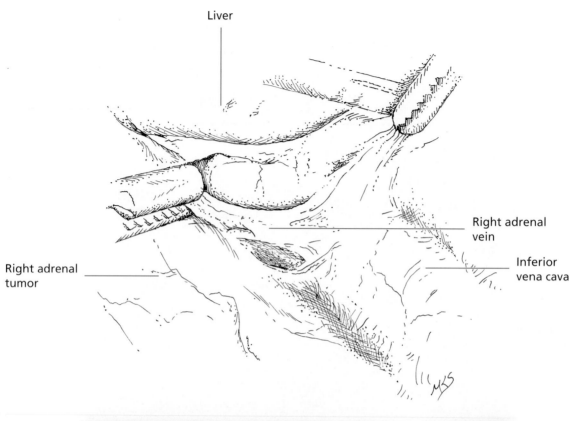

Liver

Right adrenal
vein

Inferior
vena cava

Right adrenal
tumor

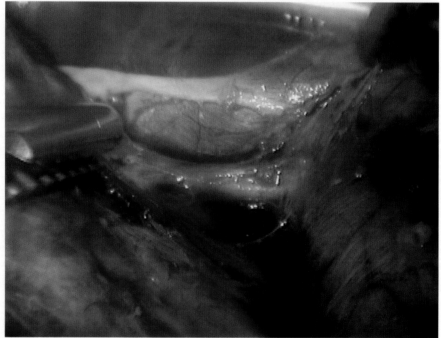

Fig. 11-21. Right adrenal vein, inferior vena cava. A right adrenal adenoma is gently being displaced laterally by pressure with a blunt grasper. The liver is seen in the background.

SUBJECT INDEX

Page numbers followed by *f* indicate figures